MENTAL HEALTH, INC.

HOW CORRUPTION, LAX OVERSIGHT AND FAILED REFORMS ENDANGER OUR MOST VULNERABLE CITIZENS

MENTAL HEALTH, INC.

HOW CORRUPTION, LAX OVERSIGHT AND FAILED REFORMS ENDANGER OUR MOST VULNERABLE CITIZENS

ART LEVINE

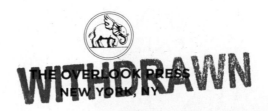

THE OVERLOOK PRESS
NEW YORK, NY

This edition first published in hardcover in the United States in 2017 by
The Overlook Press, Peter Mayer Publishers, Inc.

NEW YORK
141 Wooster Street
New York, NY 10012
www.overlookpress.com
For bulk and special sales, please contact sales@overlookny.com,
or write us at the above address.

Cataloging-in-Publication Data is available from the Library of Congress

Book design and typeformatting by Bernard Schleifer
Manufactured in the United States of America
FIRST EDITION
ISBN 978-1-4683-0837-2

*In memory of Sylvia Levine, Andrew White, Jason Simcakoski,
Rebecca Riley, Genine Zizzo and all those countless others
who deserved quality care—and never received it.*

For all those people struggling with serious mental illness and substance abuse.

*For all the clinicians, whistleblowers and reformers dedicated
to making our mental health system work for everyone.*

*For all those who shared their personal stories, research
and insights to make this book possible.*

CONTENTS

INTRODUCTION   9

1. Drugging Our Kids: Corporate Greed Joins Corruption, Apathy   35
2. Nursing Homes: Drugging Our Seniors to Death   53
3. The Secret History of the VA's Tragedies in Tomah and Phoenix   69
4. The Secret History of the VA Scandals, Part II: The Empire Strikes Back   87
5. A Marine's Descent into PTSD Hell   113
6. Stan White and the Veterans' Search for Truth and Answers   138
7. Mr. White Comes to Washington: FDA Showdown over Seroquel   146
8. Drug-Free PTSD Recovery   161
9. How LA County's Mental Health Officials Neglect Inmates and Ignore Violence   170
10. To Live and Die in LA: How DMH's Outreach Work Saves Lives, Stops Mass Shootings   185
11. Torture in Alabama   199
12. Profits and Losses from Residential Treatment: The Story of Bain Capital and CRC Health   219
13. Recipe for Disaster?: Residential Treatment Programs for Addicts and Kids   233
14. Florida: Free-Fire Zone for Killing, Abusing and Raping Kids?   246
15. Karen's Story and the Mental Health System That Never Was: Saving Families, Young People from Lifelong Madness   257
16. Why Can't We Just Do What Works?   271
17. Putting People Before Big Pharma: Overcoming the Barriers to Recovery   284

ENDNOTES   299

ASSISTANCE, ADVOCACY AND INFORMATION RESOURCE GUIDE   347

ACKNOWLEDGMENTS   350

INTRODUCTION

AFTER THIRTY-EIGHT-YEAR-OLD ARMY VETERAN STEVE TOMPKINS CAME home early one April evening in 2014, it didn't take much to set him off when he started arguing with his second wife in their home in South Charleston, West Virginia. (Tompkins's name has been changed to protect his privacy.) The hulking six-foot-four, 350-pound man was bloated and a bit dazed from the high dosages of all the Seroquel, Depakote, Lithium and other drugs his doctors had thrown at him for nearly a decade since he returned from his final tour of Iraq, but the medications couldn't quiet the depression, anger and the murderous thoughts that could explode at any time. He had been waiting for weeks to get into the specialized PTSD sixty-day unit at the Clarksburg Hospital, and could barely take all the strains in his life anymore: the fights with his ex-wife over visiting rights with his teenage kids, his despair and the stress of being constantly broke with two young children. "I was overwhelmed," he recalls. "All I was doing was throwing out red flags." So when his wife, Jolene, told him they didn't have $40 to pay someone to cut their overgrown lawn, and added that he shouldn't have spent $200 on a wood lathe, a dark cloud of rage and anguish gripped him. "I can't take this pain anymore," he declared, hurrying up the stairs to get the guns.

Tompkins moved quickly and methodically, changing into black fatigues for his final mission. He strapped on a green Army chest rig and jammed in seven extra thirty-bullet magazines to go with the AR-15 assault rifle and the .40- and .45-caliber pistols that he grabbed from his personal armory of two dozen rifles and guns; he also attached a pouch to his belt to hold even more semiautomatic rounds. His wife, their two-year-old girl and their six-year-old boy started crying when he came down the stairs and ordered them out of the house. Jolene refused, knowing that if they left, he would surely kill himself and take out anyone who tried to stop him. As they were arguing, his ex-wife called from Georgia to remind him that his thirteen-year-old son's birthday was the next day. He asked his son to come to the phone and he told him, "Hey buddy, I'll see you on the flip side in Valhalla." His ex-wife, picking up on the farewell to his son, immediately began crying and hung up the phone. Then she called the South Charleston police emergency line. About five squad cars were dispatched. The police cars pulled up outside, the cops got out of their cars and took cover, ready to train their guns on Tompkins if he stepped out of the house.

Inside, Tompkins was still urging his family to leave when Lt. Guy Amburgey, a military veteran and a skilled negotiator, called the Tompkins home, got Jolene on the phone, and tried to convince her to leave, with Tompkins following—unarmed. "He's not going to do that," she said, as recounted in the police report, and she didn't agree to leave, either. Tompkins stood nearby, looking out the window and waiting for the right moment to rush out and start shooting, willing to go out in a hail of bullets rather than go to jail or keep on living with his PTSD and unending misery. Finally, he warily got on the phone with Amburgey, who said he wanted to help Tompkins and his family, but needed him to come outside.

"Do you believe a man is as good as his word?" Amburgey asked, veteran to veteran.

Tompkins agreed, and Amburgey vowed that he wouldn't be put in a police van, but would be taken in an ambulance to a hospital. As Tompkins waited impatiently, Amburgey, talking to him with his cell phone in hand, approached the front door from the side of the house. Tompkins agreed to come out, but only if guns weren't pointed at him. As Tompkins stepped out onto the porch, arms raised, the police officers on the street started shouting commands and leveling their guns at him. Feeling betrayed, the veteran shouted, "Let's end this. Fuck you all!" At that, Amburgey whipped around to face his fellow officers and pumped his arm downward, shouting, "Put your fucking weapons down!" The two of them then resumed their negotiations and Tompkins agreed to walk to the side of the house to meet Amburgey, but not before he pulled up his shirt to show that he didn't have bullets strapped to his chest or any weapons on him. The lieutenant patted him down and found the pouch with the magazine rounds. Amburgey asked him to walk to the end of his sidewalk, sit down and wait for the medics.

At that point, Tompkins, who was as tough as anyone when he was an M1 tank crewmember fighting in Iraq, began to cry. "I've been trying for weeks to get help there and everything is full," he moaned. "It's too bad it takes something like this to get help." More than a year later, he was still waiting for admission to the special PTSD inpatient program.

· · ·

THE CONVENTIONAL VIEW OF THE STORY OF STEVE TOMPKINS—AND THE roughly 30 percent of all Iraq, Afghanistan and Vietnam vets treated by the Department of Veterans Affairs (VA) who have PTSD—is simple: Their lives would be vastly improved if there were only enough funds available so that these troubled vets could get access to the specialized care, cutting-edge medications and psychiatric care they deserve without facing long waiting lists. The VA's mental health funding, in fact, increased more than 40 percent between 2009 and 2016 to $7.4 billion a year, and thousands of new clinicians were added.

Even so, reform advocates believe that the shortage of funding for our nation's mental health system is at the root of a broader crisis—usually without acknowledging the prevalence of low quality and sometimes deadly care. For example, as the National Alliance on Mental Illness (NAMI) declares, "Services are often unavailable or inaccessible for those who need them the most." To be sure, access to affordable and trained mental health providers—from social workers to psychiatrists—remains woefully lacking: a stunning 55 percent of American counties, all rural, don't have a single mental health professional, according to the Substance Abuse and Mental Health Services Administration (SAMHSA).

The shocking arrival of Donald Trump's presidency, of course, presents an even broader barrier to mental health care. The best-known roadblock, obviously, is the potential stripping of health insurance from about twenty-three million Americans as part of the Republican drive to "repeal and replace" key features of Obamacare, also known as the Affordable Care Act (ACA). This goal was at the heart of the Republican bill that narrowly passed the House of Representatives in May 2017.

By the summer of 2017, the Republican's American Health Care Act (AHCA) fate in the Senate remained uncertain, but one thing was clear: countless Americans were still at risk of losing either their benefits or health care coverage. Just as troubling, more than 130 million people have preexisting conditions, and those with the most serious health problems could find it nearly impossible to afford private insurance under the GOP health care provisions that would lift restrictions on charging older or sicker people higher premium costs, according to the liberal Center for American Progress (CAP). In one striking CAP assessment, new rules in the Republican bill allowing insurers to charge far higher fees would cost a typical forty-year-old individual a "premium surcharge" of $8,370 for having a major depressive or bipolar disorder—and an extra $20,000 a year if the person is an addict. That's particularly grim news when over 140 people a day are dying from drug overdoses. Under the bill and planned federal waivers, even many lower-income or severely mentally ill people without coverage could well find their opportunity to enroll in Medicaid blocked in those states granted Medicaid waivers.

Amid the political furor that engulfed Washington after President Trump fired FBI director James Comey, even less media and public attention is being paid to the administration's backstage regulatory assaults on health care coverage that could harm millions of people with mental illness and addictions. These dangers remain even if a full-scale Obamacare repeal law never makes it through Congress.

The first version of the wildly unpopular bill designed by House Republican Speaker Paul Ryan drew fire from all sides of the political spectrum and won support from only 17 percent of the public. The measure was withdrawn in March 2017 because it couldn't get enough votes. But the damage to Obamacare's protections and subsidies were already well underway after Trump took office—even before Republicans in the new Congress turned to repealing Obamacare.

President Trump, administration health officials and Republican leaders have shown by word and deed their clear intentions to undermine both Medicaid and the ACA by any means at their command.

"The best thing we can do politically is let Obamacare explode," Trump told reporters on the same day that the first repeal effort failed. "It's imploding, and soon will explode, and it's not going to be pretty." The repeal campaign, whether through legislation or deregulation, also aims to wipe out Obamacare's extended Medicaid coverage in over thirty states for about fourteen million people who weren't previously covered—and almost all of them would lose their coverage under the GOP repeal bill that passed the House. Virtually *all* Medicaid recipients still remain at risk of losing either their current benefits or coverage, through some combination of federal waivers granted the states and whatever bill reaches Trump's desk.

The administration and Republican leaders have a vested interest in failure: they have done whatever they could to hasten Obamacare's demise and limit the scope of Medicaid, threatening coverage for at least four million people with mental and substance abuse disorders who were previously uninsured, according to federal and academic estimates. Even before Trump was elected, Congress passed in 2014 a little-noticed measure crafted by Sen. Marco Rubio (R-Fla.) that drastically cut $8 billion worth of reimbursement to insurance companies for losses they incurred when expanding their Obamacare coverage to sicker people, *The New York Times* first reported. A federal judge ruled against the government for its underpayment in February 2017, but that came too late for smaller companies that folded and a few major ones, including Aetna and UnitedHealth, that drastically reduced their involvement in the Obamacare marketplaces in 2017; Aetna has even announced it will leave all the ACA marketplaces by 2018.

"The entire individual market, covering millions of farmers, ranchers and self-employed people, is at risk," Timothy Jost, an emeritus law professor at Washington and Lee University, told a health care reform panel in April 2017. Citing a range of damaging steps already taken or considered by the administration, he said these endangered beneficiaries could "suffer financial instability and loss of health and indeed life if the market is destroyed."

If Obamacare were just allowed to continue, the Congressional Budget Office (CBO) found, the individual marketplaces covering twelve million people would be financially viable. That non-partisan finding also disclosed that the original failed "replacement" bill was essentially an $883 billion tax cut for the wealthiest individuals and health companies that drained $839 billion from Medicaid, but its analysis of the individual health-care market didn't take into account Trump's deliberate sabotaging of Obamacare.

The House-passed version was even more draconian than the first one that failed. The new bill gutted protections for consumers with preexisting conditions and allowed states to eliminate essential health benefits—including mental health and maternity care—even from corporate health plans. "The latest version of Trumpcare doesn't just threaten access to behavioral health coverage for those on Medicaid, it threatens access to behavioral health coverage for everyone," Rep. Joe Kennedy (D-Mass.) wrote in an op-ed for STAT, an online health news site.

Regardless of the final outcome in Congress, the Trump administration's early actions in office especially aimed at destroying the ACA on a variety of fronts. As his first executive order, he undercut active enforcement of the individual mandate needed to spur younger and healthier people to sign up; his Health and Human Services (HHS) department initially pulled $5 million in advertising designed to urge people to enroll; and the White House dithered in early 2017 about whether to support or oppose "cost-sharing" subsidies worth about $7 billion that limit such out-of-pocket costs as deductibles for the six million lower-income purchasers of marketplace plans. At first, after the first bill failed, Trump threatened to end those subsidies in an effort to blackmail Democrats into supporting a revised repeal bill. But then his administration agreed—temporarily—in April 2017 to continue paying them to avoid a government shutdown over a federal budget dispute. Without those subsidies, first challenged in a House Republican lawsuit against the Obama administration, the private marketplaces will almost surely collapse, most experts agree.

Even before these latest attacks on Obamacare, the nonstop political attacks and congressional time bombs planted by Republicans led to a stunning decline in insurers in many states. A *Vox* survey found that the number of counties with only one insurer quadrupled to 960 in 2017 compared to the previous year, leading to exorbitant premiums and potentially no coverage at all in 40 percent or more of American counties. Recent polling shows that nearly two-thirds of Americans will blame Republicans if Obamacare fails. Nevertheless, Trump is sticking by his blame-the-Democrats strategy to further undermine whatever remains of Obamacare after his agencies and the Republican Congress have artfully used their power to starve the private marketplaces of funding, incentives and support.

Although the imminent threat of a successful congressional onslaught on Medicaid's budget has diminished somewhat as of this writing, there hasn't been nearly as much attention paid to the continuing dangers posed to recipients of Medicaid even if the Republicans' frontal assaults on the program in Congress fail. Medicaid lacks the broad political support afforded Medicare, but with seventy-four million people enrolled—more than Medicare—the federal-state program is the country's leading funder of services for the most seriously mentally ill adults and children. In the harsh era of Donald Trump, they remain especially vulnerable to the regulatory schemes promoted by the hardliners now in charge of federal health agencies.

"These policies make it harder for the lowest-income people to get health care through the Medicaid program," the advocacy group Families USA notes on its web page devoted to tracking the administration's "sabotage" efforts. The new HHS secretary, Tom Price, has already signaled through rule-making and a letter to the nation's governors a willingness to grant state officials a relatively free hand to eviscerate government and private-sector health insurance programs. Administrators of both the state Obamacare exchanges and Medicaid programs have been offered far greater flexibility to limit required health benefits and eligibility for those programs.

The federal waivers Price wants to deploy are like catnip to budget-conscious officials eager to drastically cut spending. States such as Arizona, Indiana, Kentucky and Wisconsin, among others, are seeking or have already won permission to lock out Medicaid recipients if they don't pay premiums; require so-called "able-bodied" recipients to work to be eligible for benefits; limit Medicaid eligibility to five years; and test them for illegal drugs without acknowledging the deterrent effect on addicts needing treatment. As a result, new risks face all of the fourteen million recipients already added through the Medicaid expansion and millions more who could be denied coverage.

Indeed, at least thirteen million more children and adults who were already using Medicaid's behavioral health services before Obamacare took effect could find such basic benefits as medications and psychiatric care sharply curtailed or virtually impossible to obtain. In part, that's because the GOP health care bill and the Trump administration intend to place a fixed cap on all federal Medicaid spending through either "block grants" or per-person spending limits that also give leeway to states to slash their own spending on the program; these rigid federal spending limits also could prevent states from adding new Medicaid patients even in the case of a recession or a Zika-style epidemic. Even if stand-alone bills to drastically restructure Medicaid can't pass Congress now, Price and his new director of the Centers for Medicare & Medicaid Services (CMS), Seema Verma, have plenty of power to grant draconian administrators broad freedom to clamp down on the program through "Section 115" waivers.

Verma, an Indiana health care consultant who is a protégé of Vice President Mike Pence, has had plenty of practice adapting the waiver's authority to boot people off the Medicaid rolls under the guise of promoting "personal responsibility." As part of a deal with the Obama administration to allow Medicaid expansion, Verma created a "Healthy Indiana" plan that required people to make seemingly modest monthly payments—from one dollar up to a hundred, depending on their income—into a personal account to ensure coverage. But if there are any slip-ups in payments, you either get punished with higher co-pays and skimpier coverage—or kicked out of the program altogether for six months. In practice, as WFYI public radio reported, the state and private insurers too often made repeated bureaucratic mistakes that left even steadfast payers without coverage. On top of that, as USA Today reported, more than half of the low-income people who qualified for the relatively top-tier version of the Indiana program were cited for failing to make a required monthly payment, forcing them into cheaper and riskier bare-bones programs, according to a state-funded survey. State officials claim that only a small portion of them were locked out altogether from receiving any health care coverage—

regardless of the seriousness of their mental or physical health conditions. It is still being promoted as a national model for other states by Verma and the budgetary hit-squad at HHS.

The dystopian future awaiting the most seriously mentally ill people under a Trump administration can, perhaps, be glimpsed by looking at what happened when Tennessee, facing a fiscal crisis, used HHS waivers to cut over 350,000 people from the Medicaid rolls starting in 2005 and drastically curtailed benefits for others. These included limiting virtually all recipients to a total of five medications. With 35,000 of the most seriously and chronically mentally ill recipients losing all coverage, homelessness, emergency room visits and jailings rose sharply in Tennessee.

In fact, as many as half of the state's most seriously and persistently mentally ill people in some counties who were *theoretically* eligible for the state's "safety net" alternative to their lost Medicaid coverage couldn't manage the paperwork obstacles and were left to drift into oblivion. One family's obituary for their son who committed suicide explicitly blamed TennCare, as Medicaid is known, for denying him the services and medication he needed. "If you send paperwork to the severely mentally ill and require them to fill out all these forms, you're going to lose a lot of people right off the deck," says Gordon Bonnyman, the Tennessee Justice Center staff attorney who opposes such cuts and restrictions emerging now from the Trump administration.

In addition, millions of people who won coverage under Obamacare could be in for a rude surprise when their new mental health benefits either disappear or become so limited as to be nearly worthless. A little-known bonus of the Affordable Care Act is that it also mandated ten "essential health benefits" including drug and mental health treatment for all those enrolled in individual and small company plans, along with the millions of beneficiaries of expanded Medicaid coverage, theoretically offered on a par with medical benefits, a requirement known as "parity." Here's another shock: Citizens of major Democratic, pro-Obamacare states such as California and New York can't necessarily count on their progressive governors to protect them from the same sort of harsh restrictions in the proposed Republican health care bill embraced by conservative GOP governors in the South and other red states. As *Kaiser Health News* reported, the deep cuts in the Obamacare subsidies that assist Americans to buy individual and small company insurance coverage in the marketplaces could make all the plans unaffordable. So to keep insurers in their states and bring average consumer costs down, even liberal governors may have to ask for waivers allowing them to omit essential health benefits or charge far higher rates to the sickest and most disturbed people.

The far skimpier coverage that could be potentially offered is a potential deathblow especially for the most troubled mentally ill people and addicts who turn to Medicaid for help. It's disturbing that despite over 59,000 overdose deaths annually, most due to opioids and heroin, nearly three million—often mentally ill—drug addicts who got coverage for the first time under Obamacare and Medicaid could face new barriers to care; others will surely be frightened away from enrolling in Medicaid by drug-testing requirements if states win permission to do so. All these potential restrictions will be worsened by the impact of Attorney General Jeff Sessions's determination to restore maximum prison sentences for even low-level drug offenders and Tom Price's unscientific, abstinence-oriented opposition to using medically-assisted opioid treatments such as Suboxone, rejecting his department's own research findings. When taken together with reduced access to treatment, the Trump administration's extreme law-and-order response to the opioid crisis, despite Trump appointing a presidential commission to address the epidemic, could well lead to the deaths of thousands of more addicts each year.

Even the well-meaning federal parity requirements for both small Obamacare and large corporate plans are still often more a promise than a reality, due to exorbitant out-of-pocket costs and shortages of in-network mental health providers, NAMI reported in November 2016. Yet many of those reforms, too, could be further undermined in the Republican stampede to repeal Obamacare and cut Medicaid spending that is finding a new outlet in arcane agency decision-making out of the public spotlight.

"It will be disastrous," Cheryl Fish-Parcham, Director of Access Initiatives for Families USA, says of the potential passage of

Trump's Obamacare repeal in Congress. The same ominous potential remains if Republicans get everything they want through new regulations and waivers.

• • •

EVEN IF YOU RETAIN YOUR MENTAL HEALTH COVERAGE UNDER TRUMP, most people can't afford it: nearly half of all psychiatrists don't take private insurance or Medicare. As *Bloomberg News* recently reported, they're increasingly choosing to take cash-paying patients with easier-to-treat problems, forcing even more of the severely mentally ill to navigate the fragmented and overbooked community clinics in a desperate waiting game for help. Meanwhile, Medicaid enrollment remains an obstacle course even for the low-income people who qualify, and, of course, it will be virtually impossible for otherwise eligible mentally ill people to join Medicaid after rigid spending limits are enacted.

Hospital emergency rooms have already become the short-term treatment site of last resort. Too often the absence of any kind of care can lead to suicide, now the second-most common cause of death for Americans between ages fifteen and thirty-four, according to the Centers for Disease Control (CDC). Of the nation's 33,000 firearm deaths a year, over 60 percent are self-inflicted.

The nation is still reeling from state mental health budget cuts of over $4 billion during the three years after the 2008 crash. In most states, budgets still remain below 2009 levels. So if the nation would just address the funding shortage, we're told, we would go a long way towards helping the 40 percent of the nation's ten million seriously mentally ill adults who don't get any treatment in the course of a year. (Those with serious mental illness are defined by the federal government as being severely impaired during the past year by such conditions as schizophrenia, bipolar disorder and major depression.) The shortage of funds, stigma and lack of access to treatment have been singled out as the primary evils in the reform narrative offered by mental health organizations. But they generally don't pay much attention to the true quality of care or overmedication or pharmaceutical corruption of the mental health system—or of the mental health advocacy groups themselves.

Of course, there's usually little public interest in addressing mental health issues at all until there's a senseless mass shooting that shocks the country. They've ranged from the thirty-two killed at Virginia Tech in 2007 and the twenty-six killed at the Sandy Hook school in Newtown, Connecticut, in December 2012, to so many others, including the largest mass shooting in American history as of this writing: the killing in June 2016 of forty-nine patrons at a gay nightclub by Omar Mateen, a troubled twenty-nine-year-old Muslim man. He was seemingly fueled by some combination of Islamic extremism, self-hatred over his bisexuality and an undiagnosed mental disturbance. As Mateen grew up, his anger flared up regularly at classmates, his first wife, coworkers and, finally, with a legally purchased assault weapon, it took aim at all the strangers that he massacred at the Pulse nightclub in Orlando, Florida.

Unfortunately, in the first half of 2016 alone, there were nearly 170 mass shootings involving four or more people shot or killed in each incident, although there's no consensus on what portion of such killers show signs of mental illness. Estimates range from 20 percent with serious, disabling mental illnesses to as much as 60 percent, according to *The American Journal of Public Health*. Still others have been identified by Pennsylvania psychologist Peter Langman, author of *School Shooters* and creator of the Schoolshooters.info archive, as "psychopathic shooters" lacking in empathy and as "traumatized shooters" raised in abusive homes. It's likely, in fact, that most mass killers have some form of mental illness, even if many don't meet the narrow legal definition of insanity: the inability to tell right from wrong at the time of the crime.

By the time you read this, there will most likely be yet another horrific tragedy that stirs new calls for reform, new debates over whether mental illness or unimpeded access to guns is really at fault and concern from progressives that people with mental illness are being unfairly stigmatized since they are far more likely to be victims than perpetrators of violence.

After these shootings, right-wing and Republican Party leaders inevitably talk about mental health as the real issue to be addressed, rather than the truly insane lack of meaningful gun control. As usual in these and other public arguments on guns, liberals often decry right-wingers' references to mental illness as a ploy to avoid gun control, while conservatives denounce gun control as a phony ruse that will disarm regular citizens and won't stop criminals, crazy people and terrorists from getting guns. In truth, the country needs both dramatically improved and accessible mental health care along with far tougher gun control laws.

Former Arkansas Governor Mike Huckabee, a frequent GOP candidate and Fox commentator, declared after the slaying of nine at Umpqua Community College in southern Oregon in October 2015, "Do we need to do a better job in mental health? You bet we do." When Huckabee was governor, though, Arkansas received a "D-" rating on a national scorecard issued by NAMI, which remains a valuable yardstick. When conservatives talk about mental health, for the most part they're talking about tracking down chronically crazy people and forcing them to have treatment or locking them up somewhere—without bothering to think about who will pay for it all, let alone if it would be effective or helpful. (The hollowness of the right-wing's emphasis on mental illness's role in gun violence was underscored when the NRA successfully pushed—along with the ACLU and disability rights groups—for legislation that overturned in February 2017 an Obama administration regulation that closed yet another potential loophole: it required the Social Security Administration to report to the FBI background check system mentally impaired beneficiaries who were incompetent to manage their own finances.)

There is, of course, a sharp debate over the extent that seriously mentally ill people engage in violence, but they're only a fraction of all those who commit violent crimes—and they're eleven times more likely to be victims of violence than the general population. At the same time, untreated, severely mentally ill people are disproportionately more likely to engage in violence than the average citizen, and that is largely accounted for by the substance abuse that afflicts as many as 50 percent of them.

A recent controversial *Boston Globe* investigation illustrates just how inflammatory and complex the issues are surrounding mental illness and violence. It found that drug and alcohol abuse is one of the major risk factors in violence by mentally ill people, along with a lack of treatment and failure to take medications. These findings, consistent with some major psychiatric research on violence, were reported in the startling investigative series that found in June 2016 that mentally ill suspects—although some had no formal diagnoses—were involved in more than 10 percent of all homicides with known suspects across the state since 2005.

The series prompted a protest of nearly two hundred people representing mentally ill clients of state services and their allies outside the *Globe* building. They carried cards, pinned to flowers, featuring the names of some of the hundreds of mentally ill people killed over the years during treatment, including with such restraints as straps and handcuffs, and in shootings by police (149 such fatal shootings in the first eight months of 2016, *The Washington Post* reported). "They demonized us," says Ruthie Poole, the board president of M-Power, an advocacy group for mental health consumers, as they're known. The critics argued that the series also promoted the wrong kind of care: forced treatment and dangerous hospitalizations.

The real, nuanced truth about mental illness, violence and the role of treatment, this book shows, doesn't align neatly with any of the highly polarized arguments.

So even *The Globe*'s analysis of the problem, like most of the commentaries and reports about mental illness following high-profile mass shootings, focused on the lack of adequate funding and barriers to treatment. None of these explications, however, have probed deeply into the quality of care itself after people get access to treatment, outside of noting problems arising from a shortage of trained healthcare providers.

In contrast, this book explores the underlying factors driving the failures of the distorted mental health system. Ultimately, because of overspending on too many dubious, risky medications, corporate fraud and unproven therapies, fewer funds, training and clinicians are available to offer cost-effective, personalized treatments and, for some people at certain times in their lives, carefully prescribed drugs that work. For now, however, mental health care, as currently offered by most providers and clinicians, continues to be portrayed as an unalloyed good, and supposedly even more people need to receive more treatment, regardless of the actual quality. Unfortunately, the furious political debate over repealing Obamacare has obscured the hard truth that the current mental health system is such a fiasco that even having health insurance doesn't ensure good—or even safe—outcomes.

The improved access to care promised by the passage of the Helping Families in Mental Health Crisis Act, a reform bill introduced by Rep. Tim Murphy (R-Pa.) as a response to the Newtown shootings in 2012, doesn't truly address these broader failings. (Neither did Hillary Clinton's ambitious mental health plan released in August 2016, featuring such worthy goals as integrating mental and general medical health care in the same community settings.) The Murphy bill first ran into criticism from Democrats and rights-oriented mental health advocates who asserted that it overemphasized forced treatment and more hospitalization while jeopardizing the privacy of patients' records, among other concerns. After those provisions were softened, the legislation—signed into law in December 2016—now aims to improve coordination of 112 different federal mental health programs with a new assistant secretary of the Department of Health and Human Services (HHS); expand access to crisis inpatient care; and promote early prevention and screening. Yet this authorizing legislation seemed likely to be starved of the funds needed to carry out its relatively modest agenda by budget-conscious Republicans, who also oppose Obamacare's expansion of Medicaid and seek its total repeal. Nevertheless, after the mental health bill passed the House in 2016, Rep. Murphy dramatically declared: "This historic vote closes a tragic chapter in our nation's treatment of serious mental illness and welcomes a new dawn of help and hope."

These promises come too late for Janette Layne of Charleston, West Virginia. When she last saw her husband Sgt. Eric Layne alive, he had been discharged just two weeks earlier from a VA Hospital unit in Cincinnati specializing in PTSD (similar to the one Tompkins was desperate to enter) and was dozing on the couch with the TV playing while she headed upstairs to their bedroom. Because of his mounting outbursts of rage and paranoia since he first returned from Iraq, the expert psychiatrists at two VA hospitals had been prescribing Layne increasing doses of a drug cocktail for PTSD that included a powerful, risky antipsychotic drug, Seroquel. Although it's not officially approved for such "off-label" uses, Seroquel is among the most pre-scribed drugs in its class and at its peak brought in more than $5 billion a year for its manufacturer, AstraZeneca, all the while being linked to side effects ranging from diabetes to sudden cardiac arrest.

Yet even though Eric Layne kept complaining of headaches and tremors—concerns, by the way, that were discounted by the VA med-ical staff—he also gained too much weight, had trouble breathing and was so over-sedated that, according to his wife, he had become a "zombie." One month later, he was dead.

"All these doctors and medics and PhDs kept telling us that he was fine," Janette Layne says of their treatment ordeal. "We trusted the doctors."

It's a trust that's no longer warranted from the families of the more than four hundred combat veterans and other military personnel who are estimated by critics to have died suddenly after being over-medicated with PTSD "cocktails" that included Seroquel and an array of mood stabilizers. Military inquiries so far have largely blamed the seemingly mysterious deaths on suicides and natural causes—or, in a few cases, on some inexplicable "drug toxicity"—rather than looking to the way the government's own psychiatric practices are distorted by pharmaceutical industry influence. The role that the drug industry has played in these and other needless tragedies has largely been downplayed by the military and the Department of Veterans Affairs, particularly with regard to the secretive payments to VA researchers, the aggressive marketing of antipsychotics drugs for "off-label" uses like insomnia and the irresponsible, fatal use of opiates with chronic pain and PTSD patients.

Indeed, a hunger for profits has corrupted just about every con-ceivable arena of mental health care, from the overdrugging of foster care kids and the elderly to abusive teen residential facilities. Not only that, it's been abetted by what this book shows are indifferent pro-fessional associations, pharmaceutical-subsidized patient advocacy groups and government regulators that either push a drug-industry agenda or fail to halt what amounts to an epidemic of behavioral health malpractice. Already feeble oversight will be weakened further by a Trump administration determined to roll back regulations on health care and every other industry.

Mental Health, Inc. provides a comprehensive look, told through the stories of those harmed by reckless care, at the most critical mental health abuses and dangerous, ineffective practices—while probing the corporate and government obstacles to providing effective, proven and compassionate care. (The title and spirit of my book have been inspired in part by the book on corporate greed by Morton Mintz, called *America, Inc.: Who Owns and Operates the United States.*)

Despite these failures, some mentally ill people have won unexpected victories in their lives by getting smart, personalized help from programs that work. You'll meet in this book a Silver Spring, Maryland, man with schizophrenia who escaped a past stuck in an overmedicated stupor and now succeeds at the corporate job he has held for a decade; and a young college freshman in Portland, Maine, who was startled by emerging hallucinations, but received early intervention so well-targeted and so supportive that she avoided developing schizophrenia at all. Now she works as a psychiatric nurse helping others. Unfortunately, these sorts of valuable programs that helped them—for instance, "supported employment" and those based on the Portland Identification and Early Referral (PIER) model—are threatened either by hostile or inept federal agencies, as well as a chaotic mental health system.

Far more than government apathy or incompetence is involved in creating a mental health field that a presidential commission years ago justly called a "shambles." It is also largely an out-of-control, profit-driven system. The pages ahead showcase the recent trials and lawsuits targeting providers whose overdrugging or negligence helped kill their patients, and unravel the corporate and government wrongdoing that made possible the deaths of innocent people who just needed some help. The consequences of today's failed system are best illuminated by the stories of its victims told in the following chapters, as well as by snapshots of corrupt drug industry executives and academic researchers who created fraudulent marketing schemes that still needlessly kill thousands each year with medications.

• • •

DESPITE DECADES OF CRIES FOR REFORM, IT'S REMARKABLE HOW LITTLE has fundamentally changed in how we treat people with serious mental illness. Maltreatment of the severely mentally ill has been around almost as long as mental illness itself. So it's worth reviewing, in brief, the appalling story of how mental health treatment and research went off the rails before reformers and concerned citizens can start trying to fix what's wrong now.

Much of the response to madness has been driven in part by the fear and confusion felt by both the medical profession and the public over severe mental illness, especially schizophrenia. Although increasingly viewed by experts as a syndrome involving various "neurodevelopmental" disorders that manifest differently, schizophrenia is marked in part by paranoia, delusions or hallucinations that make it hard for sufferers to distinguish between fantasy and reality. Except for a few experiments in compassionate care in late eighteenth-century France and in American Quaker communities in the early 1800s, the drive to control and manage the mad can be seen everywhere—from the chained lunatics of the bedlam era of the 1700s in Europe and the US, straight through to the shock therapy, insulin injections, ice baths and lobotomies common in modern America until the mid-1950s.

This sordid record was described most notably in Robert Whitaker's *Mad in America*, but its spirit has been carried forward into the pharmaceutical era, augmented by greed, deception and fraud. That's a theme underlying the books of Whitaker and other leading critics of the pharmaceutical industry and drug-oriented psychiatry, such as Dr. Marcia Angell, journalist Melody Petersen, Dr. David Healy and Dr. Ben Goldacre.

For mentally afflicted people in the "snakepit" hospital era of the 1940s and '50s, insulin injections and other nominally "therapeutic" treatments were the norm until the spread of Thorazine and other FDA-approved antipsychotics originally developed for their ability to limit movement while patients remained awake. After being synthesized by French chemists in 1951, the drug chlorpromazine, better known as Thorazine, was hailed as a "medicinal lobotomy" and had calming effects on surgery patients and psychotics. But, as Whitaker notes, the drug's traumatizing impact started being downplayed in

1954, when marketing efforts in the US promoted Thorazine as a "wonder drug" that could essentially cure madness.

The hype surrounding the original antipsychotic drugs helped lead to the closing of many mental hospitals, leaving hundreds of thousands of severely mentally ill people out on the streets, without any better or meaningful alternatives. These trends were further fueled both by scandals about squalid mental hospitals and new legislation in the 1960s—which included Medicaid and President Kennedy's mental health act—that spurred the closing of state and county mental hospitals. In the mid-1950s, there were close to 560,000 public psychiatric beds available and by 2016, there were less than 40,000 such beds. When all public and private psychiatric beds are counted, that still amounts to less than 70,000 beds—even though nearly 400,000 seriously mentally ill people are incarcerated in jails and prisons on any given day. Essentially, then, ten times more mentally ill people are inmates than are patients in public hospitals. At other times, they may join the ranks of the people with severe mental illness who make up a third of the nation's 550,000 homeless counted on a single night in January 2016.

Others are confined with nearly 700,000 or more mentally ill people in poorly monitored nursing homes and assisted living facilities (ALFs). Nearly once a month, *The Miami Herald* reported in 2011, mentally ill and elderly residents were killed through abuse and neglect in the state's ALFs while law enforcement and state regulators looked the other way. Outside of some facilities closed following media investigations, most states have done little to crack down on these homes.

The newer generation of antipsychotics developed in the 1990s, such as Zyprexa, Risperdal and Seroquel, was supposed to usher in an era of quality care, assuming treatment could be obtained. With their potentially fatal side effects buried, these drugs were promoted as having none of the neurological side effects of the earlier drugs. The "miracle" pills were heavily marketed to virtually any agency or doctor treating people with almost any form of mental illness or distress.

The exaggerated and false claims made on behalf of these drugs by drug companies weren't fully debunked until devastating independent government-funded tests, known by the acronym CATIE (Clinical

Antipsychotic Trials of Intervention Effectiveness), were published in 2005. They publicly branded the newer antipsychotics as not any safer or more effective for schizophrenia than the older medications.

In fact, even the early tests for those newer antipsychotics (known as "atypicals") not only risked lives, but were essentially rigged against the older ones. The original schizophrenia trials did this, in part, by ramping up dosages of the old antipsychotics being studied to dangerous levels and inducing psychotic relapses through the sudden withdrawal of the patients' current meds before those in the experiments were given placebos. The suicide rates in these early trials were two to five times higher than the norm for people with schizophrenia. The experiments' dangerous subterfuges were exposed in a 1998 *Boston Globe* series led by Whitaker and in documents unveiled in lawsuits against drug manufacturers. The diabetes, weight gain and cardiac risks posed by the new antipsychotics, joined by the potentially higher risk of suicide posed by antidepressants for some youth, were well-hidden for years.

But even as drug companies have paid out $35 billion to federal and state governments in fines and settlements over the last twenty-five years for the alleged illegal marketing and sale of psychiatric and medical drugs alike, according to Public Citizen's Health Research Group, not much has changed in terms of either scientific discovery or ethics. Those penalties are dwarfed by the $711 billion in global net profits the pharmaceutical industry earned in just one decade. At least eight major drug companies, including AstraZeneca and Pfizer, had to sign two or more agreements with the federal government promising to never illegally market their drugs again. But findings of the Health Research Group and recent lawsuits show those agreements to be poorly enforced or altogether ignored. AstraZeneca, for example, shelled out nearly $2 billion in legal fees, penalties and settlement payments over government allegations of illegal marketing of Seroquel and the hiding of health dangers alleged in 26,000 liability lawsuits. That was a pittance compared to the more than $5 billion it earned, as noted earlier, in its best-selling years.

Even after all this research and controversy, neither the drug companies nor federally funded academics are significantly closer to finding definitive, overwhelmingly effective and safe medications to treat mental illness. Scientists also still haven't solved, despite promising hints from DNA and brain research, the underlying scientific mystery of madness. As the then-director of NIMH, Dr. Thomas Insel, observed in a 2010 article in *Nature*, "We still do not have a basic understanding of the pathophysiology of the disorder and therefore lack the tools for curative treatment or prevention needed for most people with schizophrenia."

Another sort of "scientific fraud" (Whitaker's term) is the development of corporate-funded pharmaceutical solutions for mental illness that rely on the cherished "chemical imbalance theory" for their claims. This posits that depression is caused by insufficient serotonin levels and that schizophrenia is caused by excessive amounts of dopamine. Leading medical journals have largely debunked this theory since the 1970s for schizophrenia (and for depression by the late 1990s) because researchers have shown that *unmedicated* people with these illnesses didn't have different levels of these brain chemicals than "normal" control subjects. Despite being widely discredited, this hasn't stopped pharmaceutical companies from marketing the theory as a solution to help boost drug sales. (The contentious dopamine argument, though, is periodically revived by some respected scientists claiming to offer dramatic new evidence for its validity.)

Many people, of course, have been helped by both antidepressants and antipsychotics regardless of how they work. Elyn Saks, a professor of law at the University of Southern California and author of the memoir *The Center Cannot Hold: My Journey Through Madness*, has praised the value of Clozaril and, earlier, Zyprexa in her life. After taking Zyprexa for the first time, she writes, "Thanks to the new chemicals coursing through my body, I experienced long periods of time in which I lived as other people did—with no psychotic thinking at all." Researchers, though, continue to debate the validity of studies that seemingly show the effectiveness—or ineffectiveness—of psychiatric medications.

By the time the independent CATIE findings appeared in 2005 deriding the superiority claims made for drugs such as Zyprexa, Risperdal and Seroquel, the marketing gold rush for the new antipsychotics was too successful to be stopped and the audience for these drugs had spread far beyond schizophrenics. (A note on language: Terms such as "schizophrenic" and "patient" are often seen as stigmatizing, but they'll occasionally be used for ease of reading.) With or without FDA approval, they were now being hawked for use with almost anyone with problems, including moody toddlers, stressed-out veterans and cranky seniors in nursing homes. A co-researcher on the major CATIE study, psychiatry professor Dr. Robert Rosenheck of Yale University, told me, "By that time, it was Katy bar the door!"

The legacy of corrupt medication research and mistreatment of the mentally ill—and troubled teens—chronicled over the years by critics of the drug industry, abusive youth treatment and psychiatry lives on today in dangerous, sometimes life-threatening, care.

In contrast to such concerns, mainstream psychiatry's most influential leaders, such as the former American Psychiatric Association (APA) president, Dr. Jeffrey Lieberman, have proclaimed that psychiatry has been "reborn" due to the introduction of what they say are safe and effective new medications. But they overlook that callous, even fatal, treatment is not just ancient history from the bygone era of hospital "snakepits." Dangerous prescribing patterns, for instance, have generally worsened in the years since the well-publicized death of an overmedicated four-year-old girl named Rebecca Riley in a Boston suburb more than a decade ago. There has been no meaningful reform of residential treatment abuses for decades, either, even after nearly ninety reported on-site teen deaths in the last fifteen years.

Beyond just chronicling the disastrous human impact of a failed and misguided behavioral health care system, this book also tells the dramatic David vs. Goliath stories of a few brave reformers who have taken on the health care and drug companies that have so warped treatment. These include whistleblowers such as psychiatrist Dr. Stefan Kruszewski, a consultant to the Pennsylvania welfare department, who was fired after reporting the deaths of kids who were killed by psychiatric drugs nearly fifteen years ago, and who later became part of Department of Justice settlements that forced $2 billion in settlements from two major drug companies. You'll also see a modern Profile in Courage in Allen Jones, a dogged investigator for Pennsylvania's

Inspector General's office who was fired and then worked as a brick-layer after uncovering a massive scheme by Johnson & Johnson to hawk its drug Risperdal by having corrupt Medicaid officials across the country buy and promote their drug with phony prescribing guide-lines. Jones's findings later led to a $158 million settlement by Johnson & Johnson with Texas that netted him about $20 million while laying the groundwork for a $2.2 billion criminal and civil settlement in 2013, one of the nation's largest health-care fraud cases.

Equally important—but often overlooked—are pioneering re-searchers and clinicians who are judiciously using medications when needed, including antipsychotics in low doses and increasingly for rel-atively short periods, as part of more comprehensive approaches that involve the support of family members and the promotion of inde-pendent living. They're challenging outmoded, drug-and-sedate prac-tices that leave 90 percent of people with serious mental illness too disabled to work.

Just as troubling, drug-based outpatient Medicaid programs are so risky and ineffective that people with serious mental illness *receiv-ing treatment* now die twenty-five years earlier than the average Amer-ican. "This is a higher death rate than experienced currently by persons with HIV and on a par with sub-Saharan Africa," said Dr. Joseph Parks, then the medical director of the Missouri Department of Mental Health. According to Parks's recent congressional testi-mony, 80 percent of the deaths are due to illnesses such as diabetes and heart ailments that can be worsened by antipsychotic use.

• • •

MENTAL HEALTH HAS BEEN IN AND OUT OF HEADLINES FOR YEARS, SUPPLE-mented by periodic lip service about reform after a tragic mass killing. Yet we should still care about fixing a system that has gone so awry, even if you or a loved one aren't struggling with a mental illness. Why? Because so many people have been damaged by a mental health system that doesn't work and is too often run like a racket. By some meas-ures, about 20 percent of Americans have some sort of mental health condition, and sixteen million adults and children face disabling men-tal illnesses and emotional disturbances. The impact is devastating.

Mental illness is the largest single cause of disability, across all categories of injury, brain disorders and illness. The most serious mental illnesses (including schizophrenia, bipolar disorder and long-term major depression) play a major role in driving more than 40,000 Americans to kill themselves each year—more than the total number of car crash fatalities and well over twice the number of homicides. Overall, the nation's suicide rate across virtually all age groups has soared to its highest level in thirty years, especially among middle-aged men and teenage girls. At its very worst, the system is so bad that roughly two million people with serious mental illness go to jail each year, cycling in and out of local jail systems that hold nearly 11 million people annually. As Miami-Dade County Judge Steven Leifman, who has pioneered model community-based alternatives to jail, points out, "Because no comprehensive and competent community mental health treatment system was ever developed, jails and prisons once again function as *de facto* mental health institutions for people with severe and disabling mental illnesses"—the "New Asylums."

The largest psychiatric facility in the country is actually the Los Angeles County Jail. Over 20 percent of its 17,000 inmates each year suffer from serious mental illnesses—worsened by guard beatings, neglect and cover-ups that have led to the convictions of over 20 current and former Los Angeles County Sheriff's Department (LASD) officials on violence-related charges. This book provides an especially close look inside the LA County women's jail, where some LASD deputies gave an account of the death of an inmate, Unique Moore, apparently due to medical neglect, in October 2014 that doesn't square with the eyewitness accounts of her jailmates. As many as fifty deputies and the department now face a wrongful death lawsuit.

Yet adding hospital beds—often proposed as the best alternative to jails or suicide—is no true solution for a system already so callous that some counties engage in "Greyhound therapy." In 2013 the *Sacramento Bee* found that not only are people just dumped on the street in California after being released from the hospital, but in Las Vegas, they were given one-way tickets to places they didn't know and then told to call 911 when they got there. Some never survived: In January 2015, for instance, a thirty-three-year-old man checked into the Texoma Medical Center in Sherman, Texas, complaining of his suicidal intention to jump off a bridge to the staff at the hospital, which is owned by Universal Health Services (UHS), the nation's largest chain of inpatient behavioral health facilities with $9 billion in annual revenue. Ten days later, according to a federal safety report obtained by *The Dallas Morning News,* he was kicked out and shown to a bus stop. The next day, he was found dead after jumping off of a Dallas bridge.

Amid today's *laissez-faire* regulatory climate and broken community care system, the tragic cycle of failed hospitalizations, homelessness and jail can cost taxpayers as much as $1 million per patient over time until, all too often, they die far too young.

Unfortunately, as this book shows, with most national mental health advocacy organizations and professional groups compromised by drug money, it will be up to grassroots members of those groups, taxpayers and political leaders concerned about waste, preventable deaths and the need for cost-effective care to drive meaningful reforms. By introducing you to those whose lives were endangered by harmful care and to the people working to make a change, it is my hope that *Mental Health, Inc.* will help bring some sanity to our understanding of a mental health system run amok.

CHAPTER 1

Drugging Our Kids: Corporate Greed Joins Government Corruption, Apathy

IT WAS OBVIOUS ENOUGH TO DR. STEFAN KRUSZEWSKI THAT THE DEATH of this behaviorally troubled seventeen-year-old boy placed in a Texas facility could have been prevented. The scholarly, fifty-two-year-old Harvard-trained psychiatrist had only recently started working as a full-time consultant to the Pennsylvania Department of Public Welfare, investigating the quality of care, abuse and fraud. The boy, writhing from a deadly seizure after being regularly plied with two antipsychotics, died in December 2002, a few months after Kruszewski assumed his post. It was only the first of several preventable, medication-related deaths—and neglect and abuse—that he flagged for his superiors before they fired him about a year later for protesting and documenting the maltreatment of children under the state's supervision.

"It was clear that they didn't want real investigations," he says. In most cases that he reviewed, his bosses didn't even bother to respond to his findings. This teenager had a history of severe seizures, Kruszewski discovered while reviewing the medical records. But the facility ignored the youth's condition by taking him off his anti-seizure medication and instead placing him on two antipsychotics: the new, heavily marketed Zyprexa and the older Thorazine. The boy was just one of thousands of kids—usually court-ordered and unable to live with their parents or family members—shipped out of state to often cheaper, poorly regulated facilities.

Children's deaths and injuries from antipsychotics at the time drew little local notice and certainly no national attention. But years before the overdrugging death of Rebecca Riley in Massachusetts became headline news, Kruszewski was exposing a dangerous pattern of prescribing that continues today generally unimpeded. *The New*

York Times reported in December 2015 the troubling account of an eighteen-month-old California boy, Andrew Rios, who had violent seizures that couldn't be controlled by an epilepsy drug. Rios was then prescribed the powerful and illegally marketed Risperdal for an "off-label" use that led him to scream in his sleep and interact with people that he saw when hallucinating.

Pharmaceutical companies have worked hard to make this wider use of antipsychotics possible. They've employed intensive lobbying of the FDA, joined by legal—and sometimes illegal—payoffs to academics, FDA advisory committee members and state officials, supplemented by countless deceptive or patently false studies. As a result, the drug industry has succeeded in driving the FDA-approved age for dispensing most antipsychotics down to as young as five years old for certain dubious diagnoses. These questionable or sweepingly applied kiddie diagnoses, such as bipolar disorder in grade-schoolers, also include the purported "irritability" of autistic children.

The use of all antipsychotics has at least doubled among children and youth since 2001, with at least seven million prescriptions—whether through Medicaid or private insurance—written each year, based on an analysis of just 60 percent of retail pharmacies. Remarkably, most of these kids don't have a diagnosed mental disorder at all. Contrary to previous optimistic reports of a drop in prescribing for those under the age of twelve, the *Times* showed that by 2014 prescriptions for Risperdal, Seroquel and other antipsychotics rose 50 percent for children two and under to nearly 20,000—even after all the major manufacturers had already paid billions to settle federal lawsuits alleging their fraudulent promotion of these dangerous drugs. In 2015, long after Kruszewski uncovered that Medicaid-subsidized Pennsylvania children were killed by overmedication, the Office of Inspector General for the US Department of Health and Human Services (HHS) reported that more than 90 percent of the estimated two million kids on Medicaid who received antipsychotics are prescribed them without the approval of the FDA—or "off-label"—and hence for fraudulent uses. Even so, federal and state Medicaid agencies today reimburse all the $1.8 billion in government spending for these drugs for all ages without question. For those who remain on Medicaid in the Trump era, overuse of these mostly generic medications could well increase because they offer an illusory quick-fix replacement for time-consuming therapy and social work support requiring adequate staffing levels.

Antipsychotics aren't the most widely prescribed psychiatric medications for children, but they are among the most dangerous. For the nearly forty-one million psychoactive prescriptions of all kinds given to US kids, close to 60 percent are for stimulants prescribed for ADHD, whose side effects can include anxiety and psychosis. Now nearly one in five high school boys purportedly has ADHD, due largely to what medical experts see as "overdiagnosis" due to faulty evaluations and social pressure to use stimulant drugs to improve school performance and control behavior. Two-thirds of those ADHD-diagnosed youths take stimulants, but the use of antipsychotics for this loosely diagnosed illness is soaring. According to Reuters, the most common diagnosis for children eighteen and under who received antipsychotics was for the unapproved use for ADHD. Indeed, a Columbia University research psychiatrist found that 90 percent of all prescriptions for antipsychotics for kids were for off-label uses, even for the privately insured.

In some ways, the roots of this pediatric drugging crisis can be found in the corrupting influence of drug company subsidies, marketing and the lack of response by state agencies to the early, potentially fatal abuses uncovered by Kruszewski and other whistleblowers. Both the state-contracted facilities and the drug companies were "exaggerating and mischaracterizing the benefits, effects and use of psychotropic drugs that lacked beneficial or positive effect," according to Kruszewski's 2004 wrongful dismissal and free speech lawsuit.

In addition, Kruszewski found at least four children and one adult died due to overmedication, with as many as five antipsychotic medications given at one time to people at facilities in such states as Texas and Oklahoma. His mounting concerns, prompted by the death of a thirteen-year-old child in an Oklahoma center, led him to write a scathing report in July 2003. The child had been given the seizure medication Neurontin, multiple antipsychotics and mood stabilizers without having any medical or psychiatric condition justifying their use. The child then died, apparently due to seizures induced by the medications.

Kruszewski's report should have been a wake-up call, not only for the state of Pennsylvania but the entire country. His preliminary assessment of the facility was truly horrifying: the children were severely overmedicated with psychotropic drugs, were housed in deplorable conditions and some were being sexually abused by the staff. Kruszewski's report warned his supervisors that children and vulnerable adults should be removed from this and other dangerous out-of-state facilities while the damaging and needless off-label prescribing of psychotropics should be halted. When he asked his agency to spend a hundred dollars on a coroner's report on each of the four deaths of children he uncovered, he was told: "That's not possible." He argued, as his report said, for the removal of those endangered clients "in order to protect other innocent individuals from morbid and mortal consequences of severe overmedication, including chemical restraints; [and] emotional, physical and sexual abuse."

On July 11, 2003, one day after his supervisor chewed him out for "trying to dig up dirt," Kruszewski was fired. The agency "didn't want to hear anything bad about what was going on," he says now. "They were just looking for a warm body to put in the position." He eventually settled a lawsuit in 2007 against the Department of Public Welfare (DPW) for $374,000, although agency officials didn't acknowledge liability.

In 2005, Kruszewski filed the first of his three lawsuits brought under the False Claims Act, or *qui tam* filings, against health-care companies; these legal actions attempted to halt the improper prescribing and other abuses akin to those that led to the deaths of children he had investigated.

Kruszewski had firsthand knowledge of the drug companies' sales schemes. As an influential psychiatrist in a Harrisburg suburb who worked primarily with adolescents and the elderly, and as a professor at Penn State Medical College, he had faced, between 2001 and 2007, a hard sell of Pfizer's new antipsychotic product, Geodon. Pfizer's sales reps wanted him to prescribe the drug off-label to kids and the elderly for a host of unapproved uses, including depression and anxiety. He began discovering the dangers this drug posed as early as 2001, and at about the same time, he rebuffed efforts by AstraZeneca to recruit him to push its antipsychotic Seroquel to his colleagues with spurious safety and efficacy claims. That, in turn, led him to secretly file his own fraud lawsuits against Pfizer and AstraZeneca, starting in 2005. (Whistleblowers' lawsuits traditionally haven't been made public until government attorneys agree to join the lawsuit and then reach a settlement.)

Kruszewski filed his lawsuits against Pfizer and AstraZeneca to prod the pharmaceutical firms to alter the way they mask their drugs' real benefits and dangers—consequences that he saw personally with all those dead and damaged youngsters under state care. His lawsuits were ultimately incorporated with other whistleblower claims as part of huge federal settlements totaling nearly $3 billion against the two companies in 2009 and 2010. (Under the False Claims Act originally passed by Congress in 1863, all the whistleblowers involved in a case are jointly awarded a fraction of the funds successfully recouped by the government as a way to encourage reports of fraud.)

While Kruszewski was discovering the ways drug company influence and indifferent agency oversight were causing needless deaths, Allen Jones, a rugged, determined investigator with Pennsylvania's Office of the Inspector General, was asked by his bosses in July 2002 to look into suspicious payments by Johnson & Johnson to a secret bank account set up by Medicaid's chief pharmacist, Steve Fiorello. By following the money trail, Jones unraveled a massive drug industry scheme to bilk state Medicaid programs across the country—under the guise of promoting cutting-edge science—with prescribing guidelines that were rigged to favor the new brand-name, risky "atypical" antipsychotics. Along the way, he uncovered a campaign, known as the Texas Medication Algorithm Project (TMAP), to bribe state officials with payments, perks and travel to spread the use of the new atypical medications for a variety of unproven and off-label uses, including for children. (An algorithm is a decision-making tree that outlines which drugs are recommended for "first-line" use with certain symptoms and mental illnesses.) His bosses covered up his findings, and then Jones was fired in 2004 for "misconduct" after leaking his evidence to *The New York Times*, eventually settling a wrongful dismissal lawsuit against the state that left him with only $1,200 after he paid all his debts.

Unable to find any professional jobs, he lost his home and worked part of the time as a bricklayer while living in his off-the-electrical-grid cabin without running water he'd built in rural central Pennsylvania years earlier. Nearly broke, he waged a lonely battle to alert officials in Pennsylvania, other states and the federal government about the menace this corrupt program posed. "I went through some tough times," he recalls about his early years after getting fired, "but if I had caved in to them in the face of what I knew about the harm that would come from this scheme, it would have diminished me so much."

TMAP was a "microcosm of how the drug companies operate: the clinical trial manipulation, the ghostwriting, the biased reporting," Jones says now.

These strategies turned these antipsychotics, which were originally approved for only 1 percent of the population (people with schizophrenia), into blockbuster drugs that still generate billions of dollars in revenue by treating a far wider array of patients, mostly off-label. With roughly sixty million prescriptions written each year for antipsychotics, according to the research company IMS Health, as many as 75 percent of adults and over 90 percent of young people take the medications for uses that aren't approved by the FDA. TMAP was the tip of the spear of the industry's successful marketing war. Yet as a result of Jones's decade-long crusade, Fiorello was sentenced to prison on felony conflict-of-interest charges for taking drug company payments—and the key government official spreading the sham prescribing guidelines, Texas mental health department medical director Dr. Steven Shon, was forced to resign in 2006 after it was revealed that he and his department's researchers received lavish trips and more than $2 million from Janssen (the pharmaceutical division of Johnson & Johnson), and other drug companies. Finally, in 2012, years after Jones filed his whistleblower lawsuit, the Texas attorney general joined him and won a $158 million settlement, which J&J offered days into a trial, partly to halt further damaging testimony. Although

TMAP has been publicly discredited, its legacy lives on in faked research that has never been retracted and continues to influence the daily practice of physicians.

All these initiatives were supplemented by a growing body of studies by researchers-for-hire that concluded that antipsychotics should be used with a newly-discovered, dubious illness in little kids: bipolar disorder. This array of drug industry-funded scientific propaganda helped set in motion a chain of events that by 2006 culminated in the tragic death of Rebecca Riley, a four-year-old foster child in Hull, Massachusetts, from a toxic amount of prescription drugs, including Seroquel.

In the summer of 2004, Carolyn Riley took her then two-year-old daughter, Rebecca, to Dr. Kayoko Kifuji, a Tufts University doctor, for help with what the mother claimed was her "hyper" behavior and poor sleep. Prodded by the mother's claims about her girl's moody behavior, the doctor kept adding more drugs and higher dosages of such off-label sedating drugs as the blood-pressure drug clonidine, Zyprexa and Seroquel. Despite warnings from the school nurse that the four-year-old girl was like a "floppy doll" and could barely walk weeks before the girl's death, Kifuji prescribed her 835 pills during her last visit. In the early morning hours of December 13, 2006, Rebecca died while sleeping in a drugged stupor next to her parents' bed.

• • •

IN 2007, LOCAL AUTHORITIES LOOKED MORE CLOSELY AND CHARGED THE girl's parents with poisoning Rebecca because they couldn't get disability payments for her. They were convicted in 2010. After Kifuji was cleared by a grand jury of allegedly abetting their crimes, she was welcomed back by Tufts as "an outstanding physician." She settled a related civil malpractice lawsuit for $2.5 million in 2013 without admitting culpability in the case.

Just as disturbing is the way Kifuji justified her actions by citing research from such academics as Dr. Joseph Biederman, a world-famous, industry-subsidized child psychiatrist from Harvard. He has been denounced by *The New York Times* as a "shill" after court documents revealed that he had solicited money from Janssen to do a study that "will support the safety and effectiveness" on Risperdal with preschoolers. Biederman's work helped fuel in nearly a decade by 2003 a forty-fold increase in the diagnosis of pediatric bipolar disorder, paving the way for Kifuji's heedless, fatal prescriptions.

The legitimacy given to such off-label prescribing of antipsychotics for children casts a shadow over the lives of many youths, particularly foster children, in Massachusetts and other states. Indeed, that's especially true for all children on Medicaid, who, according to federally-funded researchers, are four times more likely to be prescribed antipsychotic drugs. Just as troubling is that Massachusetts's Department of Children and Families (DCF) still has no capacity to monitor psychotropic drugs for kids.

Advocacy groups such as Children's Rights have forced or challenged more than thirty states, including Massachusetts, to change their child welfare policies in ways that *should* also improve psychiatric care. (Massachusetts won its case, so it has felt free to ignore cries for genuine child-prescribing reforms.) Yet very few states have made significant progress in reining in the overmedication of kids in the federal-state Medicaid program. Antipsychotic prescriptions for foster care children have leveled off since 2008 to approximately 9 percent of all the nation's 415,000 foster care kids, Rutgers University researcher Stephen Crystal reported in a 2016 *Health Affairs* study—600 percent higher than other Medicaid children. Relatively few states, he found, stirred themselves to provide psychotherapy services to these kids before doling out meds, or even measured their potentially deadly metabolic side-effects. "No state is doing a very good job," says Crystal, the director of the Center for Health Services Research. Some states, such as California, drug nearly 25 percent of their foster care adolescents into submission with the full range of psychiatric medications, although that could change with tough new state legislation passed in August 2016, spurred by a disturbing *San Jose Mercury News* series.

• • •

IN THE YEARS AFTER REBECCA RILEY DIED, ANTIPSYCHOTIC DRUG MARKETING to kids continued unabated and even won new approval from the FDA. Somehow, more high-profile deaths in Texas and Florida, and the growing alarm over the legions of kids left in a stupefied state by these drugs, didn't prompt major reforms.

In 2009, seven-year-old Gabriel Myers, woozy from two antipsychotics and an antidepressant, stumbled into the bathroom of his Florida foster home, wrapped a shower hose around his neck and hanged himself. Three years earlier, Dr. Sohail Punjwani, the physician who prescribed the off-label medications to Myers, ran experiments for Pfizer's antipsychotic Geodon on kids between ten and sixteen. Florida children became guinea pigs for Pfizer even though the use of Geodon for children has never been approved. Six kids overdosed but survived. Three years before that, in 2003, a Florida teen under Punjwani's care, Emilio Villamar, died of a heart attack after receiving cardiac-adverse Seroquel and other antipsychotics that also posed heart risks, according to a 2009 lawsuit filed by his mother. Although he received a belated warning letter from the FDA, Punjwani was never sanctioned by any state or federal agency for the deaths or overdoses, although he was arrested for cocaine possession in 2010 and entered a pretrial diversion program without being prosecuted. He defended his medical work to *The Palm Beach Post* in 2011, resenting his portrayal as a "child killer;" he also claimed he followed correct prescribing protocols in his depositions in the Villamar and Meyers malpractice lawsuits he settled for undisclosed sums.

The Palm Beach Post also found in 2011 that doctors in the Department of Juvenile Justice–run jails and homes—including, for a while, Punjwani—were prescribing enormous amounts of expensive antipsychotics, mostly to keep kids under control. Over 325,000 antipsychotic pills, including Seroquel and Risperdal, were doled out over a two-year period in jails that held no more than 2,300 boys and girls on any one day. At the same time, the four top prescribing doctors in the system were lavished with close to $200,000 in drug industry booty.

In response to the furor, the department denied that there was abusive prescribing. Six years after the scandal, however, psychotropic prescribing remains roughly the same—about 30 percent—and the juvenile agency refuses to disclose antipsychotic use or whether its doctors are receiving drug money. Florida has still largely refused to take meaningful measures to rein in such dangerous prescribing. Despite the efforts of such advocacy groups as Florida's Children First, dangers persist throughout the state. Courts are supposed to review prescribing, but it's not at all clear that such measures actually protect kids from needless medication. Yet experts see progress now that total prescribing of psychotropic medication to Florida foster care kids is down to a claimed 11 percent overall. (That assertion is derided as "bullshit" by Michael Freedland, the lawyer who successfully won settlements for the families of Meyers and Villamar.) While that low figure, if accurate, may seem promising, psych prescribing for foster care teens in Florida is still officially reported at more than 25 percent, mostly for stimulants and antipsychotics.

• • •

FORTUNATELY FOR BIG PHARMA, THE DANGEROUS OFF-LABEL PRESCRIBING for children that marked Florida and other states got an added boost in June 2009 when the FDA expanded official approval for children's drugging with antipsychotics. In 2009 and in subsequent years, their manufacturers—AstraZeneca, Eli Lilly and Pfizer—were all targeted by the federal government for illegal marketing of their drugs while they were seeking to win FDA approval to market antipsychotics to children for the same uses that the Justice Department considered fraudulent. In January 2009, Eli Lilly agreed to pay $1.3 billion to resolve criminal and civil allegations that they were promoting Zyprexa for uses not approved by the FDA, including for children and adolescents. A few months after the 2009 FDA hearing, Pfizer spent $2.3 billion in criminal and civil payments to settle allegations of fraudulent marketing of four drugs, including Geodon, while denying any civil liability; and in 2010, AstraZeneca paid $520 million for allegedly fraudulently selling Seroquel. Drug companies are legally barred from promoting drugs for off-label uses, but all doctors are free to prescribe any non-opiate drug to anyone.

But in June 2009, the companies wanted FDA approval for their drugs for teens and children as young as ten for bipolar disorder and schizophrenia, leading to their off-label use today for sleepless toddlers and distracted ADHD teens. Experts for all three companies reassured the advisory committee that their drugs "were fine for kids," despite side effects such as weight gain, prolactin increases (which causes breast growth in boys), heart arrhythmia, diabetes risk and skyrocketing pulses.

While the hearing focused on evidence supplied by the drug companies, there wasn't much interest in the testimony of Liza Ortiz, a mother from Austin, Texas, grieving over the death of her thirteen-year-old son Philip earlier that year. Suffering from some psychotic symptoms, Philip was prescribed Seroquel after other drugs failed. Four days after it was added to a cocktail of other antipsychotics, he died in the hospital. As she and her family stood in the ICU, "I saw Philip's body so stiff and rigid with seizures that his hands twisted in ways that I never thought possible," she told the panelists.

Fortunately for the drug companies, they had a champion in Dr. Thomas Laughren, the Director of the FDA's Division of Psychiatry Products. He had previously been dubbed a "double agent" for the drug industry by the Alliance for Human Research Protection (AHRP), an anti-industry group, for hiding from another advisory panel in 2004 a staff report on the suicidal side effects of antidepressants on kids, as first reported by *The San Francisco Chronicle*. (Agency officials told a congressional committee that he didn't pass along the staff findings on suicide risks because the study was "imperfect.")

In the wake of that publicity and congressional scrutiny, the FDA backed off expanding Paxil's use for kids while continuing to allow such uses for Prozac, but a stronger pediatric warning label for all antidepressants was required by the end of 2004.

This time, in June 2009, Laughren was equally willing to advance the drug companies' case for the use of antipsychotics with children. As he told the advisory panel, "We are in agreement with the sponsors that the data tend to support the effectiveness claims that they are seeking," and that the drugs were just as safe for kids as they were for adults. In the end, though, the advisory committee ruled that all three drugs—Seroquel, Geodon and Zyprexa—were "acceptably safe" and effective for teenagers and children. (Laughren became a drug industry consultant after he left the agency in late 2012.)

After a further top-level review, the FDA decided in October 2009 to reject classifying Geodon as safe for children. According to a lawsuit ultimately rejected on appeal, that didn't stop Pfizer executives from allegedly ramping up a new marketing drive in 2009 to promote the drug more aggressively to child psychiatrists—with added sales bonuses for winning higher prescribed doses—even after the FDA rejection and Pfizer's agreement with DOJ to stop unlawful marketing. Those explosive charges are contained in a whistleblower fraud lawsuit filed in 2014 by former Pfizer sales reps Alex Booker and Edmund Hebron. Pfizer has denied the allegations. In May 2016, a federal judge rejected the lawsuit. That finding was finally upheld on appeal in January 2017, largely on the grounds that the whistleblowers couldn't prove that the allegedly false marketing led to specific fraudulent billing incidents.

• • •

IN A TOXIC CLIMATE OF AGGRESSIVE, ILLEGAL SALESMANSHIP AND WEAK regulation in virtually all states, it isn't surprising that even the feckless federal government occasionally expresses alarm at the overdrugging of kids. The findings of a 2015 federal inspector general's report confirmed that poor children and foster care kids covered by Medicaid are being prescribed too many dangerous antipsychotic drugs at young ages for far too long—mostly without any medical justification at all.

Using a close-up study of nearly seven hundred claims in five of the biggest prescribing states—California, Florida, Illinois, Texas and New York—the investigation discovered that two-thirds of all prescriptions of these popular and costly atypical antipsychotics raised "quality of care" and safety concerns. One of the most troubling cases: a sixteen-year-old with bipolar disorder on three antipsychotics as part of his drug cocktail, who then went on to exhibit side effects including paranoia, hallucinations, darkly suicidal thoughts, insomnia and extreme weight gain.

Perhaps even more damning, the report found that 92 percent of all kids on Medicaid receiving antipsychotics didn't have any of the relatively limited "medically accepted pediatric conditions" supposedly justifying their use for children as young as five. So given how much leeway the industry-influenced FDA has already given the drug manufacturers to legally deploy their wares on kids, just how far outside the bounds of sensible prescribing must a doctor go to merit FDA disapproval? But most of the few media accounts and the report itself ignored an even more fundamental example of failed oversight: the federal government's lax monitoring of state Medicaid programs dispensing these potentially life-threatening medications to children.

Medicaid programs are generally all too glad to look the other way at such antipsychotic spending gone wild. This lack of rigorous enforcement is especially disturbing in light of the real-world experiences of children killed or damaged in states such as California and Texas that have been nearly as scandal-scarred as Florida. The federal government, in fact, has served as a handmaiden to deadly prescribing.

How bad is federal oversight? In 2012, both the Government Accountability Office (GAO) and ABC News reported that the federal government had touted arguably the worst prescription-monitoring program in the country, run by Texas. The state was so lax that Texas foster care children were fifty-two times more likely to be prescribed five or more psychiatric drugs at the same time than non-foster children. Yet HHS's Administration for Children and Families (ACF) lauded the Texas drugging "parameters," despite the fact that they helped turn too many kids into drooling, tremor-ridden "zombies," as foster parents reported. The parameters were subsequently revamped by state experts and replaced in 2013 with tougher standards that only began to take effect in 2014, albeit on a limited scale.

Amazingly, the guidelines panel that was originally praised by ACF was stacked with two drug company-subsidized academics who were cited in court records for helping defraud Medicaid as part of the TMAP scheme uncovered by Allen Jones. Even so, the state has made *some* progress in recent years reining in psychotropic use. State officials and even outside reform advocates proudly note that the use of such drugs by foster care kids for more than sixty days dropped to just under 20 percent. Still, the percentage of children two and under getting psychiatric drugs rose nearly 50 percent between 2005 and 2013, the years when the trumpeted reforms were put in place. Today, an alarming 62 *percent* of all Texas foster care teens are on psych meds, with nearly two-thirds of those medicated youth on antipsychotics, much higher than the national average.

"Kids' bodies aren't meant to take that many meds," says Susan Rogers, a leading reformer who served on the board of the Texas Federation for Children's Mental Health and was a foster care parent for nearly thirty years. She and her husband found that they were undermined by state-funded psychiatrists and social workers who were often indifferent to the disastrous side effects of the antipsychotics the Rogers were pressured to give youth who didn't need them. "We had a foster daughter who blimped right up on Risperdal, gaining sixty pounds, and who was so miserable she became anorexic," she recalls. "I had to buy her a totally new cheerleader's uniform."

Influential doctors throughout the state were awash in J&J money to promote the drug, the TMAP fraud lawsuit revealed. "The psychiatrist wouldn't take her off this, and I said I'm going to do this anyway even if I lose my license [to provide foster care]," she says. She even worked extra hours to ensure that the school system provided the girl added therapy.

"We were screwed by the state," she now says of the corrupted practices and rigged protocols that harmed her foster children.

Texas officials boast about the centralized monitoring role of STAR Health, a managed health care firm for foster kids that supposedly flags excessive prescribing as part of its electronic "health passports." But all that wasn't enough to protect Jo Angel Rodriguez, a troubled eleven-year-old girl who bounced around the foster care system until her death in 2009, which prompted a wrongful death lawsuit settled with Pfizer; Pfizer is the maker of the antipsychotic Geodon, linked to heart irregularities and allegedly pushed by company salesmen for use by children since 2001, according to the Justice Department. As reported by the *San Antonio Current*, Rodriguez was taken to the Laurel Ridge Treatment Center and was first given the antipsychotic Abilify, which caused vomiting and diarrhea, and then spurred the girl's withdrawn and later aggressive behavior. The solution? More drugs.

A moonlighting medical school resident offered her Risperdal, and when she refused that, the novice doctor gave her a 20 mg shot of Geodon instead, helping trigger a heart attack resulting from a cardiac arrhythmia.

The continuing dangers facing Texas foster care children shouldn't have been surprising to anyone paying attention to the dubious makeup of that fourteen-member "working group" designing the 2010 guidelines that were hailed by the federal government; two of the experts, including Dr. Peter Jensen, the founder of Columbia University's children's mental health research center, were paid by J&J to promote ghostwritten or other questionable "research" on behalf of Risperdal that helped the TMAP psychotropic guidelines to loot sixteen other state programs, according to the Texas Attorney General. (They have declined to talk to me or other journalists over the years about the allegations in the lawsuit.)

A third panelist, Dr. Charles Fischer, a child psychiatrist at Austin State Hospital, was fired in November 2011 over allegations that he had molested teenage boys during "counseling" sessions over a twenty-year period, according to a Texas Medical Board order that temporarily suspended his license. He faced accusations from as many as six former patients and one former seven-year-old neighbor, now adults, at the trial that convicted him in mid-November 2016 of multiple counts of child abuse and sexual assault. He was sentenced to forty years in prison.

Texas court documents also showed that the groundwork for spreading TMAP was laid by J&J, which spent nearly $1 million on a trio of prestigious East Coast researchers, including Dr. Allen Frances of Duke University—now known as a critic of overmedication—to craft pro-Risperdal schizophrenia guidelines and promote a forerunner TMAP. The academics promised to help the company "increase its market share." (Frances has defended those guidelines as "carefully and honestly done.")

Before the TMAP trial began in January 2012, the state attorney general outlined how what he portrayed as ethically dubious researchers—such as Jensen—helped spread the idea that Risperdal was the best of the new antipsychotics even though it was actually having horrifying effects on kids, including causing D-cup breast growth in teenage boys. The J&J marketing deceptions succeeded in large part because respected researchers put their names on studies that were actually churned out by J&J's ghostwriting firms. Others just took the cash and cooked up studies with positive results pleasing to the Janssen division's marketers. As the Texas Attorney General explained in a filing before the trial: "Defendants thus 'seeded the literature' and increased the 'noise level' in the Texas health care community," peddling false tales of Risperdal's superiority and "suitability for off-label use on vulnerable populations."

Other antipsychotic manufacturers, such as AstraZeneca, supported the TMAP scheme with funding because, as Allen Jones says, "they could see which way the profit train was moving." They welcomed the portrayal of new atypical antipsychotics in a positive light, even though Risperdal was touted as the best of the new wonder drugs.

J&J, looking to end the battering to its image it was taking in court, settled shortly after the TMAP fraud trial started. But they still faced more costly settlements. J&J ultimately paid out $2.2 billion in 2013 to settle government criminal and civil charges related to illegal marketing of the drug. Then in 2015, in the first of roughly 10,500 pending breast growth cases they faced by early 2017, a Philadelphia jury decided that the company owed $2.5 million to a twenty-year-old autistic man who had developed size 46 DD breasts as a teenager. In July 2016, another Philadelphia jury awarded a sixteen-year-old boy $70 million, a decision that J&J promptly appealed; he had been taking Risperdal since he was five—while his family was never told of the risks. The company faces lawsuits from more than 100,000 patients, although the company has won some Risperdal cases. The "warnings" section in its Risperdal label still doesn't specifically mention breast growth—gynecomastia.

Even so, the lingering, horrible effects of TMAP are still felt in the lives of young people today.

• • •

NONE OF IT HAS MATTERED TO POLICY-MAKERS. ALL THE HUGE RISPERDAL court judgments, the Texas Attorney General's revelations about the 2010 foster care panelists, and the wave of Texas overdrugging haven't changed federal officials' hands-off approach to state Medicaid and foster care programs. Part of the problem, of course, is that federal Medicaid officials insist that they don't have the legal authority to stop paying for worthless and dangerous drug uses; that's in apparent opposition to a series of federal court rulings and Justice Department fraud lawsuits. Those legal findings concluded, as in a $2.3 billion DOJ settlement with Pfizer, that the federal government has been defrauded when it's asked to pay for drug "uses that were not medically accepted indications and therefore not covered by those programs," according to the DOJ announcement.

On top of that, federal Medicaid officials have said that they can't even advise the states to stop paying for these groundless uses of antipsychotics, although states do have the option to refuse to make fraudulent drug payments. "To say 'it's not our responsibility' while 92 percent of the [pediatric] Medicaid antipsychotic use is inappropriate and killing children, that's not acceptable," counters Toby Edelman, a senior policy analyst with the Center for Medicare Advocacy, which fights to get the federal CMS agency to regulate nursing home medications that kill thousands annually. At the same time, Department of Justice attorneys spend years building cases that have led to billions in fines and settlements from the drug industry for defrauding Medicaid and illegally marketing its products to doctors and agencies.

This struggle by DOJ to recover billions in waste will never catch up with Medicaid's heedless spending on unaccepted uses of antipsychotics. "They're just pretending to address the issue of overdrugging with a wink and a nod—the Justice Department gets billions from drug companies for causing off-label uses that aren't supported by the law, while CMS is continuing to pay for these same prescriptions," crusading mental health rights attorney Jim Gottstein observes.

California, for example, is one state whose controls over foster care antipsychotic prescribing are supposed to be monitored by HHS's ACF branch under a 2011 law. But the agency has simply rubber-stamped California's and other states' slow-walked foster care medication plans—with disastrous consequences for many of its 60,000 foster care children, according to critics and youth advocates. "I was given all these medications, but I wasn't functioning," a former California foster youth, who asked to remain anonymous, told me.

California, until very recently, was typical of most states that haven't bothered yet to even develop formal plans or have only recently crafted feeble "guidelines" that are rarely enforced; Illinois, Oregon and New York are among the few states that have sought to do more. But prompted in part by the *San Jose Mercury News* series, California passed laws in 2015 and 2016 that added nurses to monitor prescribing; required doctors to try to arrange psychotherapy for their patients before giving them drugs; and expanded the power of the licensing board to investigate overprescribing doctors.

• • •

WHEN PATIENTS COME TO AN HONEST, CARING PSYCHIATRIST LIKE Kruszewski, it's hard to undo all the damage wreaked by overmedication. "About 95 to 97 percent of the children that I treat that are getting antipsychotics are given them for reasons that aren't approved by the FDA," he says. Just as troubling, he says, are the wide range of devastating side effects they suffer that aren't much emphasized in the recent federal HHS Inspector General's report or by the medical community, among them cardiac and metabolic problems, and elevated prolactin levels which cause breast growth in boys. "Imagine trying to be a seventeen-year-old black male in inner-city Philadelphia with breasts so large you should be wearing a D-cup bra—and then trying to get along with your peers," he points out. "My introduction to this was a sixteen-year-old African-American boy and when I asked him to take off his shirt, he had massive breasts. He had been prescribed Risperdal for sleep for three years by his family doctor."

After all his years fighting pharmaceutical industry fraud, it's especially disturbing to Kruszewski that neither the youth he sees, ages twelve to nineteen—about a quarter of his practice—nor their families have been warned about the side effects or even the potential benefits of the drugs they're given. Most commonly, those antipsychotics have been Risperdal, Seroquel and Abilify, given for bipolar disorder, insomnia (primarily Seroquel) and ADHD.

One of the key challenges in slowing the epidemic of overmedication, Kruszewski observes, is this dilemma: "We have to overcome the expediency of giving a prescription to solve a problem that will actually make the problem worse. As long as doctors are being expedient in their prescription writing, we can't win this battle."

The same short-term philosophy, it turns out, is actually the governing principle at most of the nation's nursing homes and other long-term care facilities housing the elderly—even if it puts patients' lives at risk. Like children, the elderly are another vulnerable population that is very profitable for drug companies.

CHAPTER 2

Nursing Homes: Drugging Our Seniors to Death

In January 2013, a historic event in modern medical care took place in a small courthouse in Bakersfield, California. Grey-haired Gwen Hughes, a former director of a nursing home in rural Kern Valley, appeared as feeble as possible when she rolled into the courtroom in a wheelchair with an oxygen pump attached to face sentencing after being convicted of overdrugging patients. Three patients died under Hughes's "care," while as many as twenty others were injured. This wasn't some serial-killing "Angel of Mercy" nurse plotting to kill patients, but a case of "convenience drugging," as then-Attorney General Jerry Brown said when announcing the arrest in 2009, orchestrated by a real-life Nurse Ratched who used psychotropic drugs to sedate patients who acted up or irritated her. It was arguably the first, and, so far, the only time in US history that a health professional was prosecuted for overmedication as part of the legitimate medical care provided.

Hughes was abetted in her crimes by Pamela Ott, the now disgraced top administrator of the hospital district; pharmacist Debbie Hayes, whom Hughes browbeat into writing prescriptions for antipsychotic drugs such as Risperdal without a doctor's permission; and staff physician Hoshang Pormir, who signed off on the scrips without evaluating the patients or seeking their consent. Despite the gauzy sales claims by TMAP, Johnson & Johnson, and their academic shills, psychotropic medicines such as Risperdal were finally unmasked for what they were: a product as potentially fatal as a gun.

Incredibly, the prescribing actions in Hughes's case are standard medical practice. Although the federal government has since 1987 barred the use of chemical restraints on the elderly by federal law, it is virtually never enforced. In fact, nearly 300,000 elderly nursing home patients a day receive antipsychotics, close to a quarter of the patient population, largely to control their behavior. One-third of all dementia patients in long-term nursing care are dosed with antipsychotics, while, according to GAO estimates in 2015, nearly 200,000 other dementia patients in shoddy, unregulated "assisted living facilities" are also treated with these drugs. Despite a decade-old FDA "black box" warning label on every bottle clearly stating that using antipsychotics for "dementia-related psychosis" can increase the risk of death, roughly 90 percent of the drugs are doled out for unapproved, off-label uses, including Alzheimer's and dementia behavioral symptoms.

"You have probably got 15,000 elderly people in nursing homes dying each year from the off-label use of antipsychotic medications for an indication that the FDA knows the drug doesn't work," Dr. David Graham, a leading FDA drug safety expert, told a congressional panel. "With every pill that gets dispensed in a nursing home, the drug company is laughing all the way to the bank," he said. "We have got so many clinical trials that show these drugs don't work that it is like malpractice to be using it."

At the Kern Valley nursing facility, no one warned the families victimized by Hughes about the dangers posed by the drugs they administered so freely. The sudden decline in health of Fanny May Brinkley, a lively ninety-seven-year-old, came as a shock to those who loved her. To Hughes, however, Brinkley apparently talked too much. She was force-fed Depakote, an anti-seizure medication with powerful sedating and weakening effects, without the consent required by state law. Usually feisty, Brinkley suddenly became "lethargic," according to her granddaughter, Tammy Peters: "I just thought it was old age." Six days later, Fanny May was in the hospital emergency room, and there she died. According to the California Attorney General's office, several others who didn't die were left to suffer in their beds, unable to eat, emaciated and drooling.

It was heart-wrenching at the hearing to see Peters, a stolid blonde woman in a gray sweatshirt and dark pants, address the judge, her voice quaking with anger and tears. The paper shook in her hands as she read from her handwritten statement: "We thought putting our grandmother in a home was what was best. We were all impressed with these people, but they calculatedly and maliciously drugged and killed our grandmother," she said. "I will never trust another nursing home to care for anyone I love again. On behalf of our family, we ask for the harshest sentence you can give."

Hughes faced ten felony charges, but she pled no contest to one count of causing harm or death to an elderly or dependent adult; in return, the nine other charges were dismissed. She was sentenced to three years in prison, the harshest sentence possible. Her colleagues Ott, Hayes and Pormir, sentenced earlier, didn't get prison sentences. After Hughes was sentenced, Deputy Attorney General Steven Muni told a local TV reporter, "I hope this sends a message to all nursing homes, and many are owned by for-profit chains, that you can't put profits over people."

• • •

THE SENTENCING OF HUGHES IN 2013 GAVE HOPE THAT CALIFORNIA'S law enforcement agencies, and perhaps even the federal government, were finally ready to crack down on nursing homes that abused the elderly. After all, since research showed that 15,000 nursing home patients die needlessly every year, that's a fatality rate equivalent to five 9/11 attacks per year. As of this writing, however, nothing has really changed. "The message providers took away was probably this: Don't do this in an obviously mean-spirited way," says Tony Chicotel, a staff attorney with California Advocates for Nursing Home Reform. Despite all the patients jammed with drug-filled needles or left to die in a stupefied state, Chicotel says that most nursing home caretakers have convinced themselves that this is somehow altruistic: "They believe they are motivated by wanting to do the right thing; the patient is exhibiting distress."

Even so, it's still not clear why the staff at Roseville Point Health and Wellness, a facility near Sacramento proud of its five-star Medicare rating, decided to give eighty-two-year-old Genine Zizzo debilitating shots of Haldol a few days into her week-long stay for physical therapy for a serious back sprain. Though Zizzo had a heart condition, she didn't have dementia or any mental illness; instead, she was an active, independent woman who drove herself around town and did her own laundry, as *The Sacramento Bee* first reported. Zizzo only required nursing home care because she tripped over a tube connected to the oxygen machine she was using for her condition. Her doctors at Kaiser Permanente, after reviewing her X-rays, recommended a brief stay at the Roseville facility.

Her daughter, Marisa Conover, a former CBS Records marketing executive, lived nearby and was especially vigilant. She not only personally checked out the nursing home before admitting her mother, but, having learned about the dangers of antipsychotics, adamantly insisted to the admissions director: "Under no circumstances and not for any reason should my mother be given antipsychotic drugs." She supplemented that request with an advanced medical directive and durable power of attorney that required her explicit approval before they could administer any treatments, with the authority to override any member of the staff, Conover says. In addition, she informed the staff before admission that her mother wasn't incontinent and shouldn't be placed in an adult diaper. That directive would also be violated.

Conover went to the facility every day, staying until visiting hours closed around midnight. As physical therapy began, her mother suffered from extreme pain. When Zizzo frequently called for help, overdrugging with painkillers began. According to Conover, Zizzo's emergency call button was moved away from her reach. When Conover left her mother at about 1 a.m. on December 7, 2012, she pinned the call button on the sheet so her mom could get the help she needed. Later that night, four staffers allegedly grabbed Rizzo from her room, placed her in a wheelchair, tied her wrists with a cord and injected her with two shots of Haldol—an event buttressed by medical records and the coroner's report.

When Conover came back later that morning, a nursing home staffer took her aside and told her, "There was an incident last night." Conover was disturbed to hear the claim, expanded in the overnight nurse's notes, that her mother was screaming and combative, and, improbably, that she had been moving up and down the hall, hitting and scratching and kicking the staff in a psychotic state. "They made her look like a Ninja turtle, and she couldn't walk anywhere by herself," she points out, as confirmed by Zizzo's medical record at the home, which showed she needed two people to assist her.

Conover speculates that her mother was injected with the drug to stop her from pressing the call button to get the attention of the staff, but no one is really sure. The facility has declined repeated media requests to answer specific questions about Zizzo's care; it's worth noting that the array of allegations hasn't been confirmed in a court of law, although the lackadaisical state health department finally confirmed in 2017 one finding: the nursing home didn't obtain proper consent before injecting Zizzo with the antipsychotic. (That same agency faced a major lawsuit filed in 2013 for failing to properly—and promptly—investigate thousands of nursing home complaints, and the court ruled against the department on these issues in the fall of 2016.)

Zizzo's decline after the injections was rapid, as she became increasingly comatose and an apparent victim of neglect. Seventeen days after entering the nursing home for routine physical therapy, she was dead.

"This was inappropriate drugging of the elderly, a *bona fide* malicious assault," Conover charges. "It's no different than using a knife, gun or bat, even if they did not intend to kill her."

The death of Genine Zizzo is a window into not only the reality of deadly nursing home care, but the lengths that government officials take to keep nursing homes and other long-term care facilities protected from any genuine accountability.

To convey progress amid a wave of ongoing death and harm, the federal government instituted two programs: the dubious Five-Star Quality Rating System for nursing homes, which relies primarily on nursing homes' self-reporting and weak state inspections; and a voluntary program in partnership with the nursing home industry that supposedly educates facilities' caretakers about alternatives to antipsychotics. Both programs are overseen by CMS, the federal agency that compiles data on health-care quality as part of its role overseeing the Medicaid and Medicare programs.

The problem with both of the nursing home assessment programs, however, is that CMS assumes that nursing homes will report their practices accurately and that state health departments will monitor violations aggressively—neither of which has been the case so far. The Roseville facility, for example, was fined by state officials only three times for modest amounts between 2004 and 2016. This *laissez-faire* response came in the face of fifty citizen complaints against the facility just since 2012. In fact, CMS used the state's upbeat inspection data to award Roseville a five-star rating early in 2017. All that should come as no surprise, considering that the California health department initially didn't substantiate a single incident of wrongdoing in the death and alleged maltreatment of Genine Zizzo, while it delayed for years responding to the appeals of the Foundation Aiding the Elderly (FATE), the Sacramento-based advocacy group that filed a complaint on behalf of Conover in June 2013—and which did not receive a reply from state headquarters until April 2017.

Yet as *The New York Times* and other media outlets have reported, building on the research of the Center for Medicare Advocacy (CMA), most nursing homes have gamed the Medicare system. According to the *Times*, Rosewood Post-Acute Rehab in Carmichael, California, was in the elite tier of five-star facilities in the country, even though it had as many as 165 complaints filed against it with the state health department in four years—and had even been fined $100,000 after a woman died following an overdose of a blood-thinning drug. As CMA attorney Toby Edelman points out, these government data sets are "fraudulent and based mostly on self-reports."

Stung by the criticism, CMS vowed to improve the star rating system in 2014 by adding additional government audits of nursing home quality claims and including the use of antipsychotics as a measurement of quality. But the nursing home industry still runs the show by apparently undermining state and federal assessments, inspections and surveys. In October 2015, roughly a year after those CMS "reforms" were announced, Al Jazeera's *America Tonight* reported that over forty nursing homes with five-star ratings *openly admitted* that they were drugging their patients at well more than twice the rate of CMS's estimated 17 percent usage rate; in some cases, up to 50 percent of patients at these top-rated facilities were being pummeled with antipsychotics.

One of the nursing homes that says it's doing better than the national average is the Roseville facility where Conover's mom died after receiving antipsychotic injections; it has reported that a mere 14.6 percent of patients get antipsychotics.

But all you really need to know about enforcement *and* the government data that consumers use to evaluate nursing homes can be found in the state health department's response to the death of Zizzo. The FATE group filed a complaint on her behalf in June 2013, alleging that the two injections of Haldol in one night left her "completely comatose in a vegetative state," and that she had been a victim of "elder abuse, dehydration, undiagnosed fracture of the spine, physical and verbal abuse." A few days after FATE complained, Conover received a call from a state health department investigator indicating the agency had no intention of seriously investigating any of the allegations.

For instance, Conover offered to send the medical records from Kaiser confirming dehydration, a urinary infection and a fractured spine, among other major problems. She also wanted to provide a letter—written by an experienced home health aide who visited the nursing home—that described the relatively few scattered dark stains on Rizzo's soiled diaper indicating dehydration, especially because it seemingly wasn't changed for days.

"Don't bother to send that," the state health official callously sniffed. "I won't be looking at it." This sort of indifferent official attitude towards Conover's concerns, as she recounts it, is one of the points raised in the nearly four-year-old appeal that wasn't answered until April 2017.

By August 2013, following this "investigation," the licensing and certification program of the California Department of Public Health (CDPH) found all the FATE allegations "unsubstantiated" and didn't find any other violations. The state agency also didn't substantiate a later complaint filed by Conover directly alleging Roseville's mishandling of her mother's urinary infection. The department didn't reply to specific allegations that it mishandled the Zizzo inquiry, but said in a statement, "CDPH takes complaints seriously and investigates thoroughly," while claiming it was working "diligently" to improve the timeliness of its inquiries. (That assertion was undermined by a January 2017 report by Disability Rights California that found that the state was "low-balling" penalties in death cases.)

This critique was reinforced by the state's final response to the appeal in the Zizzo case: It issued a "Class B" citation of $600 to

Roseville for giving Marisa Conover's mother the Haldol injections without informed consent. "It's an insult," says Carole Herman. "It's better than the original finding as 'unsubstantiated complaint,' but high-level officials in California are protecting the operator in my opinion."

At least in the case of Zizzo, the state pretended to conduct an investigation. A scathing state audit in 2014 found that the department ignored a backlog of 11,000 mostly high-priority complaints against nursing homes, including nearly four hundred cases where patients were in "immediate jeopardy" of death or injury. The audit was spurred in large part by the wide-ranging lawsuit filed by FATE in 2013 targeting the department for failing to pursue complaints against nursing homes. At the end of 2014, the director of the department and his two top associates resigned after a public outcry. (Rather than being drummed out of the health-care field, though, they've all landed plum new jobs, some with higher pay.)

The lawsuit filed by FATE was finally settled in October 2016, when a state court ordered CDPH to perform timely investigations and appeals, supplemented by a law that aimed to force the state agency in 2016 to complete new investigations within ninety days. But with numerous loopholes and a stubborn bureaucracy, long delays are still commonplace.

"There's no enforcement anywhere in the United States," says Carol Herman, the founder of FATE. "They don't really care." That indifference is also reflected in CMS's questionable five-star rating system and, as cited earlier, its highly touted "partnership" with the industry that has purportedly brought down antipsychotic prescribing in nursing homes to 17.4 percent—a figure that few, if any, nursing home reform organizations believe.

Further questions about the validity of these glowing Medicare assessments and claimed antipsychotic downturns emerged in 2014 and 2015 when a handful of the sister facilities in the same chain that owns Roseville faced new public scrutiny and criminal investigations. In addition, the federal government decertified three of that chain's nursing homes over safety questions and some deaths, barring them from receiving Medicare and Medicaid funds. Much of this new attention from federal and state agencies was spurred by a *Sacramento Bee* investigative series in 2014 looking into the chain's head, Shlomo Rechnitz, a Los Angeles entrepreneur who has become the owner of approximately eighty facilities, including the South Pasadena Convalescent Hospital, which was decertified in January 2015, three months after a mentally ill patient died by wandering off and setting herself on fire.

In response to Conover's original accusations about the alleged maltreatment of Rizzo, the *Bee* reported that Rechnitz's legal team cited the state's closing of the case, and "declined to comment further due to privacy laws protecting patients."

According to the *Bee*, Rechnitz is the largest operator of nursing homes in California. He has defended the quality of care in his facilities and noted his willingness at some sites to take in mentally ill patients whom he claims local governments don't help; his homes still serve seniors. Yet by the fall of 2015, Rechnitz's Riverside, California, facility was raided for undisclosed reasons by FBI agents with search warrants; four former staffers at two other facilities were also charged with crimes ranging from tolerating resident-on-resident sexual abuse to the death of a burn victim in a Montrose nursing home due to alleged neglect in August 2014. In August 2015, the state attorney general also charged the home itself with involuntary manslaughter. Until that criminal charge, the state government—including the health department—found no cause to cite the Montrose facility for any deficiencies or incidents for three straight years. Rechnitz and his spokesperson have traditionally cited high marks from the state for most of their facilities as a sign of their quality. (In response to an interview request in May 2016 from a Los Angeles CBS affiliate reporting on another facility death in Inglewood, a spokesperson issued this overview statement: "Mr. Rechnitz has for years been an integral part of providing quality nursing home services to Californians . . . [and] provides life-aiding services to thousands of Californians.")

The lack of any meaningful sanctions for nursing homes, especially for overdrugging, is commonplace. Indeed, in fiscal year 2012, during the first year of the vaunted "partnership" with the nursing home industry to reduce overprescribing, only twenty-five or so individual incidents of "harmful drugging" in the nation's nearly 16,000 nursing homes were cited by government agencies.

It is a common practice for regulators across a range of industries to remain on good terms with—or even advance the interests of—those they "regulate." For example, a key architect of Medicare's dubious five-star rating system, Kerry Weems, a former acting director of CMS, joined forces with one of the occasional beneficiaries of those rankings: Rechnitz. Weems signed up in early January 2014 as chief executive of a medical supply and services company, TwinMed (co-owned by Rechnitz with his twin brother Steven), that contracts, in part, with the Rechnitz nursing home chain.

• • •

THE BALEFUL CORPORATE INFLUENCE ON PATIENT SAFETY AND QUALITY of care has never been made clearer than by the drug companies' promotion of the overuse of antipsychotics in nursing facilities. That's been well documented in major federal civil and criminal settlements costing the drug firms billions over their illegal marketing, and in the very rare prosecution of a corrupt doctor for fraudulently prescribing psychotropic drugs in nursing homes.

Sometimes, despite the free rein given doctors to prescribe practically any drug for any reason, a physician can go too far and get in trouble, especially if he's been singled out by *ProPublica*, *The Chicago Tribune* and the Department of Justice. In February 2015, Dr. Michael Reinstein pled guilty to one felony charge of taking $600,000 in kickbacks from both the original maker and then the generic manufacturer to prescribe an especially risky antipsychotic drug, Clozaril, to thousands of nursing home patients in his care. It is a drug of last resort meant only for people with schizophrenia who haven't responded to other drugs, and it poses risks of fatality because it lowers the white blood cell count and causes seizures. He also agreed to pay $3.5 million as part of a federal civil lawsuit filed in 2012 for submitting 140,000 false claims for his antipsychotic prescriptions, which included Seroquel, Zyprexa and Clozaril, based not on patient evaluations, but on drug company payoffs, according to the lawsuit.

Some patients died from his overprescribing, and he has faced over a dozen malpractice and wrongful death lawsuits since 2005. Yet even as he prescribed more Clozaril than all of the Medicaid doctors *combined* in three states—Texas, Florida and North Carolina—he continued to be reimbursed by Medicare and Medicaid for nearly two decades after he was first exposed by *The Chicago Tribune* in 1993 for massive prescribing. Ultimately, over a five-year period, he raked in $55 million from Medicaid alone. Despite his guilty plea, Reinstein has remained unapologetic about his wide use of Clozaril and other antipsychotics.

Before he became a prescribing workhorse for Clozaril, AstraZeneca had already fallen in love with Reinstein, paying him nearly $500,000 for a decade starting in the 1990s to spread the good news about Seroquel's safety in over five hundred talks. He was valued by executives as potentially bringing in a half-billion dollars in drug revenues because of his heavy prescribing and salesmanship. They continued to fund his Seroquel research and pay him to promote the drug despite internal documents showing that company executives had grave doubts early on about his dubious research. One of his studies' results showed zero adverse effects from patients taking high dosages of Seroquel, while another improbably proved that Seroquel could reverse diabetes and help people *lose* weight. These prompted one executive to call them "suspect" and "hard to believe," as first reported by *ProPublica* and *The Chicago Tribune*.

Reinstein may have pushed the envelope further than most industry shills, but his eagerness reflects the aggressive marketing of the drug companies pushing antipsychotics on elderly people who don't need them. Perhaps no company has used so many corrupting methods so widely to spread its antipsychotic drug, Risperdal, as Johnson & Johnson's Janssen division. As part of a wide-ranging $2.2 billion criminal and civil settlement in 2013 for illegally marketing three drugs, primarily Risperdal, Johnson & Johnson (the creators of TMAP) admitted to the various schemes, including paying kickbacks, they used to reach nursing homes. But the company only formally accepted guilt on one criminal count.

Johnson & Johnson had an even more staggeringly ambitious plan to get Risperdal into nursing homes: paying kickbacks to Omnicare, the nation's largest provider of drugs to nursing homes. The

FDA required a warning on the drug's label stating that it wasn't safe for the elderly and told the company it shouldn't market the drug as such, but J&J didn't care with so many billions at stake. As early as 1997, as noted in Steve Brill's lengthy *Huffington Post* series, lawsuits against the company revealed Johnson & Johnson had signed an "active intervention agreement" to pay Omnicare to favor Risperdal.

Risperdal was among the first of the new antipsychotics approved by the FDA in the 1990s, and succeeding brands, especially Zyprexa and Seroquel, had to make their mark by also expanding into the lucrative seniors and nursing home market. Eli Lilly was the first company to have its fraudulent antipsychotic marketing schemes—in this case, for Zyprexa—exposed in 2006 when *The New York Times* reported on leaked internal documents. This exposé was followed by damaging whistleblower evidence included in a $1.4 billion settlement in 2009 with the Justice Department for off-label promotion; it showed just how much unapproved drugging of the elderly for such conditions as dementia was essential to its marketing game plans, including "Viva Zyprexa" for primary care doctors (borrowed from Pfizer's "Viva Viagra" campaign). For instance, for nursing home pharmacies and staff, Eli Lilly came up with a catchy slogan: a "5 at 5" campaign that urged nursing homes to administer 5 mg of Zyprexa at 5 p.m. to induce sleep in patients.

Before Eli Lilly was exposed, AstraZeneca officials had been working on cracking the primary care and nursing home market since 2001 by pushing Seroquel for dementia, according to the $520 million settlement the company reached with DOJ in 2010. They added academic polish to their marketing plans by giving doctors payoffs for putting their names on journal articles ghostwritten by the company, federal investigators found. A 2014 lawsuit filed by the Texas Attorney General charges comparable off-label misconduct in pushing the new time-released version of Seroquel, Seroquel XR, but with a greater emphasis, allegedly, on marketing to children's doctors and psychiatrists.

Whistleblower James Wetta, a former salesman at AstraZeneca, revealed in his earlier unsealed 2010 lawsuit a host of sleazy tricks used to push Seroquel on the elderly. Controlling patients by sedating them with Seroquel was a major theme of the company's invitation-only seminars for doctors, which had titles such as "Comprehensive Management of Behavioral Disturbances in Dementia." Despite the health risk, Wetta pointed out, "AstraZeneca made a marketing decision to aggressively promote its drug to physicians to 'higher functioning patients,'" as opposed to schizophrenics, including the elderly and children.

In a reply to my queries about the legal criticisms of AstraZeneca, the company's media relations director, Abigail Bozarth, said in a statement, "AstraZeneca is committed to acting responsibly and sharing information about the safety and efficacy of its medicines. AstraZeneca's policy is to promote its medicines in accordance with FDA-approved labeling and FDA regulations. Our employees are required to follow our compliance policies." She declined to comment on the pending 2014 fraud lawsuit aimed at AstraZeneca.

Even as the Justice Department plays catch-up with fraudulent marketing by drug companies, HHS and its CMS division remain adamant about continuing payments for off-label and fraudulent prescribing to seniors—just as the agency does for children. In response to an HHS Inspector General's report in 2011 decrying overmedication in nursing homes, CMS officials insisted, "Prevention of [improper] payment [is] beyond our statutory authority."

The Obama-era Department of Justice, however, showed a way forward in new fraud litigation directly against a nursing home company that could serve as a template for HHS and Medicare to finally stop paying for off-label uses of antipsychotics for unapproved uses. In May 2015, the US Attorney's office in San Francisco announced that the owners and operators of two Watsonville, California, nursing homes agreed to pay $3.8 million to settle charges that they submitted false claims for "substandard and worthless services": overdrugging the elderly. Ironies abound in this case, with a circular loop of failed enforcement. The HHS Inspector General office is charged with enforcing a five-year Corporate Integrity Agreement requiring the Watsonville nursing homes to comply with statutes that forbid fraudulent spending, including payment for off-label drugs. At the same time, the sister agency in HHS that pays for those services, CMS, has said that such fraud statutes don't apply to medications and that it has no authority to enforce such laws. Meanwhile, this same HHS Inspector General's office has conspicuously failed to enforce previous corporate integrity agreements with drug companies following multi-billion-dollar settlements for illegal marketing. These failures are worsened because the drug companies apparently didn't honestly report their marketing practices to the see-no-evil officials at HHS's Inspector General office, as outlined in new anti-fraud lawsuits against the manufacturers of Geodon and Seroquel.

But if the federal government's indifferent enforcement and its unquestioning reimbursement for fraudulent overmedication continue, as seems likely in a Trump administration, don't expect any real change that could save lives.

There are successful approaches that don't use antipsychotics for dementia patients. They've been achieved by training the nursing home staff to respond in a comforting manner to even the most troublesome dementia and Alzheimer's patients with dignity, flexible schedules based on patient preferences and empathy; if they're in pain, they're given sensible doses of non-opiate painkillers or opiates. The pioneer of this holistic model is Vermillion Cliffs, the dementia unit of the Beatitudes Campus retirement community in Phoenix, Arizona, as profiled by *The New Yorker* and *The New York Times*.

There's little reason to have faith in such a major turnaround in practices nationwide. That won't happen unless pressure builds on CMS to stop paying for "worthless" medicines, to start rewarding nursing homes for actually using gentler alternatives that can't be gamed by sham regulators, and to ensure that the HHS's Inspector General punishes violators of corporate integrity agreements.

There is one organization that could possibly bring about such a tectonic shift in federal policies and help halt those needless deaths. That is the thirty-eight-million-strong AARP, the powerful senior citizen group that is ostensibly a strong force for protecting the elderly and their benefits. Their power to shape Medicare actions and federal legislation and the views of politicians is so legendary that Medicare has become known as the "third-rail" of American politics: touch it and you die.

Until recently, though, this organization has been relatively quiet on the life-and-death issue of antipsychotic use in nursing homes. "I don't know why they haven't done more," says CMA attorney Toby Edelman. "Maybe it's because of their ties with the insurance industry?" AARP has been accused before by both liberal and right-wing groups of being too cozy with the insurance industry and, by extension, Big Pharma, which reaps so much in revenue from government programs, while AARP's licensing deals with United Healthcare allow it, indirectly, to rake in a share of federal spending on antipsychotics. Surprisingly, with more than $1 billion in revenues, over half of AARP's income has come from royalty payments from United Healthcare and non-health insurance companies for licensing the use of its respected name for prescription drugs and other plans.

Ever since AARP sided with Big Pharma during the passage of the industry-crafted Medicare Part D plan in 2003, which barred Medicare from negotiating prices and created a huge "donut hole" of thousands in uncovered costs, the organization has come under fire for placing business interests over the needs of its members. As the public interest group Public Citizen declared, "Maximizing corporate-related income and profits poses a significant conflict of interest for an organization trying to represent the best interests of its members." The organization's former policy director, Marilyn Moon, told *Bloomberg News* and the fact-checking news source *Politifact* that these potential conflicts undermine its mission: "There's an inherent conflict of interest. A lot of people there are trying to do good, but they're ending up becoming very dependent on sources of income," she said. "It's very hard for the tail not to wag the dog."

Organization officials deny there are any conflicts, and a spokesperson insists, "AARP has done a great deal to raise public and policymaker awareness." He pointed to recent AARP legal actions, a 2014 *AARP Magazine* article on overdrugging, some state testimony—and polite written requests to CMS starting in March 2014 that asked for greater education on antipsychotics and stronger informed consent procedures. But none of it has yet made an impact on federal policymakers. That mild 2014 letter, apparently AARP's first public comment on the issue to a federal agency, accepted CMS's feeble partnership with the nursing industry and its dubious statistics as a good start that should be expanded. The organization, though, didn't press for any stern measures that could slash drug and insurance industry revenues.

The organization simply hasn't mounted a full-scale attack on overprescribing at the top agencies of the federal government, or pushed for awareness through congressional hearings and TV ads or sought stepped-up enforcement through new laws. Here's a thought experiment: If CMS had a new policy that somehow no longer funded Medicare-paid kidney dialysis machines after two weeks, killing thousands, we'd probably hear about it loud and clear from AARP—and heads would roll in government agencies. That's not the case with antipsychotics.

Even so, starting in 2012, AARP joined an important, successful local class-action lawsuit seeking to enforce informed consent laws in Ventura County, California, nursing homes. Over three hundred current and former nursing home residents weren't told about the psychotropic drugs they were getting or the dangers they posed, and, as a result, some patients were needlessly injured or died.

As a result of the lawsuit, the Ventura County Superior Court granted a groundbreaking order in 2014 demanding that the nursing homes implement strict informed consent policies. Though promising, that change won't spread more broadly until the drug industry's influence on antipsychotic spending is choked off at the top of the federal government. And that won't happen until the preventable drug-induced deaths of the elderly become as politically and financially dangerous to politicians, government officials and drug industry executives as AARP has made messing with Medicare in the world of politics.

CHAPTER 3

The Secret History of the VA's Tragedies in Tomah and Phoenix

OVERMEDICATION HAD SURELY KILLED REBECCA RILEY, OTHER FORLORN children and anonymous nursing home patients. After a burst of local headlines, one could have hoped that there would have been a cry for justice and genuine safeguards. But that crackdown never happened. Instead, over the years, no one paid much attention to a wave of preventable deaths and harm caused by irresponsible, unchecked prescribing across the country. That started to change in early 2015, following the news that more than thirty patients had died needlessly at the VA hospital in Tomah, Wisconsin, that came to be known as "Candy Land."

This and other VA scandals are emblematic of the nation's entire mental health system. The documents, hearings and investigative articles exposing the array of VA scandals have offered the most detailed behind-the-scenes look at failed mental health care since the abuses of the state mental hospitals came to light over sixty years ago, but even pro-VA experts who concede some of the VA's failings say that civilian mental health care is far worse. Take senior RAND Corporation researcher Dr. Katherine Watkins, a psychiatrist who has published influential studies that found that the VA significantly outperformed the private sector on a key quality marker: appropriate prescribing for mentally ill patients. Watkins, while acknowledging the scathing conclusions of some damning independent reports on the VA's failures, told me, "Even if they do have a corrosive culture of care, even if they do have inadequate oversight and accountability, even if they do have ambiguous [clinical] policies, even if all of those things are true, they're still doing a better job than the private sector." That positive comparative conclusion was echoed in RAND's broader 2016 congressionally mandated assessment of the VA's overall quality. Despite shortages of qualified mental health staffers, RAND's assessment, which was later confirmed by a federal Commission on Care studying the VA, found "The quality of care provided by the VA health system generally was as good as or better than other health systems on most quality measures"—even though there are wide inconsistencies among VA facilities.

Looked at another way, this means that the scandal-ridden VA is actually a microcosm of what's wrong with the nation's mental health care at large, the difference being that we know far more about the VA than what's going on in Medicaid, nursing homes or foster care programs. Keep this in mind: the maltreatment suffered by these veterans could be an *improvement* over what is inflicted daily on many of the millions of mentally ill people seeking quality care everywhere from emergency rooms to community clinics, but those services haven't gotten the same intense congressional and media scrutiny as the VA.

So the story of what went wrong at the VA, from deadly wait times to veterans killed by reckless prescribing, should be more than just fodder for an ideological debate over the role of government-run health care. Liberals have sought to portray the VA's problems as overblown, as Hillary Clinton argued on MSNBC's *The Rachel Maddow Show*: "It's not as widespread as it has been made out to be." Citing some statistically questionable surveys showing veterans' satisfaction with VA care, she said, "Nobody would believe that from the coverage you see, and the constant berating of the VA that comes from the Republicans, in part in pursuit of this ideological agenda they have." It is indeed true, as reported in a 2016 article in *The Washington Monthly*, that the far-right Koch brothers, Charles and David, are subsidizing a pro-privatization agenda—one that aims to essentially replace the VA over time with vouchers for private care—through the conservative Concerned Veterans for America (CVA), part of their network of right-wing organizations. The financiers' pro-business privatization goals were supported by several members of the independent VA Commission on Care who were appointed in 2015 by the White House and congressional leaders.

Sweeping reforms of the VA were seen as a real possibility after Trump's victory, but how far they will go is still an open question. Donald Trump won the veteran vote by a two-to-one margin over Hillary Clinton because his promises to "drain the swamp" in Washington resonated with veterans fed up with failed VA reforms. But his actual reform ideas don't seem as extreme as the privatization agenda that ultimately aims to close VA hospitals and enrich corporate health care; he has proposed at times a Medicare-style option for veterans to choose freely between VA or private sector care, but that's a position that alarms mainstream veterans groups that argue it would drain resources from the VA and steer veterans away from the agency's specialized, integrated care. He also sought to fire "corrupt and incompetent VA executives."

Yet to some whistleblowers and other critics of the department, his selection of Dr. David Shulkin, a VA insider who is also not a veteran, to head the agency makes drastic, genuine change less likely. "For veterans who voted for Donald Trump, this is going to feel like a 'bait-and-switch,'" says Benjamin Krause, founder of the reform website DisabledVeterans.org. He argues, "Keeping Shulkin will keep a host of flunkies and criminals who should have been part of the whole 'drain the swamp' promise." At the same time, Shulkin, as VA Secretary, has been praised even by some internal department critics for making progress with his announced reforms; he has also demonstrated a shrewd sense of public relations by moving to remove a few scandal-ridden VA hospital directors hit by national publicity and to improve transparency about the wait times at local facilities. Yet he has done little about lesser-known, appalling health care scandals and the ongoing retaliation against whistleblowers that have continued unabated since he joined the department as undersecretary of health in June 2015. As Krause points out, "I don't know of a single instance when a VA employee has been held accountable for harassing whistleblowers."

Many liberals have discounted the VA scandals as merely some right-wing or media fabrication. Yet that stance ignores a mountain of damning reports by the VA's own Inspector General, the GAO, reputable news organizations, congressional committees—and, especially, the tragic stories of patients, families and dedicated VA workers victimized by the agency. The VA can't truly be reformed if it becomes just a political football for ideologues.

Less than a year after the dozens of wait-time deaths at the Phoenix VA medical center were first exposed in April 2014, the Center for Investigative Reporting revealed another crisis that won far less national attention: The Tomah VA hospital's chief of staff, psychiatrist Dr. David Houlihan, had recklessly overused opiates and psychotropic drugs. For years, Tomah hospital executives had brushed aside complaints, just as there was little response to the deaths of nursing home patients and foster care kids enrolled in other government-funded programs. Now, finally, a few national reporters began examining at least one government agency's role in sanctioning dangerous prescribing.

But as interest faded away, reform seemed unlikely. The few laws that passed left the agency's underlying corruption, as exposed in congressional hearings and media accounts, unchanged. And few people noticed that the roots of these new scandals lay in the medication-linked deaths of young vets such as Eric Layne in 2008, and shoddy, neglectful patterns of care. The failure that undergirds the prescribing scandals was no mystery. As Paul Sullivan, then the executive director of Veterans for Common Sense, observed a few years ago: "There's such a lack of mental health care services that service members are not treated, or their treatment is delayed, and they're only given drugs instead of the therapy they need."

The VA could have changed its approach to prescribing or provided broader, effective mental health care. Instead, it retaliated against the whistleblowers at Tomah, Phoenix and other hospitals. Rigged data, cover-ups of patient's deaths, long delays in accessing treatment and a lack of accountability were rampant. As whistleblower Ryan Honl, a secretary in the mental health unit at Tomah who quit his job in October 2014 and went public about abuses, points out, "All sorts of crazy, off-label stuff was going on to the point where people were dying, but Houlihan was never held accountable."

The VA knew about the overprescribing problems at Tomah as early as 2007, but the Inspector General didn't start investigating the alarming narcotic prescribing until 2011. He found that dozens of victims had "unusually high" opiate prescription rates and that staff dissidents were retaliated against for more than two years, including a psychologist who killed himself in 2009 after being fired for protesting overmedication. Yet the resulting March 2014 report was buried and nothing changed.

The congressional proposals to tighten prescription oversight came too late for those killed by medications at Tomah. Many of the patients had histories of addiction and some had histories of chronic pain. At a good hospital, a pain specialist would oversee their treatment. Yet at Tomah it was a *psychiatrist*, Houlihan, nicknamed "The Candy Man." A few months after the IG deep-sixed its investigation, a thirty-five-year-old inpatient in the Tomah mental health unit was found in his hospital bed dead from fatal poisoning caused by the sixteen medications his doctors had prescribed.

There were other problems. As Honl discovered when he faced a spurious internal VA police investigation long after he'd quit, "The system was slow to respond but quick to silence those who raised concerns." Nevertheless, Dr. Carolyn Clancy, the VA's interim undersecretary for health, declared to a joint House-Senate field hearing in Tomah in March 2015: "The VA will not tolerate an environment where intimidation or suppression of concerns occurs."

Today, "the VA is killing veterans and it's a national disgrace," says Honl of the agency's failure to effectively curb its life-threatening practices, augmented by its pattern of continuing retaliation against whistleblowers. (The VA has diagnosed *60 percent* of all veterans returning from the Middle East with chronic pain, plying many with opiates, even as such VA opiate prescribing has dropped about 25 percent since mid-2012.)

Yet even though the Inspector General had buried its March 2014 Tomah report, denying reality was no solution to the hospital's problems. It only increased them. In August 2014, a thirty-five-year-old Marine veteran, former Lance Corporal Jason Simcakoski, died of "mixed drug toxicity" in the VA hospital's inpatient psychiatric unit. He had just been following doctor's orders. He was already taking fourteen different medications, including high-risk opiates, benzodiazepine tranquilizers and the sedating antipsychotic Seroquel. Just two days before his death, Jason was *also* given the opiate Suboxone, typically used to reduce dependence on other narcotics. This extreme drug cornucopia was given to him despite the well-known dangers of Suboxone's potentially fatal interactions with any of the three benzodiazepines he was taking, Valium, Restoril and Serax, and with some of his other high-risk medications. "They don't value life at the VA," says his widow, Heather Simcakoski. Over the years, she says, "They took the quickest, easiest route of giving pills to patients with addictions to keep them quiet, and then send them out the door."

Jason was an addict. Yet the VA kept shipping opiates and benzos and antipsychotics by the bagful. After a near-overdose, Heather turned to Jason's father, Marvin, to begin driving over each day to bring Jason his medicine, which Marvin kept in a safe to ensure that Jason took only the number of pills prescribed him daily. Marvin also became a dedicated advocate for his son's well-being in the face of the hostility, indifference and neglect of the local VA. But the doubts of Jason's family about the "treatment" he received mounted, worsened by the apparent lack of any personalized counseling given him during the twelve years he was a VA patient before his death, except, possibly, during some of his hospital stays.

About four years before his son's death, Marvin argued with his doctors about his son's overmedication, but his views were dismissed as ignorant second-guessing. "I was always told that I wasn't their patient, even though I was his dad who truly cared about him a lot more than they did!" he told the joint congressional field hearing in Tomah less than a year after his son died, his voice quaking with an anger and pain that was still raw. "What I would like to know is if Jason was their son, would they have had him on all of these meds?" He adds now, "I truthfully don't understand why if he was addicted, they gave him whatever he wanted. When I was giving him his meds, I stood my ground."

Jason, a Marine and athlete, had lost his drive and self-esteem under the prescription barrage. His weight ballooned from 180 to 250 pounds, and he was too ashamed to go into a restaurant on those rare days he went into town, careful to order only from drive-thru windows. Near the end, he couldn't even bend down to tie his shoes. "With all these medications, he went downhill real fast," his father says.

Heather told the congressional panel in Tomah in March 2015 that Jason tried to fight his addictions in his own way. In 2013, he alerted the local police department as well as the VA's own police to the burgeoning illegal drug trade—vets selling (or "diverting") prescription pills—that took place near the hospital itself, which posed a temptation Jason wanted to avoid. "I would like to understand how and why Jason's police reports 'disappeared,'" Heather said, quietly furious. "There were reports that were made to Dr. Houlihan, the Tomah VA, the Tomah City Police Department as well as the FBI, regarding patients selling their prescriptions back in 2013, who were making so much money that they had saved enough to put a down payment on a home," she said.

After her 2015 testimony, the VA declared that its Inspector General's office—the same one that buried its earlier results—was conducting a criminal investigation. Yet in 2015, it seemed to be a pyrrhic victory. A few Tomah medical officials vilified in the press faced sanctions, such as Houlihan, who was finally fired in November 2015. After briefly having his license suspended, it was restored in April 2016. He was still practicing medicine until he agreed in January 2017 to permanently surrender his license as part of an agreement with state regulators to drop their investigation of him. He had started a new private psychiatry practice in La Crosse early in 2016. "Enjoy life again," his office's website promised. Yet, just like Houlihan initially rebounded from the Tomah scandal, there was, it turns out, little sign that the Department of Veteran Affairs could fundamentally change the way it provides mental health care if it continues to uphold a culture that has allowed irresponsible practices to flourish across the country for more than a decade.

Jason's array of prescriptions didn't get close media scrutiny—except from the Center for Investigative Reporting—but they pointed to a larger problem. Many VA and civilian doctors were willfully indifferent to the effect of the psychiatric medications marketed so heavily to them as wonder drugs for mental problems. "It is so much simpler to give a pill than to offer complex therapy as treatment,"

notes Brigadier General (Ret.) Dr. Stephen Xenakis, a pioneering former Army psychiatrist who is researching more balanced mind-body
approaches to PTSD, which avoid high-risk polypharmacy. "There's
not much difference between military and civilian psychiatric practices," he adds.

For close to two years, when his VA doctor weaned him off the
benzodiazepines and eliminated some of his other medications, Jason
made progress. He lost weight and worked more often. But in 2014,
his life and addictions unraveled again after he saw his family's dog,
Chico, run over by a car, which sent him back to the VA hospital for
a three-month stay. His behavior became so bizarre that he even ran
around one day at the hospital pulling fire alarms until he was shipped
off to the major VA hospital in Madison. He sent desperate text messages to his father: "I can't take it. I'm going crazy." The stimulants
Adderall or Ritalin worsened his mood, behavior and insomnia.
Jason's doctors had prescribed them to him for a questionable diagnosis of ADHD; it was just one of a dozen or so diagnoses they
slapped on him over the years along with bipolar disorder and PTSD.

A day after he went to the Madison hospital, he was released
with instructions to wean himself off of Geodon and the benzodiazepine Valium. Two weeks later, after lying around his home while
trying to withdraw from some of his drugs, he went back to Tomah
for a final time for his addiction and severe anxiety.

Back inside the hospital, Dr. Ronda Davis put him back on Geodon
while continuing the regimen of more than a dozen other drugs. Both
Jason and his father objected, and Marvin appealed to Davis's supervisors for a fresh look at his medication and treatment. That infuriated Davis. In a meeting with her, his son and the hospital's patient
advocate a few days before Jason died, she berated Marvin, who
worked as a building contractor. "You may know how to build houses
and pound nails, but you don't know anything about taking care of
your son," she said. It was another disturbing sign of what critics of
the medical profession see as an arrogance poisoning too many doctors who act as potentates, looking down on their fiefdoms of clinical
underlings and patients. Marvin Simcakoski later told the congressional committee, "This really hit me hard to have his doctor tell me

I don't know my son and I caused her a lot of trouble for trying to help my son who needed my help. The reason I called over her head is that my son wasn't receiving the care from her he needed." Her only "concession" to his concerns about Geodon and the array of hazardous medications was to substitute the even more dangerous antipsychotic Seroquel for Geodon.

At one point during his stay, Jason knocked on the door of Dr. Davis. The drugs were making him uncomfortable. But when she opened the door in response, she slammed it in his face. Heather, told later about the incident, was enraged. Her husband had been willing to sacrifice his life as a soldier for every American, including the physicians then caring for him. Now they could not show him even common decency. "To know that this is how they treat their patients is devastating and completely unacceptable," she testified. (Davis, whose prescribing conduct was investigated by state officials, still practices medicine. When she reached an agreement in November 2016 with the state licensing board allowing her to avoid sanctions after she took additional medical training, Davis denied any negligence or improper prescribing in Jason's death.)

On the Friday night before their next planned visit, Jason called his father to tell him he was feeling better and looked forward to coming back home for his daughter's twelfth birthday on the upcoming Monday. But the potentially toxic side effects of the newly prescribed Suboxone—recommended a few days earlier by Houlihan to his treating physician, Dr. Davis—were mixing in his bloodstream with tranquilizers. On top of that, in the morning he complained of a migraine, which he hadn't suffered from before, and they soon added a migraine medication, Fioricet, to the mix. Unfortunately, no one seemed to notice that it posed a major risk of respiratory failure, coma or death when interacting with the Suboxone that was endangering him in combination with his tranquilizers, Tramadol and the antipsychotic Seroquel.

Jason's wife, daughter and father arrived at 9 a.m. Saturday expecting to greet him as usual outside the hospital or on his floor. Told he had a migraine, they rushed into his room. He was lying on his side, his hand on his head, answering their questions with slurred, incomprehensible words. Marvin testified, "I went to the nurse's station and asked why he was so messed up and the nurse told me he will be fine in a couple of hours. We left not knowing that we would never see him alive again!"

About five hours later, they returned from their hometown more than an hour away. His dad got a phone call: Jason wasn't breathing. The staff hadn't checked up on him while they thought he was sleeping off the migraine, Heather later learned.

Hoping to see him recovered, Jason's family members met a doctor in the lobby. Jason has died, the doctor said. At first, the staff blamed a brain aneurysm for his death. "I was devastated," Heather says. "It was the most painful thing to go through after all the challenges Jason and I had lived through."

For his father, the agony remains. "There isn't a day that goes by when I don't relive that morning," he told the congressional panel. "I regret leaving my son in his room alone that morning only to get a call hours later that he had stopped breathing. I can't get that thought out of my head; I wish I would have been there for him."

Heather believes that the VA might reform Tomah, but she isn't confident that much will happen without scrutiny. "I truly believe if people stop following up with them and pushing them, it will just go back to the way it was," she says.

Despite her skepticism, Heather and Marvin Simcakoski worked with Senator Tammy Baldwin (D-Wis.) for legislation to curb and monitor opiate overprescribing, and appeared at a news conference in June 2015. The name of the bill: The Jason Simcakoski Memorial Opioid Safety Act.

At a Senate hearing, however, the VA's representatives and some senators openly wondered whether the bill duplicated current safeguards. After all that had happened at Tomah, they still asked if mandating tougher oversight was even needed.

The legislation sought to curb overprescribing in various ways. On paper, it would upgrade and strengthen guidelines and training; promote alternative, non-drug pain treatments; and ensure real-time monitoring of prescriptions and high-risk health conditions by expanding the scope of the agency's new, slow-moving Opioid Therapy

Risk Report. It was ultimately incorporated into a package of opiate abuse legislation signed into law by President Obama in July 2016.

After her return from Washington in 2015, Heather Simcakoski was hopeful but wary about the bill's real-world impact. Yet it's not clear that there will be much improvement. The VA's vaunted electronic records and drug-interaction alerts too often fail to work in practice, and drug warnings are often brushed aside when they do pop up on screen. Noelle Johnson, a VA pharmacist who was fired from Tomah in 2009 after she refused to fill high doses of opiates, told me that then—and now—the VA's outmoded software didn't flag potentially fatal opiate-benzodiazepine interactions or excessive dosages of some dangerous drugs. Pointing to software that didn't issue alerts for 1,080 morphine pills in thirty days prescribed for a patient in Tomah with "psychological pain," she also observes of the VA administrators, "My bosses tried to strong-arm pharmacists." That's a practice that she says continued at her new post as chief pain pharmacist at the Des Moines VA.

Yet in a rare example of the VA paying out for overmedication, the VA agreed to a legal settlement of over $1 million, including added benefits to the widow of former paratrooper Ricky Green, forty-three. He was killed in 2011 after getting much higher opiates and tranquilizer dosages after back surgery than he'd earlier been receiving since an injury he received in Operation Desert Storm in the 1990s. The Fayetteville VA pharmacists admitted under oath that their software didn't flag either the higher dosages or that he had a sleep apnea condition that fatally interacts with those drugs.

The VA is still coasting on its twenty-year-old reputation as a pioneer in health software. But little-noticed assessments by the Institute of Medicine, internal IT documents and the MITRE Corporation have found that the agency's electronics records software is obsolete and that sweeping upgrades are needed to "reduce frequency of adverse events and save lives," as administrators of the VA's bungled Pharmacy Reengineering Software project observed a few months before Jason died.

Heather Simcakoski remains justly skeptical about the VA's reform intentions. "The bottom line comes down to money: will the

VA be willing to spend the money to make sure these veterans are functional again?" she asks. For example, it's doubtful that the VA will truly comply with the law named after her husband. For more than a decade, the VA has not even followed its own mental health treatment and prescribing guidelines. Now this new bill relies primarily on the agency itself to monitor, train and sanction prescribers, although the VA's toothless Inspector General and the related Office of Medical Inspector have rarely been vigilant. Real prescribing reform appears unlikely.

One glaring sign of the VA's failure to strongly respond to agency abuses became clear in June 2015, when the acting Inspector General, Richard J. Griffin, was forced out of his post in disgrace after forty-three years of federal service. The Inspector General's office had responded so poorly to all the far-flung scandals since 2014 that it was brutally pummeled in congressional hearings and in media investigations, especially by *USA Today*. One of Inspector General Griffin's several low points was his September 2014 report on the Phoenix wait times which concluded that despite forty people dying while waiting for care, his office couldn't conclude that "the absence of timely care caused the death of these veterans." The original whistleblowing doctor at the Phoenix VA, Dr. Samuel Foote, blasted the report as a "whitewash." Worse, as an alliance of whistleblowers, the VA Truth Tellers, later wrote to President Obama shortly before Griffin resigned, the VA Inspector General used his office to target whistleblowers, rather than address the problems they uncovered.

The Inspector General office's debacles were spotlighted once again by the Senate governmental affairs committee, chaired by Sen. Ron Johnson (R-Wis.), which concluded in May 2016 that there were "systemic failures" in the Inspector General's response to the crisis at Tomah. The horrifying details of this so-called VA watchdog that ignored the deaths of dozens of Tomah patients were outlined in a devastating 359-page report issued by committee Republicans. In a rare admission, Sloan Gibson, the then-deputy secretary of the VA, testified at this May hearing in Tomah, "This is a leadership failure." The report also found that a culture of fear and whistleblower retaliation still continues at the facility.

The indifference to patient safety and the pattern of revenge against whistleblowers was indeed woven into the VA's warped approach to health care, raising doubts that it could be overcome by Senator Baldwin's well-meaning legislation to limit high-risk opiate prescribing and other grand reforms. As a White House report concluded in June 2014, "A corrosive culture has led to personnel problems across the Department that are seriously impacting morale and by extension, the timeliness of health care"; it blamed poor management, distrust, retaliation against concerned employees and "a lack of accountability across all grade levels."

For Heather Simcakoski, the White House report's conclusions rang true. "The officials felt protected because they're working at a government agency. They wouldn't have done anything without all the media attention," she said. "Before that, all we ever got was the staff telling us, 'We're sorry for your loss.'" The VA staff couldn't even keep the most basic promises: the nurses promised they'd send her twelve-year-old daughter, now facing life without a father, a birthday present, but never did. "They couldn't even do that," she says with a hard bitterness that hasn't yet faded. "Nobody really cared."

• • •

UNFORTUNATELY, IN THE FACE OF MORE THAN A 50 PERCENT INCREASE IN the numbers of veterans since 2006 grappling with PTSD and other mental illnesses, indifference appears to have been the default mode of the VA's approach to mental health care. That's the reality facing the roughly 1.5 million veterans receiving mental health treatment, undercutting all the statistics, hiring and training initiatives, and evolving guidelines the VA's leadership cite to show their dedication to providing world-class care. The respected Institute of Medicine reported recently, for example, that only half of veterans diagnosed with PTSD were getting the bare minimum of psychotherapy sessions, let alone getting evidence-based treatments. Equally worrisome: the agency doesn't even bother to measure patient outcomes.

Before the Phoenix and Tomah scandals, VA leaders touted their ambitious plans to implement top-quality mental health programs and they continue to make such claims. Dr. Matthew Friedman, the former executive director of the VA's National Center for PTSD and now its Senior Advisor, told me, "We promote clinical excellence." The VA has also been hailed in health reform books (such as Phillip Long-man's *Best Care Anywhere: Why VA Health Care Would Work Better for Everyone*) and in prestigious medical journals for outperforming the nation's leading hospitals in monitoring and treating medical illnesses, such as diabetes. None of those accolades has improved the agency's approach to mental health care. The Department of Veteran Affairs has not made delivering first-rate, evidence-based mental health treatment the same priority that reforming its medical care was for the agency in the late 1990s.

In April 2014, the VA scandals were exposed when *The Arizona Republic* revealed that more than forty veterans had died and, in some cases, killed themselves while waiting for care at the Phoenix VA. Yet the agency's defenders claim that once access barriers are overcome, the care veterans receive from the agency across the country is excellent.

But the new VA scandals and emerging revelations found in lawsuits, whistleblower complaints and previously downplayed or buried Inspector General reports undermined those cheery assertions. The unfolding data-rigging and quality of care scandals spurred at first new VA investigations into more than ninety VA hospitals, as well as DOJ federal criminal probes into forty of those sites, although those investigations seemed to be leading nowhere by 2016. On top of that, the Center for Investigative Reporting showed that in the decade after 9/11, the Department of Veterans Affairs paid $200 million to nearly 1,000 families for wrongful deaths. There would doubtless be far more lawsuits, but the agency is protected by its narrowly legalistic counterattacks against grieving families and court rulings that limit the department's liability.

The VA's administrative practices have also incentivized endangering patients' lives. The agency's approach across many of its facilities has been to reward administrators and staffers with cash bonuses who meet faked performance and safety goals, to protect wrongdoers and to punish employees who object to unsafe conditions, corruption and rigged data. In 2013, nearly $300 million in extra pay and bonuses were given to top executives and other employees who, investigators later found, often fabricated claims that they met the official wait-time and quality goals.

A leading recipient was one of the very few officials fired in the VA debacle, Sharon Helman, director of the Phoenix VA Health Care System where dozens died waiting for treatment. But she was fired for failing to disclose that she received a trip to Disneyland and other gifts from a lobbyist—not for the delays. A court later ruled that the VA had to return the initial $5,000 garnished from her wages, even though she collected over $41,000 in bonuses awarded for her bogus "outstanding performance" through 2013. Her lawsuit contesting her termination as unconstitutional remained pending in federal court throughout 2016 until an appeals court sided with her in May 2017. She had seemed early on likely to win—until she was sentenced in May 2016 to two years probation for taking thousands in gifts from the lobbyist—because a sloppily written new 2014 law didn't grant her the right of an administrative appeal. (She still pursued the civil lawsuit after being convicted in criminal court, and the appeals court overturned her firing when it agreed that the new law unconstitutionally restricted her right to appeal to the independent Merit Systems Protection Board [MSPB]. That board for civil service employees seemed likely to uphold the basis of her original firing.)

New bipartisan legislation has been introduced in Congress to expedite the VA Secretary's authority to fire any of the department's more than 300,000 employees. It's a measure that its backers hope will now pass constitutional muster—although it's opposed even by some whistleblowers who worry that it could be turned against them and, of course, public-sector unions. (Hypocrisy alert: the unions, including the American Federation of Government Employees (AFGE), framed their opposition to the bill as standing up for dissident employees, but whistleblowers, including Brandon Coleman, told me that the unions did little or nothing to protect them. "They offered no help," Coleman says, and when he finally went public with his concerns, his local AFGE president denounced him for being "foolish" by going to the media.)

The groundwork for this latest "accountability" legislation was set in motion when the Justice Department announced in May 2016 it would not contest Helman's claim to get her job back—and the VA openly declared in June 2016 it would no longer use the enhanced firing authority granted the agency as part of the sweeping $16 billion 2014 reform legislation.

Yet in 2014, after scandal engulfed the agency, the VA spent nearly half of its millions in bonuses on the same people it rewarded the previous year. The same pattern continued through fiscal 2015, *USA Today* reported, with senior executives averaging $10,000 each in bonuses amid a bounty of $177 million to nearly 190,000 employees. That untrammeled, brazen largesse was unleashed even as hundreds of its 312,000 employees were directly linked to the use of the secret waiting lists that caused patient delays in at least 110 major hospitals, 70 percent of all those studied in June 2014 by the agency. The same wide-ranging internal audit by the Veterans Health Administration—the VA division directly in charge of health care—discovered that 121,000 veterans were still being victimized by delays lasting more than ninety days for their first appointment. The 2014 survey looked at more than half of the VA's 1,053 hospitals and clinics then in operation.

Few VA staffers were punished or lost their jobs, but many who created these waiting lists throughout the VA system were handsomely rewarded for their schemes. "VA's sordid bonus culture is a symptom of a much bigger organizational problem: the department's extreme reluctance to hold employees and executives accountable for mismanagement that harms veterans," now-retired Rep. Jeff Miller (R-Fla.), then the chairman of the House Veterans' Affairs Committee, declared in 2014.

But most of the congressional reforms turned out to be little more than window-dressing. The 2014 legislation, although designed in large part to shorten wait times, actually allowed by 2016 a 50 percent increase in veterans who waited more than a month for primary care. Even the agency's feeble Inspector General found in April 2016 that veterans were waiting as long as seventy-one days for primary care appointments—while officials were still gaming the system by starting the clock when they called back veterans with available times, not when veterans first requested care. More than two hundred veterans died while waiting for care in 2015 at the Phoenix VA alone.

In a well-publicized response to such concerns, Secretary Shulkin unveiled a new website, accesstocare.va.gov, in April 2017 that purports to show the average wait times for patients at VA facilities around the country and how they compare to nearby private-sector hospitals, along with the percentages of veterans expressing satisfaction.

Some reformers have applauded this departure from past secrecy and his other reform gestures, including Brandon Coleman, a prominent Phoenix VA whistleblower who won a settlement from the federal government. "I'm cautiously optimistic," he says of Shulkin, citing such actions as the quick removal of the director of the DC VA hospital in April 2017 after the Inspector General reported unsafe conditions there, and the new website that at least acknowledges some long wait times. Nevertheless, he points out its limitations: "Internal figures are never accurate with the VA." After quickly checking with fellow dissidents in a few VA hospitals, he found some significant discrepancies between the new website's claims and the reality on the ground, but not as bad as the flagrant fakery during the height of the 2014 VA scandals. Look, for instance, at the Shreveport, Louisiana, VA hospital, where Shea Wilkes, then a mental health administrator who was busted back down to social worker, exposed in 2014 thirty-seven wait-time deaths among those people on a secret mental health waiting list of 2,700 patients. As a result of exposing these deaths, Wilkes was subjected to a contrived criminal investigation by the VA's Inspector General that drew national attention; his courage helped spur years of complaints about long waits and the bullying behavior of director Toby Mathew that finally led to Mathew's firing in April 2017. Yet the VA's access website reported in the spring of 2017 that the wait time for new primary care appointments in Shreveport was a still-problematic forty-five days, when the reality for some clinics, Wilkes notes, was that it took as long as sixty days. And while the VA has been able to provide some same-day crisis mental health services, as it promised, all too often at his and other hospitals, he says, patients can't get prompt, regular counseling: "The one thing the VA is very good at is throwing pills at the problem."

Even when wait times seem to be reported honestly, as in the unusually long eighty-seven day delay for new mental health appointments in April 2017 at a clinic in Santa Fe Springs, California, it's another sign of just how far the VA under Shulkin still has to go to keep its promises to veterans. Having seen VA secretaries come and go, all ignoring problems and shielding wrongdoers, Wilkes has a somewhat jaundiced view of Shulkin: "He's talking the talk, but will he walk the walk?"

So it was an open question how much impact the ambitious 2015 VA mental health legislation, the Clay Hunt Suicide Prevention for American Veterans Act, would actually have. The law aims to improve access and quality through the use of peer outreach programs, the recruiting of more psychiatrists and annual independent assessments of the VA's mental health care. Worthy goals, but it's not clear that these plans will fare better than other promises and guidelines that have crashed against the rocky shores of the VA's stubborn bureaucracy. In recent years, destroying the reputations of whistleblowers was a higher VA priority than improving services. Doctors, counselors and even a few bold executives discovered this after they came forward to try to stop fraud or save patients' lives.

CHAPTER 4

The Secret History of the VA Scandals, Part II: The Empire Strikes Back

AT THE PHOENIX VA MEDICAL CENTER, CHIEF FINANCIAL OFFICER Tonja Laney should have been honored for helping expose fraud and the undermining of patient care. Instead, after she assumed her post in 2012 and soon started raising questions about apparent financial fraud by a top administrator, she became the target of harassment. It included bizarre, poison-pen allegations that she was having sex orgies with black men inside her office; these were initially concocted by racist colleagues outraged that she was divorced, had biracial children and was dating a black man. The mounting workplace hostility became so severe that she even attempted suicide by overdosing on OxyContin at one point.

Three VA-led inquiries in 2012, 2013 and 2014 found that the smears against Laney were indeed baseless. The harassment campaign against her was ramped up again in May 2014 after she told investigators from the VA's Inspector General about fraud at the hospital and barriers to patient care. She was thrown out of her office the next day, demoted and, a few months later, even faced a trumped-up criminal charge—later dismissed—of stealing government property (she'd kept two copies of letters from her previous VA post). Remarkably, in April 2015, a national VA board that was sent by the new VA Secretary, Robert McDonald, to supposedly investigate the Phoenix wait-time deaths and other scandals instead asked Laney, "Did you have threesomes in your office?"

Meanwhile, for nearly a decade, staff and patient complaints about real, life-threatening problems that had caused hundreds, if not thousands, of deaths due to fatal delays, negligent care and prescription drug overdoses had been ignored throughout the country. As a spokesperson for the Phoenix VA concedes, the Laney inquiries were a "distraction," while still contending that the allegations against her were so serious that they had to be investigated multiple times.

Laney has a more sensible view: "I wish the VA cared as much about the wait times as they did about my [fabricated] sex life," she says.

If this happened to a top executive at the Phoenix VA, imagine the fate of lower-level whistleblowers and average patients struggling to get decent health care at VA facilities that did not fall under such intense national scrutiny. As a result of such attacks, there's a high cost paid by both patients and the thousands of honorable VA employees— whether administrators, clerks, social workers or doctors—when staff morale and the opportunity to do their best work are under sustained institutional assault.

Until July 2015, when the Department of Justice belatedly filed its first indictment against a VA administrator for falsifying records, that criminal charge against Laney remained the sole criminal filing brought to court against any employee at any of the VA's scandal-scarred facilities. Unfortunately, in the absence of either accountability or transparency at the VA, we'll never know the precise count of all those who needlessly died because of the delays.

Although Laney believes there has been some progress made in reducing the long wait times at the Phoenix VA, she says, "There is a systemic problem: You can't improve access and care for veterans unless you improve morale for employees." And despite public vows by then-VA Secretary McDonald and his deputy, Sloan Gibson, that they would protect and encourage whistleblowers, Laney, along with several other prominent whistleblowers, never heard back from them after seeking help. (McDonald and Gibson were still in charge before Trump's inauguration, but they both left their jobs early in 2017.)

Even after Laney had been reinstated to her CFO post in September 2014, and after the federal MSPB ruled in October 2015 that she had indeed been retaliated against, the harassment continued. Hospital executives occasionally delayed paying Laney's checks, cut her staff 50 percent and forced her to work overtime without added compensation. Finally, amid the unrelenting abuse that worsened her military service-related depression and her PTSD, she took a leave without pay early in 2016 and retired in June, at age forty-one, unable to work again. She is filing a lawsuit against the VA for the decades of lost earnings she faces, while expecting to receive additional damages from the MSPB. No officials at the VA have ever been punished or lost their jobs because of their campaign against her.

"It was clear that the retaliation was never going to end," she says.

For the VA's clinical staff throughout the country, such persistent harassment is especially damaging: it is a direct attack not just on them but on their ability to care for their patients and broader efforts to improve quality. In Phoenix and at other hospitals, dissidents such as Brandon Coleman kept getting punished just for trying to save lives. A bearded, blunt-talking addiction therapist at the Phoenix VA and a disabled Marine Corps veteran with a blown-off left foot, he filed a formal federal whistleblower complaint in December 2014. With his own past as a meth addict who came close to shooting himself in 2005 in a cemetery, he was especially alarmed that the understaffed ER was allowing suicidal or homicidal patients in crisis—often brought over by addiction counselors—to simply wander off the site. One patient killed himself in the parking lot after being ignored by the staff.

"It crushes me personally when a veteran successfully commits suicide," he says—and since 2011, at least six of the addicts he counseled killed themselves until he was pushed out of his job early in 2015. All told, Coleman has said of veterans' care, "There are dozens and dozens who commit suicide in the Phoenix area each year." After going public with his concerns in January 2015, a successful, specialized year-long outpatient program he ran in the evenings for addicted veterans with criminal convictions was shut down; he was forced to take administrative leave; and he was then investigated for purportedly threatening a colleague, actions that hospital officials claimed were unrelated to Coleman going public with his concerns.

All these ginned-up VA assertions were shattered when an independent federal agency, the Office of Special Counsel (OSC), sided with Coleman in May 2016. It offered him a generous, undisclosed financial settlement that allowed him to pay off all his debts and help his kids buy a home and cars. He was reinstated as an addiction specialist at an outpatient clinic unaffiliated with the Phoenix system, and was able to restart his life-changing program for addicted vets. During more than a year of forced leave, he became an informal leader of the nation's countless VA whistleblowers. He says now, "I kicked the VA in the nuts and I won my case." Today, he rides around in a prized new classic car, a blue 1968 Mustang, with a license plate that reads, "THX VA."

Coleman's fierce advocacy on behalf of the VA's truth-telling insiders has earned him a national platform as a witness before Congress, as a regular interview subject on TV and, in late April 2017, on the stage at VA headquarters when Donald Trump signed an executive order establishing a new office at the VA to investigate employee misconduct, including retaliation against whistleblowers. Even as he stood there behind the President, an unbowed, imposing man who felt no need to cut his pony-tail and proud to be a representative of the hundreds of employees punished for exposing wrongdoing, he was all too aware of how hollow the new "Office of Accountability and Whistleblower Protection" could prove to be if people like him aren't involved.

As he later told Shulkin after the ceremony and the viewers of *Fox and Friends,* "If they don't bring whistleblowers to the table, this is just going to be another dog-and-pony show; we've already got a lot of agencies inside the VA that are supposed to protect whistleblowers and none of them do it." Equally worrisome, many whistleblowers were concerned that this new office will be yet another instrument of retaliation and cover-ups as the Inspector General's office, a similar accountability group within the VA and the Office of Medical Inspector (OMI) have all turned out to be, regardless of their ostensible missions. Even so, while standing on the stage with the President and later sharing photos as a dad of three Marines with Vice President Mike Pence, also the father of a Marine, Brandon Coleman recalls, "It was the first time as a whistleblower that I actually felt that I'd really won."

But there usually isn't a happy ending for other whistleblowers. They are now targeted with apparently greater ferocity by the VA's leaders since most national media outlets have turned their attention away from the VA scandal and the Phoenix hospital where it all began.

"I still get two to four calls a week from VA whistleblowers [across the country] I have never met who are crying, scared and losing their careers all for merely telling the truth," he says. "It has not stopped because the VA has never been made to stop."

So patients at VA sites such as the Phoenix and St. Louis hospitals (where the chief of psychiatry, Dr. Jose Mathews, was forced out in 2013 after reporting that suicidal patients were ignored by staff) continue to see honest, dedicated clinicians get punished and removed from their posts. The agency has done virtually nothing on its own to rein in those who engaged in clinical misconduct or harassment. In reply to questions about the rarity of such reforms, a VA spokesperson pointed to the Office of Accountability Review established in 2015 to focus on senior executives that "ensures leadership accountability for improprieties" and its cooperation with the independent Office of Special Counsel on whistleblowing retaliation complaints. (That same VA accountability office, though, refused in January 2016 to confirm all but one of the major acts of administrator retaliation against Brandon Coleman and buried its mild report on his case for ten months.)

To be blunt, it's hard not to conclude that all these accountability sound bites from federal officials are just noble-sounding bromides that haven't changed the most poisonous culture in the federal government. VA's true scorn for both veterans *and* whistleblowers was most recently underscored by the revelations in February 2016 of horrifying scandals at the chaotic VA Medical Center in Cincinnati. It was bad enough that thirty-four whistleblowers had to turn to the Scripps News Washington Bureau and its affiliated local TV station, WCPO, to expose such longstanding problems as surgeons being pressured to use blood-and-bone splattered instruments as "sterilized" for operations by the hospital's acting chief of staff, Dr. Barbara Temeck, who then denounced them as "picky" for raising objections. Meanwhile, she raked in over $300,000 a year as both an administrator and thoracic surgeon without doing any surgeries, and essentially shut down the orthopedic surgery, neurosurgery and prosthetic limbs units to save money by sending veterans into the wilderness of the Choice program to wait as long as nineteen months for surgery. Yet she wasn't even *demoted* until she was exposed by the Scripps organization for improperly prescribing opiates to the wife of her regional supervisor, Jack Hetrick, who eventually retired before being fired. (She denies any wrongdoing.) The VA's leadership was doubtless aware by 2013 of dangerous hospital conditions after a Cincinnati congressman complained about dirty surgical instruments soon after Temeck's arrival— and the hospital staff started reporting hundreds of dangerous incidents in internal documents compiled in 2015, later obtained by Scripps and WCPO.

Yet even though Secretary McDonald, a former CEO of Procter & Gamble in Cincinnati, was personally warned by the whistle-blowers about hospital conditions in a letter about five months before the story broke, he did nothing. In fact, in January 2016, supervisor Hetrick and hospital chief Temeck were *awarded* $12,500 and $5,000 in bonuses, respectively, *USA Today* reported. A month later, while forcing out Hetrick and Temeck from their jobs after the publicity, McDonald and Dr. David Shulkin approved an initial OMI "inspection" that found no safety problems. That investigation didn't bother to interview any of the public whistleblowers; it also ignored 581 separate "quality events"—including bone-contaminated instruments— affecting 16 percent of all the hospital's surgeries, outlined in that fiscal 2015 report obtained by Scripps. Finally, McDonald and the new regional supervisor publicly vowed to protect whistleblowers who provided more information. But just two days after this offer was made to a surgical tech, Scott Landrum, who went public with his safety concerns for the first time at a televised community meeting in April 2016, he was threatened by the VA hospital with being fired. During Secretary McDonald's reign, the VA evaded questions about this scandal that flourished on the watch of the new VA secretary, Shulkin, when he headed the VHA division.

Now that Shulkin is in charge, the department is defiantly standing by its earlier findings and responses: "The VA OMI and other reviews of sterile processing practices at the Cincinnati VA Medical Center affirmed that high quality, safe services were and continue to be provided to veterans. No personnel actions were taken as a result of these reviews," a spokesperson said in a March 2017 statement. This brief, dismissive response to a locally reported scandal that received virtually no major national attention is perhaps the best sign yet that the VA remains fundamentally broken and unchanged.

So in the absence of a genuine crackdown, about two dozen current and former employees who went public as whistleblowers first joined together in June 2015 to form the informal reform alliance "VA Truth Tellers." The group prods the agency to get serious about improving care and transforming its bureaucratic culture. "Until the VA starts terminating the bad actors, everything else is just fluff around the edges and accomplishes nothing," Ryan Honl told *USA Today*.

The VA and its defenders have never really acknowledged these harsh realities, so it's difficult to understand how, for instance, the VA's latest suicide prevention plans announced in 2016 can truly succeed. These include providing meaningful same-day treatment access for veterans with urgent mental health needs at 1,000 different facilities. The Clay Hunt suicide prevention act does require a third-party assessment of the VA's efforts by December 2018 and each year thereafter, with the evaluators selected by the agency itself. Unfortunately, there are several groups, such as the Joint Commission for hospitals, that have a reputation for rubber-stamping whatever facilities pay their way, so it's unclear how the public will be able to prevent the agency from gaming or even evading the Clay Hunt Act.

• • •

IN THE CONTEXT OF THE USUAL WASHINGTON RESPONSE TO A SCANDAL— the ritual sacrifice of a few top officials as scapegoats to appease a rabid media—the lack of even an ersatz response after Secretary Eric Shinseki was forced out in May 2014 has been staggering. In June 2015, over a year after dozens of needless deaths were exposed at the Tomah hospital, the national VA finally responded with vague proposals that included "listening sessions," but took no effective actions that would prevent future Tomah administrative scandals.

Following the prescribing excesses, Tomah officials also said they were following tougher new DEA guidelines on opiate prescribing that, some veteran advocates say, are harming patients with legitimate pain issues. That's because patients are now required to see their doctors in person once a month for refills—a near-impossible task amid the backlog and delays throughout the VA system. Equally troubling, the VA's crackdown on opiate prescribing—a swing from one extreme to another—may be contributing to an increase in heroin and illegal opiate medication use among veterans, as well as suicides from pain-wracked veterans going through unmonitored withdrawal.

Veterans are twice as likely to die from accidental opioid overdoses as non-veterans, the VA reported in 2011. As chronicled in Sam Quinones's book *Dreamland*, by the late 1990s, the VA joined with leading medical organizations and the drug industry in promoting the unproven notion that opiates were "virtually non-addictive" when used to treat chronic pain. As secret corporate records disclosed in litigation showed, the VA's pain management team became a propaganda arm for the drug industry, fueled in part by a $200,000 grant from Purdue Pharma, the manufacturer of OxyContin whose executives pled guilty to "misbranding" the drug's addictive dangers in 2007. The department's pain experts released a "Pain as the 5th Vital Sign Toolkit" for clinicians in 2000, then joined with DOD in 2003 in issuing guidelines spreading the industry's fraudulent message: "Repeated exposure to opioids . . . only rarely cause addiction." Helping spread the gospel of opioids for chronic pain was psychiatrist Rollin Gallagher, who testified in 2002 against restricting OxyContin before the FDA and worked as a consultant for Purdue and other narcotic manufacturers before becoming the VA's deputy national program manager for pain management, a position he still holds as of this writing. In response to questions from *The Austin American-Statesman* in 2012, he said, "I am not influenced by the pharmaceutical industry in my work," noting that he hasn't received drug industry funds since 2006 and claiming he advocates safer pain management.

The department started backing away from its freewheeling prescribing of opiates only a few years ago with new initiatives that led to approximately a 25 percent drop in opiate prescribing, although it doesn't track veterans who have turned to heroin or illegal prescriptions as a result of the cutbacks. Meanwhile, the agency has promoted more holistic approaches to pain. But even with these assorted reform pronouncements, the number of veterans with opioid-use disorders increased 55 percent over five years by 2015—and there are still few signs that any clinicians or administrators associated with reckless care faced any strong sanctions. Ignoring these deadly failures and the Tomah scandal altogether, Shulkin, in an opinion piece he co-authored in *JAMA Internal Medicine* in March 2017, shamelessly painted the VA as a national role model: "The VA has been able to address opioid overuse and pain management in a comprehensive manner." Yet back at Tomah, the doctors, administrators and nurses who played a role in the deaths of Jason Simcakoski and over thirty other veterans weren't initially disciplined, and not even a single dollar was deducted from anybody's paycheck. As Ryan Honl, the original Tomah whistleblower, observed in mid-2015 with undisguised bitterness in an email: "Houlihan is still on paid leave. No one disciplined. Not a single person whatsoever. Nothing." (The doctor's paid leave lasted until he was finally fired in November 2015, and, of course, he was back in business treating patients until recently.)

• • •

THE VENOMOUS BUREAUCRATIC CULTURE ALSO REFLECTED THE VA'S LONG-standing failure to actually implement and monitor their sweeping mental health plans. That's the inescapable conclusion drawn from the findings in recent years of even the agency's own insipid Inspector General office; an under-reported federal court ruling in 2011 that condemned the VA's "unchecked incompetence" in mental health care; and the daily tragedies and barriers to quality care that veterans endure. It was a commonly cited—and tragic—statistic that twenty-two military veterans take their own lives each day, based on the VA's own analysis of the data. A more recent, comprehensive July 2016 VA report placed the suicide rate at twenty a day, with 7,400 veterans killing themselves a year—a rate that is an alarming 21 percent higher when compared to civilian adults. Meanwhile, every month nearly 1,000 veterans attempt to take their own lives. By some measures, that's more than one attempt every half hour. Roughly two-thirds of veterans who commit suicide are over fifty, the VA has reported. But an updated analysis showed a 44 percent increase in the suicide rate of male VA patients between ages eighteen and twenty-four in a recent three-year span.

One problem could be the VA's troubled Veterans Crisis line. Reports mounted in 2015 about a hotline system that often placed distressed callers on hold or shifted them to voicemail. One suicidal thirty-year-old Illinois veteran, Thomas Young, called the VA crisis line in July 2015, but no one answered. Wracked with despair, he went to the nearest rail lines outside a suburban Chicago Metra stop and waited for a train to run him over. His body was found on July 23rd, leaving behind a wife and two daughters to mourn him. "The next day, the veteran's phone rang—it was VA's emergency line returning his call," according to the revelations at a 2016 Senate hearing reported by the conservative *Daily Caller*. *Military Times* found that some hotline staffers are still answering as few as one call a day even after a new hotline director was forced out in June 2016 after only six months.

The VA promised to build a new satellite Veterans Crisis Line site in Atlanta by October 2016 to create "redundancy" and add two hundred more responders. The VA asserted in an April 2017 congressional hearing and statements to the press that the problem of busy suicide calls rolling over for waits as long as thirty minutes had basically been solved, with claimed rollover rates of under 1 percent. Members of Congress were skeptical, and hidden problems remain: Benjamin Krause, a critic of the VA, recently reported on his DisabledVeterans.org website that a disabled veteran, Rob Matthews, recounted being transferred to an overseas operator with a foreign accent, not an American, when he called the crisis line during a family emergency. "It made me feel like I was sold out, and I have a loss of hope due to the response I received," Matthews said.

All such failures are emblematic of broader patterns of indifference and shoddy care in the VA system—yet it's worth recalling that it's still better than what most mentally ill *civilians* receive. As many as half of Iraq-Afghanistan war veterans suffering from PTSD and depression, along with other illnesses, get treatment from the VA, according to a RAND Corporation study and recent VA reports. But only a portion of them get "minimally adequate" mental health care, RAND found—and that was based on the VA's own hyped statistics.

The end result of such neglect can be seen in both the rising numbers of suicides and accidental prescription drug deaths. Starting in 2012 and continuing through today, more active duty soldiers die from suicide than in battle. Roughly 4,400 service members and over 75,000 veterans killed themselves between January 2005 and the end of 2015, according to the latest available findings. On this front, however, the VA is essentially better than no treatment at all: since 2001 the rise in suicides of veterans who manage to access VA care rose just under 9 percent, while the suicide rate for those who don't use VA services or receive no treatment at all increased by 39 percent.

Women veterans are especially vulnerable to deficiencies in a VA system that was created primarily for men, and commit suicide at an increasingly high rate. An important VA study released in 2015 found that although women veterans commit suicide at somewhat lower rates than male veterans, their suicide rates were six times the rates of women without service records—and nearly twelve times higher than civilians for female veterans ages eighteen to twenty-nine. That's often because of the trauma resulting from the high rate of sexual assaults in the military.

It's small comfort that the increased rate of suicides was far higher among female veterans who couldn't bring themselves to access a VA controlled by a male-oriented military culture. A scathing 2014 report by Disabled American Veterans on the failure of the VA and other federal agencies to provide adequate services to post-9/11 female war veterans concluded: "Nearly 300,000 women veterans are put at risk by a system designed for and dominated by male veterans."

In practice, what this all means is that the increasing numbers of women veterans will likely be exposed to much of the same neglect and roadblocks to receiving quality care that men have endured for years.

• • •

EVEN AS SUICIDES GARNER MOST OF THE PUBLIC'S ATTENTION ON MILITARY mental health issues, the prescription drug deaths of veterans such as Eric Layne and other West Virginia veterans in 2008 were early warning signs of a related health-care disaster that has never been seriously addressed. Neither the Department of Defense nor the VA has conducted a full-scale inquiry into the numbers, scope and specific causes of accidental overdoses due to prescribed psychiatric drugs, although the opiate crisis has obviously drawn considerable attention. But independent inquiries by veterans' advocates, a leading academic researcher and a few media outlets have uncovered disturbing trends in mental health prescribing. By some estimates, reform advocates charge, over four hundred active-duty soldiers and veterans died in their barracks or at home from antipsychotic-related sudden cardiac death by 2014. As one reformer, neurologist Dr. Fred Baughman, contends, until military leadership limits the availability of antipsychotics, antidepressants or prescription polypharmacy, such deaths will likely continue.

A few rigorous studies suggest that thousands of veterans have been killed by accidental prescription drug overdoses in the last decade. One of the few scholarly reports on accidental overdose deaths of veterans, by University of Michigan and VA researcher Amy Bohnert, used 2005 data to conclude in 2011 that 1,013 patients receiving VA services died through unintentional overdoses, mostly from prescription medications. Legal opioids, at nearly a third of the accidental overdose deaths, were the most common substances involved, while nonnarcotic psychiatric drugs and sedatives were involved in 22 percent of the deaths she studied. Strikingly, the risk of prescription drug deaths including opiates was highest among mentally ill veterans even without a "co-occurring" addiction diagnosis, her follow-up research showed.

Remarkably, in 2014 across the entire US population, nearly 50 percent more people—almost 16,000—died from psychiatric drug overdoses than from heroin. According to the CDC, the psych med fatalities were led by benzodiazepines and other sedatives, although nearly 19,000 people were killed by prescription opiates.

As of 2016, the VA hasn't released more recent overdose data, but because veterans were already dying from drugs at twice the rate of civilians in 2005, the annual number of veterans' deaths hasn't climbed as much as the civilian plague, Bohnert told me. Even with the scant available information from the agency, it's still reasonable to assume that the number of veterans dying from accidental overdoses annually is nearing 2,000, if not more. Just the striking 272 percent increase in the VA's legal opioid prescribing between 2001 and 2012, according to data obtained by the Center for Investigative Reporting, should be a source of concern.

In some localities, the potentially deadly spike in prescribing was far worse. *The Fayetteville Observer* discovered that in the Fayetteville, North Carolina, area, the VA's prescriptions for the opiate hydrocodone shot up 4,100 percent in 11 years by 2012, with nearly 48,000 patients on that drug alone. National trend data from the CDC is just as alarming: The number of accidental overdose deaths for all people at least doubled between 2005 and 2016 to over 59,000 a year, mostly due to prescription opiates and heroin. Heroin use has increased nearly 500 percent in a decade.

"Mental health providers need to assess and address the risk of death from accidental [prescription] overdose among patients with psychiatric disorders in addition to risk for suicide," Bohnert, an assistant professor in Michigan University's psychiatry department, recommended in *The American Journal of Psychiatry* in 2012.

Yet despite new drug safety initiatives, few in the VA are successfully implementing such preventive steps for psychiatric medications, or keeping a systematic public count of these tragedies. They represent far more than numbers on a spreadsheet to Heather Simcakoski and the other widows and families left behind.

Of course, prescription drugs, if poorly monitored, could on their own drive veterans to suicide. These potential dangers have been established since the 1990s when class action and wrongful death lawsuits exposed that manufacturers hid those risks for some patients taking such fraudulently marketed drugs as Paxil and the discredited cure-all Neurontin.

All these controversies have played out amid the raging debate among medical experts over the risk of increased suicide and the medical value of antidepressants. Those suffering from depression may just have to look to their own experience with medications and weigh the conflicting advice and competing "meta-analysis" overviews, even with the knowledge that many of those authoritative conclusions are undermined by corrupted drug industry studies. The arguments for and against antidepressants, as marshaled in books by such authors as

Dr. Peter Kramer and Irving Kirsch, shouldn't deter those with depression from consulting with an empathetic psychiatrist who will take any concerns about side effects seriously. Ideally, people grappling with depression should decide in collaboration with their doctor whether such medication is the best course. While it does seem that the benefits of appropriately prescribed antidepressants outweigh the risks for adults with major depression (with up to 70 percent of patients experiencing a significant reduction in symptoms), there isn't a consensus on whether those drugs are effective for mental illnesses such as anxiety, moderate chronic depression or major depression in children and adolescents.

The case for medicating the young with antidepressants took another blow in the fall of 2015, when *The BMJ* (formerly *British Medical Journal*) re-analyzed previously hidden data in GlaxoSmithKline's notorious Study 329 on Paxil for adolescents with major depression. *The BMJ* researchers found that the drug was ineffective and that the study failed to disclose that youth on Paxil were as much as *eleven times* more likely to engage in seriously suicidal behavior than those on placebo.

The published data on all antidepressants for young people is nearly as troubling as that found in Study 329. For children, adolescents and young adults up to age twenty-four, the risks of suicidal behavior and aggression in clinical trials are reportedly at least twice as great with antidepressants when compared to placebos, according to a 2016 *BMJ* overview and other studies, although some young people clearly benefit from those medications.

In a situation similar to the wave of off-label prescribing of antipsychotics, many adults who probably could be helped by antidepressants aren't getting them at all, while those who likely don't need them are receiving them unnecessarily. Even as the use of antidepressants among those twelve and older has increased roughly 400 percent since the late 1990s, a remarkable August 2016 study in *JAMA Internal Medicine* and other reports have found that most people taking the drugs don't have mental illnesses justifying their use. Meanwhile, remember, suicides have soared to a thirty-year high across most age groups. By analyzing recent patient survey data, a Columbia University team discovered that less than 30 percent of people with signs of depression were getting treatment, including antidepressants, while Columbia University and Johns Hopkins researchers concluded in separate studies that close to 70 percent of those who received antidepressants never had major depression, generalized anxiety or obsessive compulsive disorders that could offer a rationale for the prescribing. Dr. Mark Olfson, a professor of psychiatry at Columbia University Medical Center, told NPR about the unnecessary prescribing, "There are simpler forms of psychological interventions that can be adapted for primary care," including counseling and exercise—rather than turning to antidepressants first.

Given this upsurge, it's especially necessary to vigilantly track side effects, because as many as one out of every hundred patients may experience violent and homicidal thoughts, leading a few people to commit murder. In 2001, a jury awarded $6.4 million to the family of a man who killed his wife, his daughter, his granddaughter and then himself after taking the antidepressant Paxil made by GlaxoSmith Kline. (Such lawsuits have sharply dropped since the FDA required black-box warnings about increased suicide risk for teens and young adults, starting in 2004, while adding other warnings on the risks of aggressiveness, mania and hallucinations.) But the dangers continue: British documentary filmmaker Katinka Blackford Newman in her recent book, *The Pill That Steals Lives*, profiled murderers without previous histories of mental illness who became delusional and violent after taking antidepressants. She began the book after she recovered from a psychotic decline that went on for a year after taking Cymbalta, which initially led to her hospitalization after stabbing herself with a knife and wanting to kill her own kids—even though she wasn't even clinically depressed when she began using the medication.

Whatever the final truth about the risks and benefits of using antidepressants, careful monitoring is especially vital with young people receiving these psych drugs. That's precisely what is generally missing in busy public clinic settings. There's rarely time, encouragement or rewards for careful prescribing in the real world of public mental health systems, whether funded by Medicaid or run by the VA and military.

The danger to mentally ill veterans continues, despite all the hearings and initial media scrutiny. For example, in 2014 the GAO found that a software error in diagnostic coding led the agency to omit "major depression" entirely in the records of a third of the patients the GAO reviewed. The VA didn't fix the error until after the GAO issued its report based on a sampling of thirty cases, but the mistakes in these patients' medical records before the "fix" was implemented have been left intact. These sorts of errors still affect an unknown number of other veterans, possibly tens of thousands. As a result of this and other record-keeping flaws, the department—and its harried clinicians often just doling out drugs or downplaying suicidal signs—still doesn't have accurate information about all the veterans burdened by this depressive disorder that can be a prelude to suicide.

• • •

THE VA'S LEADERSHIP HAS NEVER FULLY ACKNOWLEDGED ANY MAJOR FAILures in the agency's approach to the wave of suicides, even after all the shocking news stories about veterans shooting themselves, driving off cliffs and hanging themselves after being denied treatment or disability benefits. Nearly a decade ago, there was little done nationally after Lucas Senescall, a depressed Navy veteran, hanged himself in his garage with an extension cord in July 2008, three hours after being turned away by the VA medical center in Spokane. As first reported by the *Spokane Spokesman-Review*, in a one-year span starting in July 2007, twenty-one veterans in the Spokane area were publicly reported to have killed themselves, fourteen of whom had received care at the VA. (The full scope of the suicides by Spokane patients was undercounted by the VA under the watch of the hospital director, Sharon Helman, who was transferred to another facility in 2008—until she took over the Phoenix VA in 2012 and began faking wait-time outcomes. She apparently continued undercounting VA suicides in the Phoenix area as well, *The Arizona Republic* found.) Under a local media spotlight and facing a raft of potential lawsuits, the Spokane Veterans Affairs Medical Center grudgingly increased its suicide-prevention efforts.

Yet the sort of concerted initiatives undertaken in Spokane were either missing in most VA hospitals and clinics, or done in a way that only appeared, on paper, to comply with whatever new guidelines were put in place. Less than a third of Iraq and Afghanistan war veterans with PTSD even receive specialized mental health care treatment from the VA, according to internal agency documents obtained by Veterans for Common Sense (VCS) that were even more damning than the RAND Corporation findings.

In court filings and at a trial resulting from a 2007 lawsuit, the attorneys and leaders of VCS, joined by Veterans United for Truth, made a compelling case for immediate court-ordered relief. The veterans groups showed that 1,400 veterans died in one six-month period while waiting for their disability claims appeals to be heard. The lawsuit also highlighted that as far back as 2005, the VA Inspector General found some VA health facilities were improperly "gaming" and falsifying wait-time information. But that didn't set off alarms in Congress, the VA or the media until the Phoenix VA scandal almost a decade later.

The only strong ruling in favor of the veterans' lawsuit came in May 2011 when a three-judge Ninth Circuit appeals court panel upheld the merits of the lawsuit and declared that delays in providing care deprived veterans of their constitutional rights, opening the way to court-ordered injunctive relief. "VA's unchecked incompetence has gone on long enough," Judge Stephen Reinhardt wrote for the majority. "No more veterans should be compelled to agonize or perish while the government fails to perform its obligations." The public and Congress didn't start to respond to that failure until the Phoenix scandal broke open three years later.

Unfortunately, the VA didn't see any of these tragedies or the lawsuit as a wake-up call. Instead of responding directly to the rising tide of suicides or the striking failures demonstrated in the lawsuit, agency officials fought the case on narrow technical grounds for six years. Their assertion: the courts lacked the constitutional authority to order the VA to institute reforms. While the VA's lawyers were arguing against making any improvements in court, numerous veterans in Tomah and Phoenix and across the country were dying in increasing numbers because they couldn't obtain quality care in the VA system.

In 2012, the full Ninth Circuit agreed with the VA's constitutional arguments and overturned the Reinhardt ruling, saying it was up to Congress to repair the VA. The VA eventually triumphed in the Supreme Court in February 2013, when the court refused to hear an appeal of the lower court decision.

The lawsuit did spur the VA to create its now-failing crisis line in 2007. It also helped create momentum for a new law in 2008 enabling most veterans to receive free VA medical care for up to five years after their discharge from a combat zone, in part to accommodate the long wait times for disability claims the lawsuit and congressional hearings exposed.

Yet the VA remained a disaster zone. Before the issue became a high-profile national scandal in 2014, the evidence of the agency's deadly failures was clearly laid out in that early VCS lawsuit and Inspector General reports, coupled with media accounts. Even as early as 2009, the Inspector General found there wasn't a single suicide prevention specialist at any one of the agency's approximately eight hundred community-based outpatient clinics, where most veterans get their health care.

The VA's reluctance to respond in an effective manner to veterans' mental health needs was originally considered a byproduct of Bush administration attitudes that saw veterans with PTSD as malingerers and fakers. But all that was supposed to change with the election of the dedicated young president, Barack Obama, in 2008. Within a few years, however, a few progressive veteran groups' leaders, influential media outlets including *The New York Times* and even some Democratic members of Congress were openly critical of the mounting signs of a VA in disarray, unable to respond to the rising demand for mental health services.

The VA's resistance to giving timely treatment and accurate PTSD diagnoses was abetted by the military's policy of booting out active-duty troops with cooked-up diagnoses and the denial of PTSD claims. Those actions, in turn, limited those veterans' ability to get disability benefits or receive long-term free health care from the VA; that's because the military classified them as not having any "service-related" illnesses.

By 2010, for example, at least 31,000 service members were discharged under the vague diagnosis of having a preexisting, lifelong "personality disorder" instead of a service-connected mental illness, such as PTSD. These sorts of bogus diagnoses, including "adjustment disorder," prevented veterans from collecting their full disability benefits, and limited their opportunities to access in many cases either free health care for life or specialized PTSD treatments at the VA. (It's not widely known that veterans of the Iraq and Afghanistan wars are entitled, in theory, to five years of totally free health care after they leave the military, as long as they weren't dishonorably discharged, but after that point they could face some out-of-pocket costs for VA treatment if they are classified as not being injured physically or mentally during their military service.) In 2015, the GAO found that the Department of Defense still engaged in shady diagnostic practices that misclassified service members, robbing them of veterans' disability payments and the full scope of VA health care.

Some of those suffering from genuine service-related psychiatric conditions may also engage in misconduct—such as smoking marijuana while in the military—that brands many with an "Other Than Honorable" (OTH) discharge that bars them permanently from any VA health care unless they successful appeal their classification. In 2014, three veterans groups, including Vietnam Veterans of America, joined a class-action lawsuit on behalf of tens of thousands of veterans who developed PTSD during their service but received an OTH discharge; indeed, PTSD wasn't even a diagnostic category until 1980. The lawsuit led the military to loosen its standards in allowing discharge upgrades for veterans of all ages with PTSD, but DOD's appeals process is still so onerous that in the Army, for example, only 164 veterans applied for an upgrade in 2015.

And after tens of thousands of veterans have been branded with the OTH discharge by the military, they're then confronted by the VA's own barriers. About 125,000 veterans who served since 2001—over 6 percent of all post-9/11 vets—are still receiving such "bad papers" discharges, and the VA hasn't reviewed their cases. As a result, according to a 2016 report by Harvard Law School's Veterans Legal Clinic and the Swords to Plowshares advocacy group, the VA has largely ignored a federal eligibility law allowing the agency to take into account these veterans' mental health conditions and offer them care. "In most cases, the VA refuses to provide them any treatment or aid," the study concluded, obstacles that contributed to their committing suicide at twice the rate of other veterans. In the face of mounting public pressure, Shulkin, the new VA Secretary, announced in March 2017 that the agency would begin offering mental health services to OTH veterans at VA emergency rooms, the counselor-staffed Vet Centers and the Veterans Crisis Line. But as Bradford Adams, the supervising staff attorney at Swords to Plowshares, points out, the VA is already doing that for any veteran. In fact, the ballyhooed reforms don't extend to offering psychiatric or neurological care. "These veterans need services, not lip service," he says.

What's especially cruel is that these misguided discharges and diagnostic ruses can force veterans who have been kicked out of the military to pay back their enlistment bonuses, which can be as high as $40,000. That burdens them with debt as the traumatized veterans struggle to find jobs. In addition to financial difficulty, the black marks of an OTH discharge, or getting severed from the military for having a spurious "adjustment" or "personality" disorder, can prevent them from landing jobs.

On any given night more than 300,000 jobless veterans of all ages, mostly men, are living on the streets or in shelters. Meanwhile, the questionable psychiatric discharges alone save the military $4.5 billion in medical care and are used to save the government $8 billion in disability compensation payments, according to the Vietnam Veterans of America.

Even though wait times have worsened and the rigging of the VA's appointment system is well known, there hasn't been a comparable challenge to the related statistical gamesmanship on the supposedly shrinking disability backlog. The VA claims it has slashed first-time physical and mental disability claims delays by over 80 percent to just under 100,000. In fact, the actual number of total pending claims has grown to nearly 1.5 million because the VA simply wasn't counting appeals and other disability-related claims, including 480,000 appeals that have been pending for more than four years, according to Gerald

Manar, the recently retired director of National Veterans Service for the Veterans of Foreign Wars.

Tens of thousands of other disability claims never even made it into the VA's cumbersome disability system to be counted as part of the backlog. For instance, as CBS News first reported in February 2015, Rusty Ann Brown, a claims reviewer for the Oakland VA system, found that 13,000 "informal" letters from veterans asking to apply for disability benefits were stuck in file drawers without a response between the late 1990s and 2012. "Half of the veterans were dead that I screened," she told CBS News after she and a team were finally asked to review them. Yet, at hearings in March 2015, the VA undersecretary in charge of the Veterans Benefits Administration (VBA), Allison Hickey, still insisted, to the disbelief of legislators, that there were no problems at all. But the independent OSC concluded in October 2016 that the VA retaliated against Oakland whistleblowers and covered up its massive failures.

The sloth-like response of Hickey's agency to veterans in need stood in sharp contrast to her efficiency in approving $400,000 in moving-related expenses for two regional directors who were accused by VA investigators of scheming to get easier jobs at the same salaries. (Another scathing Inspector General report led to Hickey's resignation in October 2015, but the two accused VA scammers were returned to their high-ranking posts in 2016 by administrative judges after being demoted.)

• • •

THE SAME SORT OF INACTION AND LACK OF ACCOUNTABILITY GUIDED THE VA's response to new laws passed in the wake of the original VA scandal. Even legislative reforms that passed Congress in 2014 and early 2015—designed to address the lack of access by veterans to care—are already being undermined.

Spending for the Choice section of the legislation, which allowed veterans to go outside of the VA if they couldn't get access to a nearby VA facility, was shaved to $10 billion by the time the program took effect in August 2014. But veterans' advocates say that if fully applied, the plan would actually cost closer to $50 billion. Although the legislation passed with near-unanimous bipartisan support, it only proved how much ideology trumps meaningful reforms at the VA and throughout the mental health system when partisan interests are at stake.

At first, it seemed that the most ludicrous part of the Choice plan was the VA's attempt to limit its use to veterans who did not have a VA facility within forty miles of their home "as the crow flies." After Jon Stewart excoriated that idea on *The Daily Show*, the VA changed its policy by allowing "forty miles" to be calculated by driving distance. That doubled the number of veterans who could be served—and potentially doubled the program's costs to $20 billion.

But the Department of Veterans Affairs didn't stop its efforts to prevent patients in need, especially those with PTSD, from going outside its troubled system. Their leaders initially claimed that few veterans were interested in enrolling in the Choice program at all.

But the Choice program as run by the VA posed dangers to veterans far greater than even the agency's spin or semantic disputes over how far a crow flies. The new program designed to help veterans get speedier help outside the VA turned into a logistical nightmare that blocked veterans from getting care for months. It was also seen by critics as a boondoggle for two corporations: Tri-West Health Care Alliance, which landed a $72 million VA no-bid contract in twenty-eight mostly Western states, and its eastern US counterpart, Health Net—on top of the billions they were already contracted to receive for running an earlier network of specialized private sector "Community Care" providers. As exposed in September 2016 by CIR's national radio program, *Reveal*, Tri-West raked in added bonuses from the Choice program every time one of their temp staffers, mostly without medical experience, called a veteran. But instead of being rewarded for actually arranging timely care, different staffers sometimes placed calls over and over again to the same veteran. Total health-care costs to the VA soared as well, but because the Choice program is funded by a separate federal revenue stream, nobody seemed to care. (The company and VA leaders say that implementing the complex program on a ninety-day rush schedule forced by Congress added expenses and problems, now basically fixed.) Yet some Tri-West workers were so ignorant, *Reveal*'s Lee Romney reported, "One gal told me the rep sitting next to her thought PET scans were for pets."

In charge of both the Community Care contracts and the newer Choice program, the $9.5 billion combined VA windfall for Tri-West and Health Net had disastrous impacts on the health and well-being of veterans, according to the VA's Inspector General, *The Arizona Republic* and NPR, among others. *Reveal* demonstrated how the VA's top-down, outsourced approach to the Choice program caused horrific problems in Alaska without a full-time VA hospital in the state. The *Reveal* investigation focused on those needing vital medical care, but the same roadblocks clearly affected those requiring specialized mental health care in a system so short of clinicians. Although the state had a well-run, informal network of non-VA providers, after Tri-West took over, it continually bungled getting treatment authorizations to community doctors. As a result, a disabled Alaskan veteran like Daryl (who didn't give his last name on air) suffering with PTSD and chronic pain had to wait months for medical care and physical therapy for his back and arm. His arm became so weak that he lost his job as an airplane mechanic. Daryl aptly dubbed the program, "No Choice."

The Choice contractors also came under fire from NPR and some state officials for delays in funding and arranging timely mental health care. Clinical psychologist Cher Morrow-Bradley in Jacksonville, North Carolina, for instance, found that Health Net delayed paying her for the sessions with vets for close to a year; the company refused to answer NPR's questions. With Health Net in charge of much of the eastern and central US, at least two states, Maine and Montana, have withdrawn mental health services from the VA Choice program and scrambled to find other funds to pay for them, NPR reported.

Amazingly, the VA has continued to pay close to a billion dollars a year each to Tri-West and Health Net while only recently making some improvements in the Choice program. In fact, as noted by the conservative *Daily Caller*, Tri-West paid a $10 million fine in 2012 to settle Justice Department charges that it defrauded the Pentagon by not passing along its savings on provider costs to the government. Despite the fraud charges—disputed by Tri-West—the VA signed up the company in 2013 to that multibillion-dollar contract to help oversee the Community Care program that was a "precursor," also poorly run, to Choice, according to multiple Inspector General reports.

This time around, objections from the Alaskan members of Congress led the VA to scale back Tri-West's role in interacting with veterans—first in Alaska, then in a few other locations. But even as the contractors remain responsible for paying claims, the VA is planning to return far more of the scheduling authority back to the VA centers that generally got away scot-free with rigging wait times in the first place.

When he headed the VHA overseeing this mess, Dr. David Shulkin, although conceding some problems, told NPR in 2016 that the program was "working well" in many places. But instead of effectively resolving the disaster, first as the head of VHA and now as Secretary, he has touted instead a few dozen contract changes and four minor congressional amendments, while pinning his hopes on a broader legislative package that will create "Choice 2.0" that's still stalled in Congress, although a short-term extension passed early in 2017. As late as a March 2017 congressional hearing and in interviews, Shulkin and his top deputies were still disputing blistering recent reports by the GAO and the VA's Inspector General that found months-long waits for Choice enrollees and a stark absence of any meaningful oversight of these outsourced programs; the VA leaders claimed that the reports used faulty assessment methodology and were based on outdated information that doesn't reflect the most recent reforms. "The VA has no reliable data to measure how long the entire [appointment] process takes," the GAO's director of health care, Randall Williamson, told the House Veterans Affairs Committee in March 2017.

In response to these reports, Dr. Baligh Yehia, the Deputy Undersecretary for Health for Community Care, doubled down on the claim that the watchdogs' findings were mistaken, used obsolete methodology and were outdated. He only concedes, "This program has design flaws and we're redesigning Veterans Choice."

As media accounts of the Choice fiasco increased, though, the VA, echoing some VA Commission on Care findings on expanding civilian-sector care, still sought other ways to restrict the sort of outside help veterans can seek. The agency proposes to oversee an integrated, "high-performing network," but it would still limit veterans with mental illnesses from going outside the VA if their nearest facility offered timely access to "specialized behavioral services."

One such haven of purported excellence is the Phoenix VA's Outpatient PTSD Clinical Team. Yet this VA system still has far to go in terms of quality and outreach: In May 2015, yet another troubled veteran killed himself in the parking lot of the Phoenix VA.

Other improvement initiatives don't offer much more grounds for hope. Senator Baldwin's opiate prescription reform proposal, cited in the previous chapter, could limit medication excesses if enacted, but it doesn't address most of the abuses in psychiatric drug prescribing, especially involving antipsychotics. For example, years after the FDA in 2011 added new warnings about heightened cardiac risk posed by the antipsychotic Seroquel in interactions with at least seven categories of drugs, the VA still hasn't bothered to warn its clinicians about those dangers in any high-profile alerts. In short, the VA has done nothing in practice to truly limit off-label prescribing of Seroquel despite the troubling number of deaths linked to the medication, often in combination with other prescription drugs.

Those were essentially the same mild, unenforced off-label policies in place when Eric Layne, an Iraq veteran who had served with his wife Janette in the National Guard overseas, started his regimen of Seroquel, Paxil and Klonopin in the summer of 2007 to deal with his increasingly tempestuous PTSD symptoms. "Eric was told that he would get his life back once the VA got his medications right," Janette remembers. But that never happened. By October, he was suffering from incontinence, severe depression and continuous headaches as he became more listless and gained weight. He even fell asleep with food in his mouth. He lost his job later in the fall and entered an eight-week residential program for PTSD in Cincinnati where his high doses of medications were supposedly monitored. When he finally returned from the VA hospital, they talked about possibly seeing a doctor to investigate the side effects of the medications.

He never got the chance. Three months later, after he came back disoriented and drugged from the special PTSD program at the Cincinnati VA in January, he was dead.

The surviving West Virginia family members hoped that the

federal government would learn from the experiences of veterans such as Eric Layne and rein in the use of psychiatric medications. But it soon became clear that neither the FDA nor the VA was really influenced by such tragedies. Looking back, it sometimes seems as if agency officials were trying out in small markets a scenario for hiding scandals and deaths, with sham Inspector General reports, pro forma expressions of regret and a reluctance to hold anyone accountable or to change prescribing practices. These tactics all played starring roles in West Virginia before they took the production national in response to the furor over Phoenix and Tomah.

CHAPTER 5

A Marine's Descent into PTSD Hell

CORPORAL ANDREW WHITE, A MARINE CORPS VET FROM CHARLESTON, West Virginia, wasn't supposed to end up like this. At twenty-three, he'd gone from leading his Junior ROTC color guard in his spiffy dress blues to skillfully defusing explosives and serving as a lead Humvee gunner in Iraq to becoming another traumatized veteran scrambling for help.

When Andrew decided to join the Marines shortly after graduating high school with honors in May 2003, he was following the example of his two older brothers: William, a non-commissioned officer in the Navy now in his forties, and Robert, who was based in Fort Bragg, North Carolina. His father Stan White says, "His brothers were both career military, and Andrew really looked up to Bob and he chose the Marines. I think because he could prove himself as a Marine," marking out his own path. That strength clearly derived in part from his father, a formidable retired high school administrator whose pain and anger over his son's death can still be traced in his long, determined face that seems even more resolute with his white Fu Manchu-style mustache.

When in battle, with his brother as a role model, despite the danger and without complaint, Andrew jutted through the roof of the vehicle and exposed himself to enemy fire in the desolate, windswept deserts of western Iraq, handling the mounted machine gun with steely resolve.

In May 2005, though, whatever outward coolness he displayed in battle couldn't conceal his shock at the violence he encountered when he took part in the massive Marine campaign known as "Operation Matador" to retake control of insurgent-held areas. Flooding the area with 1,000 soldiers, supported by helicopter gunships and jets, the Marines swept through surrounding towns, largely going after elusive foreign insurgents allied with Abu Musab al-Zarqawi, an Al Qaeda leader behind many suicide bombings in Iraq and the founder of what later became known as ISIS. During the Matador campaign, Andrew was part of a large convoy leaving Al Qaim on patrol. While standing with his machine gun at the top of the Humvee, he was ordered to fire on muzzle flashes from near the roadway. A rocket-propelled grenade, or RPG, then came whistling past his head. "This was terrifying, and he felt he was almost killed and still might be killed. He believed he should return fire in the direction of the RPG firing, but he didn't," the VA psychologist noted in Andrew's 2007 medical chart. "He had a flashback related to this on July 4th this year, and experiences intrusive thoughts and images as well as trauma dreams related to this trauma."

But the fighting only got worse, searing more horrifying memories into Andrew. The next day, an armored personnel AmTrac carrier near the town of Haban was carrying a squad of reservists from Lima Company in Ohio when the vehicle ran over an explosive device that turned it into an inferno. Four Marines were burned to death inside. Ten other men were seriously wounded, and Andrew saw it all from his perch as a Humvee gunner. The hellish vista was even more disturbing because inside the AmTrac, undergirded with tank-style treads, were rounds of explosives that were "cooking off," sending weaponry and orange flames skyward. White was deeply shocked, feeling both horrified and powerless at once because all he could do was watch; he later told a VA psychologist that for years afterward, he at times experienced vivid flashbacks about the incident.

He also remained forever plagued by one night mission in his Humvee. As a gunner and combat engineer, his confusion in the dark, bleak desert was compounded by night-vision goggles as his team provided protection for an eight-wheeled Stryker fighting vehicle in their convoy. The Humvee was about one hundred meters ahead of the Stryker when that vehicle was blown to pieces by an IED that Andrew and others had apparently missed. A GI in the Stryker was killed, and the shock was so great that White continued having intrusive thoughts about it for years.

Even so, everything seemed fine at first when Andrew and his two closest buddies from the reserve unit that served in Iraq, Jacob Towner and Seth Montgomery, came back to Camp LeJeune. It was September 2005, and the southern weather was still warm enough so that when they were given a twenty-four-hour leave from the base, they headed straight to Topsail Island in North Carolina to unwind. Years later, when Shirley White, a short, sweet-tempered woman with a voice still husky from loss and regret, looks at the early photo of Andrew, broadly smiling in his green fatigues moments after they first saw him come back to Camp LeJeune, she points out: "You can see he's in good spirits. He's glad to be home."

The good feelings didn't last long. He came home to Cross Lanes on a Saturday evening. On Monday, the Whites were at an IHOP in Charleston, talking about how pleased they were that Andrew was home safe, when they got the phone call no parent ever wants to hear. Shirley's cell phone rang, and Cathy White, Bob's wife, said, "We lost Bob." Reeling from the shock, they could only ask, "Are you sure?" Stan and Shirley rushed back home, placed some calls and started making arrangements to drive down to Fort Bragg, where Bob's family was located. Andrew White took the news very hard, but he didn't say much about it. Bob's death at age thirty-four came so suddenly after Andrew's return that visitors in those first days couldn't help but notice that he hadn't even finished unpacking: his Marine duffel bag was still on the screened-in front porch.

Ten days later, when Bob's body was returned to Fort Bragg and funeral services held, Andrew was so upset by it all that he had to leave the chapel several times. He never really got over his brother's death and gradually unraveled. By the time he joined a veterans' support group in February 2007, it quickly became apparent to social worker Debbie Linzmaier and some others there that he could benefit from a professional evaluation at the nearby Kanawha City clinic. After one of those early visits, he got his first psychiatric medications.

Within a year, he was dead.

• • •

ANDREW ULTIMATELY RECEIVED NINETEEN DIFFERENT PSYCHIATRIC, PAIN-killing and other drugs during the months he sought help. By the end, there wasn't much left of the six-foot-one young man with short-cropped black hair, six-pack abs and laconic manner who had once been filled with so much promise.

Initially, the prescriptions seemed reasonable enough. He was given the antidepressant Paxil and a low dose of an older generation antidepressant, trazodone, used for its non-addictive sedating effects.

Soon enough, though, Andrew became yet another victim of the military's clueless health practices and the corporate marketing that promoted Seroquel's off-label use with PTSD patients—and even for active-duty soldiers. The VA was in the early stages of an initiative to cut down on prescribing for PTSD patients receiving potentially addictive benzodiazepines, such as Klonopin, Xanax and Restoril. Yet it was also allowing the mostly off-label use of Seroquel, the most sedating of antipsychotics, to skyrocket more than 770 percent between 2001 and 2010, although the number of patients covered by the VA increased only 34 percent, the Associated Press reported.

For active-duty troops, the growth in antipsychotic use, including Seroquel, was even more astonishing. Dr. Richard Friedman, a professor of clinical psychiatry at Weill Cornell Medical College and a regular op-ed contributor to *The New York Times*, revealed as part of a series of important columns on military drugging that antipsychotic prescriptions increased by 1,083 percent between 2005 and 2011. He noted in 2013 that it was probable that almost all such prescribing was off-label, because the military is supposed to screen out enlistees with the serious psychiatric disorders treated by antipsychotics. Doctors may be prescribing different types of psychotropics, he theorized, "for off-label use as sedatives, possibly so as to enable soldiers to function better in stressful combat situations," joined by a fifteen-fold increase in stimulant prescribing to wake them up for battle the following day. Yet this roller-coaster prescribing pattern may well have contributed—with the addition of such stimulant drugs as Adderall—to a rise in these medication-addled soldiers of the brain chemical norepinephrine, which is released by stimulants. This chemical also naturally surges during combat as part of the fight-or-flight response, he pointed out, helping sear memory of a traumatic combat event in the brain. The upshot: "A soldier taking a stimulant medication," he suggested in 2012, "could be at higher risk of becoming fear-conditioned and getting PTSD in the setting of trauma."

His research showed that the prevalence of PTSD within the US military increased over a thousand-fold to 22 percent by 2009, although he made clear that no causal link had yet been firmly established between stimulant use and the skyrocketing PTSD rates. Yet his hypothesis was apparently confirmed in 2015 when Pentagon researchers studying nearly 26,000 soldiers reported that those prescribed stimulants were five times more likely to have PTSD. So it seemed likely that all the off-label use was actually helping create a new market of PTSD sufferers primed for using antipsychotics after they were discharged.

Seroquel also became the VA's second-largest drug expenditure—after the blood-thinner Plavix—in 2007, the year Andrew was first prescribed it back home. More than four years after his death in 2008—and the deaths over time of hundreds of other veterans and soldiers taking Seroquel for PTSD symptoms, usually with other medications—the VA was spending $150 million annually for mostly off-label uses of Seroquel while the drug was under a patent. Costs dropped for the medication after it lost its patent protection in 2013. Even so, the number of VA prescriptions written for the drug dipped only slightly even in the face of FDA warnings about Seroquel's cardiac risk; a damning 2011 *Journal of the American Medical Association* (*JAMA*) study on the ineffectiveness of antipsychotics for PTSD; and payouts of over $1 billion by AstraZeneca in settlements by 2011. (These resulted from nearly 30,000 lawsuits against the company for allegedly hiding the drug's health dangers, including diabetes, along with several federal and state anti-fraud settlements.) Despite all that, Seroquel still remains the most heavily prescribed antipsychotic in the VA system, with nearly 800,000 prescriptions annually—more than twice as many as Abilify, the nation's most prescribed antipsychotic.

As purchases of antipsychotics by the VA and the Defense Department exploded after 2001—overwhelmingly for medically unapproved uses—so have the number of state-side young soldiers and veterans found "dead in bed" or "dead in barracks" who have often been taking Seroquel along with other prescriptions. These incidents have been chronicled by advocates for veterans in updated spread-sheets, but no government agency tracks them. Especially in the VA, there have been no major initiatives yet to halt or even to systemati-cally study these preventable deaths. (One exception: in 2012, DOD's US Central Command decided doctors needed a waiver to prescribe Seroquel to soldiers in combat zones.)

Andrew was no match for such bureaucratic forces. On his sec-ond visit to a nurse practitioner for a key medication review, he was clearly irritable, nervous, his legs shaking constantly. So he was given the powerful, sedating Seroquel as a substitute for the milder tra-zodone. What's particularly striking is that no other, relatively safer drugs designed specifically for insomnia were ever tried on White—including a non-benzodiazepine drug approved in 2004 by the FDA, Lunesta. "The trazodone is ineffective and will switch to Seroquel be-cause of the levels of suspicions he has and the agitation, irritability," the nurse, no expert on psychiatric medications, noted nonetheless.

But at the time Andrew visited that professional in 2007—and, long after his death, through 2016—there were virtually no pub-lished controlled, independent studies that showed any "statistically significant" value in using Seroquel for PTSD or long-term insomnia. *All* remotely positive results about antipsychotics for trauma were found only in studies written by researchers who had been subsi-dized by AstraZeneca and other drug companies. Indeed, most of such AstraZeneca-funded sketchy research on PTSD didn't even bother to compare Seroquel to anything else. But Andrew's first VA prescriber heedlessly switched him to Seroquel to help his "mood" and sleep anyway.

All the drug company's off-label marketing was paying off for AstraZeneca, as the Department of Justice found by tracking its sales tactics that it eventually cited in 2010 in the $520 million settlement. As Dr. Marvin Schauland, the osteopath and psychiatrist who became Andrew's final prescriber at the Huntington VA hospital, points out, "The drug companies pushed these new drugs for everything from alopecia to hemorrhoids to lumbago." Back in 2007 and 2008, Schauland notes, "The drug company salesmen could come into the VA to glad-hand us and give out samples." The VA didn't start limiting on-site visits by drug company reps until 2012, but there are still no meaningful limits placed on marketing to the VA's doctors through such lures as fancy seminars with meals led by influential local physicians.

The 2010 Justice Department settlement with AstraZeneca outlined some of the various sleazy strategies the company used to influence everyone from family physicians in the community to VA psychiatrists to prescribe Seroquel for such unapproved uses as PTSD and anxiety. AstraZeneca paid the settlement without acknowledging wrongdoing.

Seroquel remains off-label for PTSD, anxiety, insomnia and depression in youth, but virtually no one in clinical practice at the VA appears to be paying attention. That's in large part due to the effectiveness of the alleged illegal sales techniques that the company has deployed since 2001 and that the Department of Justice first highlighted in its April 2010 settlement agreement.

These shady gambits haven't stopped, according to the new 2014 whistleblower fraud lawsuit filed by the Texas Attorney General against AstraZeneca concerning alleged misconduct since 2006, the last year covered in the 2010 anti-fraud agreement.

Despite all the salesmanship underway before and after Andrew's death in February 2008, the VA's own widely-flouted official guidelines didn't support using antipsychotics for PTSD symptoms. But, in practice, the agency sanctioned the off-label use of antipsychotics with PTSD patients. "The evidence for using antipsychotics with PTSD patients isn't very good, and the potential side effects can be deadly, really," says Dr. J. Douglas Bremner, the chief of Emory University Medical School's Clinical Neuroscience Research Unit and one of the world's pioneering researchers on PTSD.

Andrew was started at a relatively low dose of Seroquel: 25 mg. That soon escalated, ultimately rising to 1,600 mg, twice the upper limit considered safe for use with people with severe schizophrenia. In fact, that dosage was more than *five times* the dosage used in the dubious schizophrenia studies first submitted by AstraZeneca to win FDA approval for that limited use of the drug in the late '90s. "In those studies, they were using relatively low doses, but VA doctors are using Seroquel like a nerve pill, giving it out like Valium or Librium," said Dr. John Nardo, the former director of the psychiatry residency at Emory University—who died in March 2017—and a retired psychiatrist who had published perhaps the most in-depth scrutiny of the shoddy Seroquel research with schizophrenics. "These doses being given to veterans are astronomical and since some of them have been killed, there's nothing I know of in *any* research to indicate that those kinds of doses are rational. The VA has exerted no upper limit on this medication," he observed.

Yet all this was done to Andrew without any sign that the doctors at the VA or others he eventually consulted ever took seriously the risks the drug posed: extreme weight gain, diabetes and even sudden cardiac arrest, among others. In fact, in over two hundred pages of VA medical records reluctantly released to the White family after his death, there is no indication that any VA staffer he dealt with knew about the findings of the agency's own *VA/DOD Guidelines for Management of Post-Traumatic Stress.* Adopted in 2004, they said there was "insufficient evidence" to recommend using antipsychotics for PTSD. The latest version of the guidelines hasn't changed that weak—and ignored—cautionary note for Seroquel.

As of 2016, the VA still had not created any high-profile alerts about the dangers posed by Seroquel, especially relating to the risk of drug toxicity it poses when mixed with other medications. At the grassroots level today (and back in 2007, when Schauland took charge of prescribing for Andrew), clinicians either didn't pay attention to the unenforced VA treatment guidelines for mental illnesses, including PTSD—or didn't even know they existed. "There's no set drug regimen for PTSD," Schauland claims, "so you to try to make a regimen to fill the needs of the patient." Yet even in the VA guidelines in effect when Andrew sought treatment, there were *some* prescribing recommendations. For instance, only the serotonin-based antidepressants were viewed as having significant benefit then for PTSD. The latest version of the guidelines has been expanded to include, among other medications, the beta-blocker Prazosin as having some benefit, while the VA labels antipsychotics as having "unknown benefit" at best.

Whatever the treatment guidelines said on paper, for Andrew, the VA's indifference to safe prescribing was only worsened by the lack of well-proven, personalized cognitive therapies for PTSD available to him at VA clinics, although they may fail half the time. For example, one of the most relatively effective, thoroughly researched treatments is Cognitive Processing Therapy, which trains the veteran to pay attention to and challenge the emotions generated by past traumas. In White's medical records, except for one brief notation in the last week of his life, there's virtually no hint that local VA personnel knew such therapies existed or that they should be used to help him. Schauland, who was in charge of his care, says, "I couldn't do psychotherapy because I was just there for meds. That's what the psychologists were for; I thought patients were going to groups or individual therapy." It's a telling sign of the VA's continuing failures that no health-care provider took responsibility for ensuring that Andrew got appropriate care, including targeted psychotherapies for PTSD.

It didn't matter that the agency's mental health handbook had recommended evidence-based behavioral treatments since at least 2004. That's because there have never been any full-scale efforts to implement them, despite various grand pronouncements by VA leaders to do so. White's sporadic counseling sessions were little more than superficial check-ins on his current status, supplemented by occasional medication reviews by psychiatrists, including Schauland. "The therapists weren't trained to deal with PTSD," declares West Virginia veterans' advocate Tom Vande Burgt. Vande Burgt's therapist, for instance, often used the time to just chat about problems in her own marriage.

Meanwhile, even the VA's lackluster Inspector General repeatedly confirmed the lack of widespread adherence to effective PTSD treatment strategies by the VA's mental health providers. Shirley White recalls that, just a day before his death, Andrew visited a Ph.D.-level psychologist, the only one ever assigned to him: "He's a year into treatment and this is the first time they *talked* about strategies."

In truth, smaller and rural clinics were especially prone to neglect the VA's own therapy guidelines, the Inspector General's office has found over and over again, in part because of the difficulty in recruiting mental health practitioners. Yet both in big cities *and* rural areas, the Inspector General reported in 2009, less than a year after Andrew's death, "At present we are unaware of a system by which the Veterans Health Administration [the VA's lead health-care division] reliably tracks provision and utilization of evidence-based PTSD therapies on a national level." There has been little improvement since then, despite the hiring of more therapists.

So, despite the recent scandals and public critiques, it still remains disturbing that so little has changed since White endured the VA's inept care. After seeking treatment back in 2007, Andrew only got more Seroquel and increasing dosages of Klonopin, Paxil or other antidepressants—and little actual therapy. The medications just kept increasing even though he also told the clinic staff about continuing to drink heavily on most days, while declining to enter alcohol treatment. But the prescriptions he was given couldn't quell his nightmares, increasing irritability, anxieties and pent-up rage. "I want to kill people," he admitted at one thirty-minute session, while being quite concerned that he'd lose control if he returned to Iraq.

The only service offered by the VA that provided any comfort to Andrew was the weekly voluntary support group, led by the well-liked, dedicated social worker Deborah Linzmaier. (She declined to be interviewed.) It provided a safe space, understanding and some basic information on PTSD for those like-minded veterans struggling with the illness, but not personalized therapy.

But as the months wore on, Andrew faced more bad days. Although he dated a hard-partying girlfriend, a bartender, in the spring, he also ended up drinking as many as thirty beers in a night, moving in with her for several weeks and ultimately losing his job as a cook at Famous Dave's. By that summer of 2007, he and his parents realized he was quickly going downhill, forgetting medical appointments, losing his short-term memory and becoming increasingly irritable. Yet the prescription drugs were doing little for him except causing noticeable side effects: tremors and a steep weight gain, eventually to 220 pounds, soon to be joined by the horrifying early growth of breasts and testicular shrinkage. "There wasn't really any significant problems with side effects," claims Schauland, who began treating him in late July. "He was *not* obese; he was a pretty good-sized man."

In contrast, "Every side effect Seroquel has, Andrew had. Every one of them," Shirley White observed. But the doctors at the VA reassured him—and later her—that there was nothing to worry about. The doctors who examined him sporadically noted the complaints in his medical records, but glossed over them and didn't connect them to the Seroquel he was taking.

By now, Andrew's nerves were all but shot. After a vet he knew from Iraq died in a car accident on the way to work, his depression only deepened, causing him to burst out into tears at odd times during the day and reminding him again of the death of his brother Bob. "The littlest thing makes me cry," he told a counselor during a sudden walk-in clinic visit in July 2007. He also admitted that he was only sleeping two hours a night and was wracked with "horrible nightmares." The drugs he was taking were still not working, he felt. Just as troubling, his days were sometimes disrupted by the waking nightmares of flashbacks triggered by unexpected noises, whether they were fireworks outside or mysterious sounds in his house that kept him as vigilant as the nights spent patrolling the perimeter at Al Qaim.

He was desperate enough for more or better pills that in July, on the same day as his local walk-in session, he drove to the mental health clinic sixty miles away at the VA Medical Center in Huntington. Once there, the social worker arranged for a quick medication review by a physician, who restarted him on Paxil, discontinued use of two other sedating meds but ramped up the dosages of Seroquel to 200 mg a day. Most critically for his future safety, though, they also gave him 25 mg tablets of added Seroquel and noted, in writing, "Take one-half tablet by mouth twice a day as needed."

As needed—whenever he felt he needed some more. This was a risky approach for a PTSD patient who often couldn't remember when or if he took his meds, who was desperate for relief and would soon get Seroquel refills mailed to him via the VA's mail-order service like clockwork every thirty or ninety days, enough to eventually fill a large shoebox. Ultimately, "he had a drawer filled with Seroquel bottles," Shirley White says bitterly. "He had an excess amount from the VA."

Yet the added medication couldn't erase the harsh memories of his tour of Iraq. All this was exacerbated by his increasing isolation in his room, playing the online multiplayer shooter war game *Halo* on his Xbox with an obsessed, furious intensity. His parents could hear him shouting at the futurist shooters he confronted on-screen, "Get the motherfucker!" His bedroom became his hiding place to retreat from the world, and as he told one VA counselor, "I'd like to crawl in a hole for a month and then come out and things would be better." But he wasn't, of course, able to shield himself from the world outside that was assaulting his nerves.

After hours, with his drinking compounding his short temper, getting into arguments and fighting became almost inevitable. One Saturday night in mid-July, he went out on the town with a hard-drinking friend from work. In a parking lot outside a bar, they got into an argument over who was in good enough shape to drive. In the ensuing fistfight, Andrew was beaten up, with his ribs and back so badly bruised that he had to go to a local emergency room, getting a few days' worth of Vicodin in the process. He came home later that day, recounting what happened without any contrition or shame. "That's one of the things that this does to you," Shirley says. "There's no remorse. Things just happen."

Still, in some ways, the incident seemed to be a wake-up call for Andrew that he hoped would lead to positive changes. He started cutting ties with his drinking buddies. Shirley says, "He's thinking, 'I need to disassociate myself from this. I want to try. I want to do better.'" Over the next few weeks, still experiencing the torment of PTSD flashbacks, sharp physical pains when he breathed and an inability to sleep, he switched his care from the local clinic and went to the Huntington hospital for medical and mental health evaluations. He hoped to get better quality treatment at the hospital.

That decision led to even more changes in his meds and the ultimate addition of more Seroquel. His initial evaluation at the Huntington hospital was conducted by Schauland, an osteopath-cum-psychiatrist with a past history of drug addiction and an apparent fondness for stockpiling 19,000 dosage units of narcotics and other prescription drugs at his home, according to Minnesota medical board records and a DEA investigation. At the time he saw Andrew White, he had faced state investigations instigated by the Minnesota medical licensing board—and already had his Drug Enforcement Administration (DEA) authority to prescribe controlled substances revoked in February 2007. Schauland, in his own view, had done nothing really wrong in failing to file the needed paperwork on his stockpile of medications.

Seroquel, despite its growing reputation as a street sedative with addictive potential—it was nicknamed Suzie Q—isn't a "controlled" medication requiring a valid DEA registration. That category includes narcotics or, in Andrew's case, the benzodiazepine Klonopin that Schauland prescribed. In need of psychiatrists, the local VA hired Schauland in June 2007, regardless of its purported policy of refusing to employ doctors who had faced DEA sanctions. West Virginia, though, permits its doctors to prescribe controlled medications without personal DEA registration as long as they have a facility's DEA authority; all licensed doctors in the US can prescribe regular, non-controlled medicines that aren't monitored by the DEA without needing a DEA permit. Schauland, in sum, wasn't breaking any state or federal law despite his questionable background and untrammeled prescribing after being hired by the Huntington VA.

But the Huntington VA, it turns out, has long exceeded the VA's already excessive 20 percent national average rate of prescribing ineffective, off-label antipsychotics like Seroquel for PTSD patients. In practice, it did little to rein in doctors like Schauland, who prescribed as they saw fit for patients such as Andrew. Still, although Schauland temporarily discontinued Seroquel for Andrew in July 2007 and started him on Klonopin again, Andrew continued after this July visit using the earlier prescribed Seroquel pills the hospital staff had reassured him could be taken "as needed." A few weeks later, Schauland then authorized higher doses of Seroquel to pacify Andrew's complaints about sleep. Schauland also viewed the drug as having other useful benefits: "Andrew had a wild and wooly side and I was trying to calm him down," he says.

Yet a few days after the July 2007 visit with Schauland, the sedating effects of Seroquel became dangerously obvious: he came home from his restaurant job on a Wednesday evening and slept thirty-six hours straight through to Friday. His parents frantically tried to rouse him, but Shirley recalls, "We could not wake him up." They were so worried that Stan White checked in on him periodically to make sure he had a pulse and was still breathing. His parents, adept at discovering any alcohol abuse, knew their own son well enough to know that he hadn't been drinking for a few days, so they grew far more concerned about his medications. Andrew managed to drive himself to the Vet Center, and with his mother on the phone, they were patched through to a clinical social worker at the hospital. At one point, defending why he was taking the sedative Klonopin during the day, he explained, "It mellows me out and keeps me from wanting to stick a knife in someone's face at work."

Shirley White was, perhaps for the first time, being given a raw glimpse into the turmoil sweeping across her son's mind. With Andrew's permission, Schauland encouraged her to monitor his sleep patterns and dispense his medications. But the medical staff brushed aside her growing concerns over the prescriptions themselves. "Mother believes he is having effects from all of his sedating medications—could be alcohol withdrawal," the social worker noted dismissively. "I can recognize his drinking," she says now. "He didn't hide the things he was doing."

In an intense phone call with the psychiatrist that same day, the pro-medication Schauland emphasized to her the importance of monitoring his prescriptions. Shirley asked, justifiably worried for her son's safety, "Is he taking too much of his medication?" Schauland discounted that risk. The doctor also made it sound as if the VA really cared: "I conveyed to her that VA services will be available to be helpful and supportive of her efforts in her son's behalf," he wrote in his notes on August 3, 2007.

Unfortunately, that turned out to be a hollow promise. The VA's doctors just gave him more pills for his back pain, and, all too soon, more Seroquel.

As Shirley remembers one hospital visit, the medical doctor sought to ease his reported back pain with more meds but didn't do much else. "I can't see anything wrong," the doctor told Andrew.

"I can't see any problems that you're having, but here are some pain pills that should help." The doctor then simply grabbed samples of Vicodin for Andrew without bothering to warn him about interactions—or even recording the painkillers he dispensed in his medical records. The next day, Andrew tried to get himself admitted as a psychiatric inpatient.

His request was denied by a hospital psychologist who viewed him as stable enough, while also noting dryly that individual therapy "may be beneficial." Yet he never was given access to that sort of therapy until a week before his death. Later that day, he had a critical psychiatric appointment with Schauland that set him on a pathway to his death; this psychiatrist who had promised Shirley that the VA would help her son decided instead just to increase his medications. So a week after Seroquel helped put Andrew under for thirty-six hours, and knowing his history of sporadic heavy drinking, on August 8, 2007, Schauland still went ahead and resumed his prescription of Seroquel at 600 mg. That was nearly the maximum recommended dose for people with *schizophrenia,* and it was used as an unproven, unapproved treatment for what Schauland noted as "mood and sleep" in his records. "You use the patient as the rule of thumb," he explains now. "You start with low dosages, then watch out for side effects. If there were any problems, I would have cut back the dosages."

A few days later, with all these drugs back in his system, he was driving to the Vet Center in his brand-new red Mustang on a straight stretch of road when he plowed into a car in front of him that was clearly signaling to turn. "My reaction time was off," he told his parents later. He'd been so proud of the car, bought with a car loan two weeks earlier. Now, with the car being towed to the shop, he called his mother, who drove him to the emergency room so that doctors could examine the new back and neck pain he was experiencing. He also received more Vicodin for his pain after the ER doctors screened him for any alcohol or illegal substances, and all the tests came back negative. It was another sign that he didn't fit the caricature used in the VA's subsequent spin campaign—accepted by most mainstream news outlets—to essentially blame the deaths of soldiers like White on their own rampant substance abuse.

The car accident just worsened his depression and isolation, and hastened the final, medication-fueled descent to death. His physical and mental health deteriorated as the VA gradually ramped up his medications, with the side effects of extreme weight gain and male breasts becoming more obvious. His hands and feet were shaking with uncontrollable tremors as well, but there were no positive trade-offs to justify the gradually increasing dosages of Seroquel and other drugs. They brought no new calm or stability in his life.

Instead, he almost never left his room now, retreating into his world of *Halo* and other video war games until the early morning hours, the sounds of recorded gunfire echoing through the house. His nerves were more on edge, his sleep worsened, and he took almost all his meals alone in his room. From August 2007 until the day he died, he only shared a meal with his family twice. Yet in August and September, he had close to twenty different medical, psychiatric and psychological appointments, often accompanied by his mother. The periodic half-hour or so therapy sessions largely consisted of Andrew telling social workers about his anxiety, depression and insomnia, with little being done about it except doctors increasing his medication dosages.

Getting *access* to care itself didn't turn out to be Andrew's problem with the VA; it was getting access to effective, personalized and evidence-based treatments from an agency that couldn't keep its promises to its wounded warriors. After a thorough review of his case, the final decision that he was 100 percent disabled by PTSD and qualified to receive approximately $2,500 a month in disability payments wasn't reached until roughly two years after he returned from Iraq.

Yet, essentially all that any medical professionals continued to do for Andrew was to encourage him to increase his medications. By September 2007, he was taking an astonishing 1,200 mg of Seroquel a day, along with other medications. "Is it safe?" Andrew asked during one clinic visit, and the clinicians there blithely reassured him he had nothing to worry about. "He appeared to tolerate it, and he seemed to be okay," Schauland adds.

Andrew's parents knew he needed more specialized help than the local VA system was providing, but their efforts to get him treated at the residential PTSD unit in the VA's Clarksburg, West Virginia, hospital were stymied by the agency's Catch-22 rules. Even as the national VA was tacitly encouraging the use of antipsychotics and Klonopin with PTSD patients, the Clarksburg PTSD residential unit declined to admit patients who had been prescribed those very same drugs by local VA doctors. "They refused to take him because he was on medication," Stan White says. Prodded by the VA's Inspector General, the hospital ultimately altered its absurdly restrictive policy after Andrew White died.

As Andrew continued to unravel in that fall of 2007, his parents started to look outside the VA system for psychiatric help for their son, where they found the area's most highly recommended psychiatrist for treating PTSD, Dr. Lawrence B. Kelly. Kelly was also, in the eyes of Big Pharma marketers, an influential medical "key opinion leader" (KOL) worth paying to hype their drugs, according to recent corporate disclosures. It wasn't until its settlement with the DOJ in 2010, though, that AstraZeneca began to stop paying doctors to tout Seroquel for the sort of off-label uses that contributed to Andrew's death. Kelly declined to comment or answer phone calls on his receipt of drug payments, although records show he received roughly $30,000 from drug companies in 2010 through 2012.

But in 2007, when Shirley accompanied Andrew to some initial visits, no major companies disclosed their payouts. So there was no way of knowing for sure why this expert doctor joined the VA in thinking that the best solution was to increase Andrew's Seroquel dosage up to 1,600 mg under his direction, along with Paxil, Klonopin and other meds. While White did talk about his nightmares of all those dead Iraq bodies during those sessions, he got little else from his treatment except more side effects. These included severe constipation and a plummeting libido in addition to weight gain and glandular effects. Still, the switch to the new psychiatrist also seemed to offer a few glimmers of hope: he began planning a trip to the beach in the summer, a small but important sign that he was looking ahead to the future.

When the PTSD group he had been regularly going to began falling apart in mid-November 2007, one of the few stabilizing forces in his life was yanked away. "He lost contact with that weekly regimen of meeting with his friends," Shirley White says. "He didn't have anywhere to vent."

There was never any reason given by VA officials as to why the support group was closed down. But Linzmaier was encouraging veterans to apply for benefits at a time when the agency's *de facto* policy was to downplay the seriousness of PTSD and to thwart veterans' access to care—a point later confirmed in the scathing federal appeals court ruling in 2011 decrying the VA's "unchecked incompetence" in failing to deliver timely mental health services to veterans in need.

In January 2008, Andrew was involuntarily committed to the decrepit Mildred Mitchell-Bateman Hospital in Huntington, West Virginia. Andrew ended up there after he had gone on a bender that included cocaine, triggered by a notice from the Marine Corps that he had been discharged on medical grounds. When he returned home, he holed up in his room with his Xbox and video war games, all his stress and frustration building throughout the weekend. By Monday, he was breaking items, hurling his Xbox controller at the TV and throwing his CDs across the lawn from the porch. A frightened Shirley White called a few friends that night to calm him down and convince him to get emergency help. But his rage spiraled out of control while waiting for hours to be seen at the nearby Charleston hospital, and he began threatening to kill a doctor who told him to simmer down. White's original interest in admitting himself voluntarily had so backfired that the hospital's medical staff, clueless about how to deal with PTSD patients, filled out a mental health warrant to commit him involuntarily.

A 2008 state investigation report cited the Bateman mental hospital for overcrowded conditions and inadequate psychiatric care, but it was still operating unimpeded at the time Andrew was committed. Even then, after the decision to commit him on January 16th was reached, the disarray, ineptness and shortages in the local mental health system—common across the country—became evident once again. With no hospital bed anywhere, it wasn't until the early morning hours when the court officers shipped him to Bateman in Huntington, which didn't have space either, but reluctantly admitted him as the referral option of last resort.

It became clear enough that the degradation he felt at being committed to Bateman didn't speed his recovery. Instead, they slapped on new diagnoses and altered his medications yet again. He was now deemed to have bipolar disorder with psychotic features *and* PTSD. The doctors at Bateman stopped the Paxil and, with an eye towards boosting his chances of getting admitted to the restrictive Clarksburg PTSD program, took the risky step of suddenly stopping the anti-anxiety benzodiazepine he was taking, Klonopin. Unfortunately, that was a highly dangerous move that not only can induce panic attacks, psychotic symptoms and seizures, but can also lead to mistaken psychosis diagnoses—as apparently happened to White while at Bateman—all resulting from failing to gradually, carefully wean patients off the drug over several weeks. The medical staff also lowered his dosage of Seroquel to a still-dangerous 800 mg.

Unfortunately, while Andrew was in the hospital, the deadly risk posed by taking Seroquel in combination with other drugs wasn't apparent to the Whites—even after Eric Layne, a member of Andrew's support group, was found dead on the couch by his wife on January 26th. Shirley White first learned of Eric's death when she was on her way home from visiting Andrew. At the time, Eric's family believed his death was due to kidney failure, but nobody really knew for certain.

Andrew's parents, though, made a decision not to tell him about Eric's death while he was still in the hospital. "I think we just thought he would handle it better when he was home," Shirley recalls.

But if Eric's death was a tragedy for all who knew him, the news was especially frightening and mysterious to fellow members of his support group, in part because he died just a day after being discharged from the residential PTSD program at the Cincinnati VA hospital. "He was the first one of us to die, and it was a shock," says support group member Chris Tharp, who had even made plans with Eric to go the driving range together when he got back. "We didn't know anything about medication," he says.

Once Andrew learned what happened to Eric, Tharp recalls, "It took him off guard and messed him up psychologically." Andrew even joined in the search for answers but didn't connect Eric's medication use with his own. "By the time we came up with conclusions," Tharp says, "it happened to Andrew."

The day after his discharge from Bateman, Andrew, still lacking any effective treatment but somewhat more relaxed, returned again to the snares of the VA's hit-or-miss strategy for dealing with his PTSD. On February 2nd, joined by his mother, Andrew traveled to the Huntington VA hospital to meet with both a senior psychologist, Robert Huwieler, and his lead psychiatrist, Schauland, to start what was supposed to be, at last, a definitive treatment plan. He first saw Huwieler, who had thoroughly evaluated him the previous August for his PTSD disability claim. Even with all the medications he'd been prescribed, Andrew, restless and nervous at this session, was still reporting flashbacks and regular nightmares from his time in Iraq. Huwieler concluded that his condition had been marked by a "progressive worsening over time."

One obstacle, Huwieler noted, was that he had "extremely limited coping skills" for managing his PTSD symptoms. One key reason for this inability, of course, was that until then, no professional at any VA facility ever bothered to teach him such elementary coping strategies as using slow, deep breathing during stressful situations.

Still, Huwieler showed a willingness to bend the rules for Andrew. He agreed to see him personally each week rather than relying on the VA's scheduling obstacle course. Huwieler's plan for Andrew: "Participate in individual cognitive-behavioral psychotherapy to learn and apply coping skills . . ."

"We had to beg—honestly beg—to get him that extra treatment," Shirley says.

But it would prove to be too late. In the final weeks of Andrew's life, his medications were adjusted yet again without regard for the risks involved. "If you are going to see us, it's us only," Schauland told Andrew. He had not seen White since October 2007, when he had increased his Seroquel dosage to a breathtaking 1,200 mg. "A fair amount of de-compensation has transpired," Schauland later wrote in his notes about this February session, without raising any questions about his own prescribing strategy or the VA's therapeutic failures. Schauland reinstated his previous drug regimen with the doses slated to be escalated: Paxil, Klonopin and, for now, Seroquel at 800 mg.

With the new treatment plan in hand, Andrew, the VA's clinical staff and his mother were all optimistic. "I really thought he was going to get better," Shirley White says. "We were very upbeat on his last visit to Drs. Schauland and Huwieler."

The next week, Huwieler met with Andrew privately while his mother waited in the car. He came down the steps afterward with some new hope and the first tangible coping technique he was ever provided: a rubber band around his wrist. "He had on the rubber band, and it was suggested that any time he started thinking about Iraq, that he was to use that rubber band and snap it, and then that would bring him back to now," Shirley recalls. "That was one of the strategies." It was meant as one of the "grounding" methods used in cognitive therapy for a PTSD sufferer plagued by intrusive memories.

When they returned home that Monday afternoon, he was smiling a bit more than usual as Shirley left to go to the Sylvan Learning Center franchise she and Stan owned. Stan was working at a Canaan Valley, West Virginia, resort for the ski patrol. With a snowstorm underway, Shirley returned home that night much later than usual. Knowing how anxious Andrew got when she wasn't home on time, she called to reassure him three times on her way home.

Yet when she got back, "he seemed to be doing well," she says. He was speaking to his younger sister on the phone for about a half hour, talking about his plans for a dinner date with one of her friends the next evening. While Shirley stayed up late painting cabinets for a renovation, he chatted easily with her, asking for a twenty-dollar loan for tomorrow night's date and making plans to meet Shirley at the cell phone store near her job at 1 p.m. the next day.

It was getting late. About 10 p.m., she doled out, as usual, his prescribed medications, including Seroquel, but they continued talking until 11:30 p.m., when Andrew said he felt tired and started getting ready for bed. Nothing seemed particularly wrong, although his mother told him he looked very pale. Andrew just laughed it off. Since he often took their pet cat to his bedroom to help relax during his restless nights, she asked, "Do you need the cat to come up and spend the night?"

"No, actually I feel pretty mellow this evening," he said, heading up the stairs in his pajamas and T-shirt. That turned out to be the last time she ever spoke to him.

The next morning, on her way out to work, she stopped by his

room to put the twenty-dollar bill on his dresser drawer and turn
out the bedroom light. Nothing disturbed the heavy snoring that
typically marked his medicated sleep. At work at the Sylvan Center,
she started calling before noon to the house phone and then his cell
phone to make sure he would be awake in time for their appointment. With no answer, she soon started calling the numbers again
and again, and was growing increasingly frantic. She then called on
a neighbor to check on him. The neighbor went over to the house
twice, pounding on the front door and his bedroom window without
getting any response.

"I think something's wrong," she told Shirley by phone at about
3 p.m.

Shirley rushed home in her car, hoping that her worst fears
weren't coming true. When she ran into the house and up the stairs
to his room, she found her youngest son Andrew lying on his side in
his bed, deathly still and facing the wall. It was mounted with pictures
of his Marine buddies, his Xbox controller and the white dress Marine
cap he once wore with pride. She cried in anguish at what she saw: it
was obvious that he had stopped breathing and was almost certainly
dead. She called 911 anyway, but the paramedics couldn't revive him.
Even today, this shy woman—who has gone public in a crusade to
change the VA's mental health treatment of veterans—breaks down
in tears at the memory of those final horrifying moments that ended
her son's long struggle to get effective help. All she will say about it
now is: "It's painful."

Less than three years after Andrew returned from Iraq, their second son was dead, too, killed at twenty-three in his own way from the
after-effects of the wars in which both sons fought. The agony of their
loss would only be compounded by not knowing for certain what had
killed Andrew. After the paramedics had finished their work, Andrew
was pronounced dead at 4:09 p.m. on February 12, 2008.

Shirley called Stan on the slopes at Canaan Valley to tell him the
terrible news. Still reeling from the phone call, he also thought about
the mysterious death of Eric Layne, a fellow member of Andrew's
PTSD group, barely two weeks earlier. They were both taking a similar
array of medications, but Stan thought the fault could just as well lie

with other risks of the war. "I had a suspicion in my mind that it could be chemical poisons from weapons of mass destruction," he recalls.

The role Andrew's prescription drugs played in his death, though, soon became more evident. Because Andrew died at home in questionable circumstances, the police showed up to scour his room and seize the drugs—all legally prescribed—they found. Stan White's suspicions were heightened when the Marine casualty officer dispatched the next day to help the Whites prepare for the funeral told him some more disturbing news. "By the way, there's another soldier who died whose funeral we did a couple of weeks ago, and I think there are some similarities there," he told Stan and Shirley. Indeed, there were: Corporal Nicholas Endicott from nearby Logan County died in his sleep January 29th while being treated for PTSD at Bethesda Naval Hospital. Like Layne and White, his drug cocktail included Paxil, Klonopin and, of course, Seroquel, the VA's unofficial sedative of choice for PTSD patients. "We had three right there," Stan White says, all living in the same area and dying within weeks of each other. A week later, he reached out to the mother of Nicholas Endicott, sharing the pain of their sons' deaths and asking questions about the VA's prescribing practices they would soon take public.

As for Schauland, he now says, "I feel as badly as I can, it was devastating, but I complied with the patient's needs. People were trying as hard as they can with this young man." As he told investigators from the VA Inspector General's office after White's death, "If I had done anything that I could look back and say was a mistake, I would tell you, but I can't." In Schauland's view, "I don't think he was overmedicating."

Yet as Dr. Grace Jackson, a former staff psychiatrist at Bethesda Naval Hospital who reviewed records of Andrew and Eric Layne's treatment at my request, points out, "None of these people should be dying. Any sensible physician should know they're far enhancing risks with polypharmacy of any kind. These are potentially lethal combinations."

For both Eric Layne and Andrew White, though, the risks they faced from their prescribed drugs were heightened by their apparent sporadic use of non-prescribed painkillers, an all-too-common practice in West Virginia. It wasn't until the release in April 2008 of the autopsy report for Andrew, for example, that his parents learned that he had relatively small amounts of methadone in his bloodstream along with appropriate levels of Paxil and Seroquel. If taken by itself, the amount of methadone alone almost certainly wouldn't have killed him, but the report from West Virginia's Office of the Chief Medical Examiner concluded that "combined drug intoxication" was at fault.

"We were never warned that Andrew shouldn't take Seroquel with painkillers," Stan White says. "Seroquel enhances the side effects of methadone, and it is the catalyst, the culprit, that causes cardiac arrest." The FDA, but few VA doctors, knew about a major study in 2007 showing that Seroquel sharply raises the blood plasma levels of methadone and hence the risk of a deadly heart arrhythmia interaction, yet it took until July 2011 for the warning label to be quietly revised. The VA still has not publicly warned any clinicians in the years since about Seroquel's cardiac risks or potentially fatal interactions with tranquilizers and painkillers—even in West Virginia, which had been ravaged by opiate overdoses. But one common misconception—still promoted by military leaders, including then-Army Surgeon General, Eric B. Schoomaker—is that the growing number of military prescription deaths is just like the celebrity overdoses of performers like Heath Ledger or Whitney Houston: "a consequence of the use of multiple prescriptions and nonprescription medicines and alcohol," Schoomaker said in an interview, just four days before Andrew died.

That's true enough—up to a point. "They're being called multi-drug intoxications," says Dr. Fred Baughman, a longtime critic of psychiatric overprescribing. "But that's a way to point the finger and blame the soldiers themselves." But these drugs' effects are not like a standard drug overdose that produces a protracted coma-like response that can allow the victim to be discovered and saved, Baughman and leading medical journals say. Instead, an atypical antipsychotic like Seroquel can induce sudden cardiac arrest: a rapid, pulseless condition that often causes brain death in under five minutes. Atypical antipsychotics have been identified in over one hundred studies since the 1990s as perhaps the single riskiest class of drugs for inducing a particularly dangerous form of arrhythmia known as the prolonged QT interval, named for the measurement of time between the "Q" and "T" waves of the heart's electrical cycle.

In some ways, the grassroots challenge to the military's prescribing policies began at the military funeral held near the White family's church. Memories of Andrew's service to his country were evident everywhere, from the grieving faces of the young veterans who knew him well to the American flag taken from his casket, ceremonially folded by the uniformed Marine officer and then handed to the Whites. Yet to Stan White, the determination to find out the truth behind Andrew's death became another way to honor his son. After his son's funeral, he made a pact with his wife: "I wanted to find what really caused Andrew to die, and to keep someone else from going through this." He adds with quiet understatement, "I thought I owed that to Andrew's memory."

With three similar deaths within weeks, he recalls, "I was already seeing a pattern." He soon discovered at least two other Seroquel-related deaths in just West Virginia. The diligent online news research of support group co-founder Diane Vande Burgt (the wife of the National Guard vet Tom Vande Burgt) and others soon found nearly three hundred suspicious, probable sudden cardiac-linked military deaths across the country. By following up with as many families as they could reach, she, Baughman and Stan White seemed to be doing a more thorough investigation of these deaths than any federal agency.

Unfamiliar with the ways of Washington, Stan nonetheless took it upon himself in the months after Andrew's death to contact his local congresswoman, Rep. Shelley Moore Capito, and the influential Sen. Jay Rockefeller, then the chairman of the Senate Veterans Affairs Committee. "I wanted a congressional hearing to find out, if there is five dead in West Virginia and that's a large sample from a small state, it's got to be bigger. Let's find out what it is, and the best way to do it is to get a congressional hearing," he says. His quest for truth and answers, it turned out, was only just beginning.

CHAPTER 6

Stan White and the Veterans' Search for Truth and Answers

At first, Stan White wasn't really sure what had killed his son and the other returning veterans. "I had a suspicion in my mind that it might be chemical poisons from weapons of mass destruction, or it might be Agent Orange," he says. But after speaking to Janette Layne, Eric's widow, then Cheryl Endicott, the mother of Jason Endicott, who was found dead in his bed in late January at Bethesda Naval Hospital, Stan White was moving closer to his final conclusion: "It absolutely was the drugs." Layne, White and Endicott had died within three weeks of each other. Soon, Stan and Shirley learned about other suspicious deaths in West Virginia, and, eventually, other grieving parents from around the country began contacting them.

The families of the three veterans soon got a chance to air their concerns in March 2008 on WOWK-TV in Charleston. At the time, all the families were still waiting for toxicology results, but they knew that all three of the men's prescriptions included the same combination of Paxil, Klonopin and Seroquel. "Are these three medications—is there any connection with the three of them? Did those three react? Or is there some foreign substance these guys picked up overseas?" Stan White asked on camera. In the first of several public declarations he would make over the years, White pointed out, "You're always expecting and fearing when your children are at war that they're not going to make it back. But they don't come back and lie in the bed, go to sleep and die. That doesn't happen. That's not supposed to happen."

Looking back, this short local broadcast was one of the first news accounts in the country addressing deadly psychiatric prescribing to soldiers and veterans. But until the Tomah VA opiate deaths were exposed in 2015, the issue never emerged as a major national scandal. In May 2008, Julie Robinson of *The Charleston Gazette* became arguably the first journalist in the country to write about the early signs of a psychiatric medication crisis apparently causing veterans' deaths in West Virginia or anywhere else in the nation. By this time, Stan White had learned of eight similar medication-related deaths in the nearby tri-state area of Kentucky, Ohio and West Virginia. Robinson identified by name a fourth West Virginia victim, twenty-two-year-old Derek Johnson of Hurricane, who died in his sleep on May 2nd; he had been taking the same combination of Paxil, Klonopin and Seroquel that was given to Layne, Endicott and White. He was also taking a prescribed painkiller for a back injury he suffered in a car accident the week before his death, even though his wife warned the ER doctor about other drugs he was taking that were known to have deadly interactions with opiates and other painkillers. The night before he died, Johnson called his grandfather Duck Underwood to come pick up Derek's five-year-old son, one of three young children he and his wife Stacie were raising. Underwood came by, but there was no answer when he first knocked—until he heard Stacie screaming that she couldn't wake up her husband.

Ray Johnson, Derek's father, told Robinson, "I want to know the cause of death. Stacie said he was fine that night. Everything was normal. He kissed her goodnight and went to sleep."

Stan and Shirley White met the Johnson and Underwood families at Derek's funeral and offered to help them in their own search for the truth of what happened. "When I talked to his family about Derek, I realized it was the same old story," White told *The Charleston Gazette*. "It was all too familiar. He was taking those same drugs as the others."

After that, other families started contacting Stan White from West Virginia and other states. In addition, Baughman, a retired California neurologist who was best known for denouncing ADHD diagnosis and medications as a "fraud," found the *Charleston Gazette* article online in June and realized its broader national implications. "This struck me as really different, a unique occurrence: four similar deaths of guys found dead in bed in the same area," he recalls. "None of these guys were suicidal and none of them overdosed," he points out, in terms of taking higher than prescribed dosages of the drugs. As a researcher, he had seen a peer-reviewed article in *Expert Opinion on Drug Safety* first published online in March 2008, reviewing the extensive medical literature since 2000. The troubling meta-analysis was headlined: "Sudden cardiac death secondary to antidepressant and antipsychotic drugs." He reached out to Stan White to flag for him the evidence for dangerous psychiatric prescribing that Stan and Shirley saw firsthand with Andrew's death. By June 2008, he issued a press release denouncing the lack of informed consent and the polypharmacy that caused what he called a "cluster of veterans' deaths." He pointed out, "The more drugs given simultaneously, the less the science and the greater the risk of injury and death."

Baughman never managed to win much media interest over the deaths of veterans caused by medications. But over time, he and some West Virginia veterans' families, led by the research of activist Diane Vande Burgt, worked to compile through news accounts a list of veterans and soldiers dying suspiciously in beds and barracks, a list which eventually grew to over four hundred. Over the years, he also launched a drumbeat of letters to Senate leaders and committee staffers, network TV producers, medical journals (only a few which were published) and the VA Inspector General's office asking them to take seriously the issue of cardiac risk of antipsychotics, nearly always starting by pointing to the tragedies in West Virginia. His argument, backed by medical citations on the cardiac risks of antipsychotics and polypharmacy, was blunt: "There is an epidemic of sudden deaths occurring throughout the US military."

His determination—and that of Stan White and other concerned families—to get to the bottom of what led to the medication-linked deaths didn't seem to be matched by the VA's Inspector General's skewed inquiry into the West Virginia deaths. At first, it seemed to the Whites that the agency was doing a thorough job. The investigators spoke to the families at length; interviewed all the VA health-care providers including those at the Huntington VA, the Charleston community clinic and the Cincinnati VA medical center where Eric Layne was treated before he died; and reviewed medical, autopsy and toxicology records.

But when the report focusing on the White and Layne deaths was released in August 2008, it became clear that other institutional priorities were more important than solving and preventing the deaths of veterans. It would take a few years before the full scope of the deliberate omissions and distortions in the report became even more apparent. In retrospect, it can be seen as a dry run for the Inspector General's cover-up and inaction in response to the deaths at Tomah.

Eventually, a half-billion-dollar federal settlement in 2010 with AstraZeneca and an emerging research consensus prodded AstraZeneca itself to reluctantly change its warning labels to concede Seroquel's cardiac and diabetes risks, which it had previously downplayed. At the time the VA Inspector General did its review of the two veterans' deaths, though, Seroquel and other new-generation atypical antipsychotics were already implicated in "QT prolongation" and sudden cardiac deaths in nearly seventy medical studies.

Yet the Inspector General's report's central finding was that the treatments Layne and White received met "community standards of care," supplemented by a claimed wide-ranging review of the medical literature that concluded there was no link between Seroquel and other leading antipsychotics with sudden cardiac death. This conclusion was reached despite the known dangers being widely cited in the research literature at the time that the Inspector General's medical consultant, Dr. Michael Shepherd, helped prepare the dubious report. Its findings completely ignored the most salient medical research *and* the VA's own prescribing guidelines that said there was no evidence supporting the use of antipsychotics for PTSD. Among the studies ignored: the comprehensive review of over 120 studies on the cardiac risks of all psychotropic drugs—the one from *Expert Opinion on Drug Safety* that Baughman cited in his June 2008 press release and flagged for Stan White. It also recommended that electrocardiograms be given before antipsychotic treatment begins and checked during the course of treatment to ensure patient safety. If those recommended ECGs were given as the research indicated to Andrew White and Eric Layne, the risks of arrhythmia could have been flagged and they might still be alive today.

In contrast, out of the numerous studies on antipsychotics' cardiac risk since Seroquel was approved in 1997, the VA only cited the safety reassurances in one (1) out-of-date study, published in 2001, concluding that there was "no association" between the atypical antipsychotics and cardiac risk. The VA also leaned on that archaic study to contend that agency officials were "unaware" of any recommendations to use ECG monitoring with young patients receiving Seroquel. Even the co-author of that 2001 study, Columbia University cardiology professor Dr. J. Thomas Bigger, doesn't defend the study's obsolete conclusions today and declines to discuss it, and would only tell me, "There's been more research on that topic since then."

"They turned a blind eye to the medical consensus," says Baughman of the Inspector General's conclusions on the cardiac risk of antipsychotics. The most telling sign of a research cover-up, he contends, is the failure to mention the most thorough review then available on the topic: the *Expert Opinion* review, published several months before the IG report. "It took an overt act of omission to miss this article," he says, noting how widely cited it was in the medical literature. Dr. Stephen Xenakis, a former Army psychiatrist who believes that appropriately prescribed psychiatric drugs can be helpful for PTSD along with psychotherapy and thorough medical workups, is just as blunt as Baughman about this IG report's failings: "They cherry-picked the studies. They find the information that justifies what the VA is doing," a "protective" pattern he's found throughout the Inspector General's work over the years.

The VA's main finding that the treatments Layne and White received met "community standards of care" wasn't particularly credible, either—especially if their care flouted the VA's own guidelines. Dr. Grace Jackson, the former Navy psychiatrist and author of *Rethinking Psychiatric Drugs*, says after reviewing the IG report and White's prescription history, "This is a whitewash that sanitizes his [White's] medical records. It's a complete embarrassment: the way these drugs were used was overkill." Xenakis agrees: "I wouldn't have treated those soldiers with high doses of antipsychotics. It's not appropriate: There's a risk of sudden death."

In fact, as the Inspector General's legal counsel, Maureen Regan, concedes, the term "community standards of care" in the report isn't a scientific judgment, but merely a legal term used in malpractice lawsuits. "It's the standard measured under tort law: what a reasonable practitioner would do in like or similar circumstances," Regan says. But, as Jackson points out, giving PTSD patients like White up to 1,200 mg of off-label Seroquel in defiance of the VA's own guidelines is a "very dangerous community standard of care." In fact, given how wildly overused antipsychotics are in civilian and VA settings, the risky prescribing that played a key role in the deaths of Layne and White "does sort of fit with community standards," Xenakis says ruefully. Still, Jackson observes that for PTSD patients, "I don't think it's reasonable or prudent to give a neurotoxin like Seroquel unless you absolutely have to do it."

The VA Inspector General's office not only wouldn't permit me to interview the consultant Shepard, claiming patient confidentiality, but declined to reveal what medical guidelines or scientific research the VA reviewed before releasing its report. The same blanket claim of confidentiality applied to the VA offering any scientific justification for VA doctors plying Andrew White with levels of Seroquel that were as much as 50 percent higher than that maximum recommended dosage of 800 mg for schizophrenics. Even when I presented her with a confidentiality waiver from Andrew White's parents, the IG's counsel, Regan, wouldn't answer questions about the VA's care of Andrew White or even acknowledge that the report reviewed the treatment of Andrew White and Eric Layne, who are listed only as Patient A and Patient B. "We don't discuss the cases of individuals who are the subject of our investigations," she said. End of story.

But it didn't prove to be the end of the story for Stan White and other families seeking answers—and changes in military and VA treatment practices. And the VA's conclusions, no matter how shoddily prepared, had lasting consequences. It meant, in practical terms, that the surviving family members of Layne, White and most of the few hundred other young soldiers and veterans who have died after taking Seroquel had few grounds for filing a lawsuit against the government. And it helped pave the way for thousands of more soldiers and veterans to be exposed to Seroquel as a sleep aid on the battlefield or as a treatment for PTSD after coming home. "I don't know what standards the VA was meeting if Andrew got such high dosages of Sero-quel," Stan White points out. He and Shirley believed, in the end, that the IG report didn't really answer the questions about the deaths of their son and Eric Layne.

Regardless of its shortcomings, members of Congress accepted the Inspector General's conclusions discounting the dangerous pre-scribing that helped kill White and Layne. That, in turn, undermined any initiatives to hold the VA accountable for its practices, or any further probe of these soldiers' deaths and the overprescribing of an-tipsychotics to veterans in general. One aide to then-Senator Jay Rockefeller, the legislator who asked for the Inspector General inves-tigation, insisted to me, "The VA took this very seriously. The VA faces a major challenge with suicides and PTSD, but it has done a lot of efforts to improve mental health care for veterans." The staffer added, citing the mixture of prescriptions with alcohol, "I'm sure the VA physicians tell their patients not to drink, and this important ad-vice is ignored." But this blame-the-victim perspective common in Washington doesn't reflect the absence of alcohol in the toxicology findings for Layne and White—or the reality that, in too many of the deaths of soldiers such as Cpl. Nicholas Endicott, they were just fol-lowing the doctor's orders.

Stan White, dressed in his best dark blue business suit and armed with a folder thick with letters from grieving relatives, urgently sought to convey the need to protect our soldiers and veterans from deadly, substandard care when he went with his wife to the offices of each member of the House and Senate veterans committees for the first time in April 2009. He visited about forty in all.

Reading those letters now is like walking through a graveyard of despair and naive hopes for a meaningful response, distress signals from the not-so-distant past that went unheeded. "These are our he-roes we are mistreating," Derek's grandmother pleaded. With rare ex-ceptions, White only got to meet with the congressional aides who listened with polite concern as he made his case.

"I'm Stan White from Charleston, West Virginia," he told them. "I've lost two sons in the military. One was killed in battle. One died from medication for PTSD. Through my research, I've found numerous others: I think that's a problem. I want someone to investigate it. Here is my evidence, here are my charts." He then gave them his carefully prepared folder of research, news clippings and letters. During that first visit to Washington, he presented a list of over fifty suspicious deaths gleaned from news accounts and public records found by White and his allies. By 2016, the list would grow to over four hundred soldiers and veterans.

In a plea that now seems at once so sensible and heartfelt, the cover letter with his packet declared, "We believe that the DOD and VA need to provide more counseling and therapy for our veterans. Most important is the need for research as to why the combination of these medications seems to lead to so many deaths."

Citing a recent wave of salmonella-poisoned food, he said at the time, "When six people die from contaminated peanut butter, the factory is shut down and there's a massive recall. But when we find at least fifty-one military men have died in their sleep, no alarm seems to sound." He, for one, would keep trying to sound the alarm, but what he discovered about the influence of the drug industry in Washington would truly shock him.

CHAPTER 7

Mr. White Comes to Washington: FDA Showdown over Seroquel

THERE WAS LITTLE SIGN THAT ANYONE IN CONGRESS OR THE VA WAS really listening to Stan and Shirley White. Still, they and other West Virginia families, joined by a handful of medical experts and reformers concerned about Seroquel's effects, attempted to convince the FDA to at least not *expand* the drug's use.

During their visit to Washington in April 2009, the Whites attended a hearing in which the influential FDA Psychopharmacologic Drugs Advisory Committee was considering a request from AstraZeneca. The company wanted to considerably expand Seroquel and its extended-release version, Seroquel XR, beyond its approved use for schizophrenia and bipolar disorder. The suburban Hilton ballroom was packed with nearly three hundred people, mostly AstraZeneca and other well-tailored drug industry officials and doctors. The handful of voting members of the committee listened to the largely pro-industry FDA experts and polished AstraZeneca scientists make their case for broadening the drug's use to cover anxiety and major depression.

The Whites, overwhelmed by it all, were pointed to assigned seats and waited with some other aggrieved victims and critics of the drug, including Janette Layne, for their allotted three minutes near the end of the meeting to offer their appeals. The final decision would be made by the full agency. Despite the FDA's (loosely enforced) conflict-of-interest rules, these advisory panels tend to support the goals of drug companies and their findings are generally approved by the FDA.

In fact, less than a week before the April 2009 hearing the Whites attended, the *Philadelphia Inquirer* reported that Dr. Jorge Armenteros, the chair of the committee was, in fact, a longtime paid speaker for AstraZeneca who had promoted Seroquel and also sought to drum up more AstraZeneca cash by proposing new research on Seroquel. Armenteros held this chairman post for five years without any challenge until the newspaper contacted the FDA for comment shortly before publication. Suddenly, the FDA determined that Armenteros and four other drug-industry subsidized researchers sitting on the committee shouldn't be allowed to vote on AstraZeneca products, and were hastily replaced by temporary members, some also with past ties to the drug industry.

These revelations emerged from documents that were uncovered during lawsuits filed on behalf of thousands of plaintiffs who developed diabetes while on the drug. Armenteros, who had published research on the value of antipsychotics for such off-label uses as ADHD, wasn't available for comment. Philadelphia attorney Steve Sheller told the *Inquirer*, "The industry is infected with greed. You can't trust the approvals, you can't trust the studies, and now you can't trust the FDA."

By the time the FDA advisory committee met in the spring of 2009 to discuss the company's request for approval to market the drug to millions of potential new patients with depression and anxiety, AstraZeneca's Seroquel research and safety claims were essentially thoroughly discredited—except, it seemed, in the eyes of the FDA.

A year later, the company would be forced to pay a half-billion dollars to the Department of Justice and twenty state Medicaid programs for hiding Seroquel's dangers in its alleged illegal marketing campaign. Even in the months leading up to this FDA hearing, the company's skewed research on Seroquel was becoming a major scientific scandal. For instance, as a result of still more findings from the 19,000 pending liability lawsuits against AstraZeneca, released internal documents showed that AstraZeneca buried studies showing harmful effects back in the 1990s, when the FDA first approved Seroquel for schizophrenia. As *The Washington Post* reported, in a damning August 1997 email regarding the never-published "Study 15" that showed 45 percent of patients had significant weight gain, AstraZeneca executive Richard Lawrence praised company physician Lisa Avantis for putting a "positive spin" on this "cursed study" by masking the weight gain: "Lisa has done a great 'smoke and mirrors' job."

Just as disturbing, *The New England Journal of Medicine* reported in January 2009 that patients receiving the atypical, new generation antipsychotics, including Seroquel, faced a risk of sudden cardiac death that was over 200 percent higher than those who weren't using the medications—even higher than the better-known risk posed by the older generation of antipsychotics. The lead author, Dr. Wayne Ray of Vanderbilt University, told *The New York Times,* "The implication of this study is that physicians need to do a very careful cardiovascular evaluation prior to prescribing these drugs"—while using the lowest possible dosages if treatment moves forward. Years later, those practices still haven't been adopted by the Department of Veterans Affairs.

Ray attended the April 2009 hearing and the committee granted him permission to give a presentation that warned about expanding the drug's approved uses. But before he could make his case, the committee was briefed by that wily ally of the pharmaceutical companies, the FDA's Dr. Thomas Laughren, who by June of 2009 would also help make the case that Seroquel was safe for kids.

Now, as Laughren and other FDA officials prepared to spin the findings on Seroquel before this advisory committee, it was especially relevant that he had in 2004 reportedly misled another FDA advisory committee about the safety risks arising from the expanded use of antidepressants for kids.

So in April 2009, Laughren had a new chance to shape the findings on another drug, Seroquel, and help advance the pharmaceutical industry's agenda yet again. Yet with the scathing publicity over rigged Seroquel studies, along with the spotlight on FDA employees and advisors who were seemingly colluding with the drug industry, this advisory committee had good reason to appear a bit more cautious while deciding if it would give AstraZeneca everything it wanted.

What AstraZeneca sought was a way to make more money by winning FDA approval for first-line "monotherapy" treatment with its newer extended-release drug, Seroquel XR, for depression and anxiety. An added bonus for the company: Seroquel XR's exclusive patent wouldn't expire until 2017, roughly five years after regular Seroquel's patent expired, opening up the competition to generics. A second preference, but still enormously lucrative, would allow the drug to be used as an "adjunct" therapy if other FDA-approved drugs weren't fully successful; the potentially deadly Seroquel could be, with the FDA's blessing, used to "augment" the effects of other medications. All of this would expand Seroquel's potential market from less than 4 percent of the adult population with schizophrenia and bipolar disorder to nearly 10 percent of adults with generalized, unrelenting anxiety disorder, or those with major depression. (That latter diagnosis was defined by a seriously disruptive bout of depression lasting more than two weeks in the previous year.)

The increased sales opportunities could potentially add over fourteen million new FDA-approved patients, not counting millions of more off-label customers eager for stress relief. With the added appeal of Seroquel's heavy sedation, the FDA's full-throated approval of the drug for anxiety and depression could ensure that its future earnings would dwarf the nearly $5 billion a year it was on track to earn in 2009. The retail cost of Seroquel XR was then over $12,000 per patient a year for just two pills a day.

Perhaps chastened by all the recent scandals, and facing an impossible-to-ignore *New England Journal of Medicine* study on cardiac risk, Laughren was essentially forced to acknowledge the potential safety risks of the drug. Yet he still accepted at face value the array of AstraZeneca's subsidized research on Seroquel's effectiveness for anxiety and depression. While telling the panel the drug was safe enough for its current uses, he cited possible metabolic and diabetes risks; the tremor-filled neurological disorder tardive dyskinesia; and the new findings of sudden cardiac death associated with atypical antipsychotics.

Before the committee could make its decision, or critics could raise concerns, a series of smooth AstraZeneca scientists made their case. This new set of company experts—replacing the earlier researchers disgraced by their exposed emails—blithely continued the same sales job on the drug's safety and effectiveness, all buttressed with impressive-seeming PowerPoint slides. The only adverse effects to worry about for some patients were such modest side effects as dry mouth and dizziness, they reassured the panel. The drug certainly couldn't kill you, they argued. Yet the company's own data showed that nearly seven times as many people who used the medication died during drug trials compared to those on placebo, but since far fewer people received placebos, the *rate* of death was about the same, they contended. (By April 2005, though, the FDA had already warned that all antipsychotics had a 170 percent higher risk of death for dementia patients than placebos.)

Stan White's speaker number was soon called, and when he stood before the panelists, he was, like all the other members of the public, only allotted three minutes to funnel all his frustration and pain into testimony that might sway them. After explaining how his son died from a combination of drugs that included Seroquel and that nearly ninety other veterans and soldiers had died up to that point while taking the drug, he said, "My belief is that overuse of these medications has caused our soldiers and Marines to die."

His wife Shirley emphasized in her brief talk the betrayal she felt. "He was told, and I as his mother was told, 'These medications will not harm you,'" she said. "I trusted the doctors to do what was best for my son, and he died in his sleep."

There was little sign that the panelists were paying much attention as the families spoke. In the end, the advisory committee didn't accept Seroquel as a first-line drug for depression and anxiety, but approved its use as an adjunct treatment for depression. This paved the way for AstraZeneca to legally enter a new market potentially as lucrative as the one dominated by Abilify.

• • •

PART OF THE VA'S ONGOING RELUCTANCE TO SERIOUSLY REIN IN THE HIGH-risk, off-label prescribing of antipsychotics stems from the influence of the drug industry on both the agency's top researchers and its local doctors charged with caring for troubled veterans. That's a pattern, of course, affecting virtually all of mental health care. For instance, some of the earliest work that pushed Seroquel on veterans came from Dr. Mark Hamner, the director of psychopharmacology research and PTSD clinical care at the Ralph H. Johnson VA Medical Center in Charleston, South Carolina. With the support of AstraZeneca, he co-authored a series of papers boosting Seroquel and launched additional research on the drug. The results were apparently so unimpressive that most were never published in a medical journal. With AstraZeneca funding, he reported in February 2003 an uncontrolled—or "open label"—study in the *Journal of Clinical Psychopharmacology* that found in a short trial of Seroquel that it produced "significant reductions in core PTSD symptoms" and only mild, "transient" adverse events. Even while lawsuits were revealing damning evidence against the drug, Hamner remained on the bandwagon for the drug.

When I first spoke to Hamner in 2011, he denied that the funding he had received from AstraZeneca over the years—which he declined to reveal and wasn't required to be disclosed publicly at the time—had any impact on his research or talks about the drug. "I don't think it does at this point," he said.

In 2004, Hamner appeared on an AstraZeneca-funded panel at the American Psychiatric Association talking about broadening the use of atypical antipsychotics beyond then FDA-approved uses. He cited preliminary studies showing positive benefits with Seroquel and other antipsychotics, especially Risperdal, as an adjunct treatment for PTSD. Although he mentioned the possible metabolic risks, he said of his own studies on Seroquel at relatively lower doses, "From a safety standpoint we did not see changes in weight . . . or significant changes in vital signs."

AstraZeneca was apparently pleased with Hamner's work in this field because it funded directly or served as a "collaborator" with the VA on two additional twelve-week studies that he conducted measuring Seroquel's impact on PTSD symptoms when compared with a placebo. Neither study was published in a medical journal until some of the underlying data finally made it into print in 2016, and for nearly a decade or more the studies' outcomes were known only to Hamner and presumably AstraZeneca. For years, the results weren't even listed on the federal government's voluntary clinicaltrials.gov website.

AstraZeneca and its allied researchers were just following the common industry practice of hiding as many side effects and poor outcomes with their drugs as possible. The results of roughly half of all clinical trials are never published anywhere, often to mask disappointing or alarming results about a drug or procedure; that has prompted a worldwide campaign of over six hundred medical organ-izations and journals, led by Alltrials.net founded by *The Guardian* columnist Dr. Ben Goldacre, to force the registration of all trials and the disclosure of all results. But Hamner told me in 2011 that he was in the process of readying both studies comparing Seroquel to a placebo for publication. When asked why he hadn't published the re-sults of his VA-based research, he insisted, "There is no pressure or anything like that from AstraZeneca not to publish. Certainly we are being very careful about the analysis."

The analysis shouldn't have taken years to complete. Even the more complex of the two twelve-week studies only had twenty-five patients started on Seroquel, had a drop-out rate nearly twice that for the placebo *and* the outcomes were known by 2006. That study meas-ured Seroquel's impact against a placebo as an adjunct treatment for patients with severe PTSD who weren't helped by Paxil alone. Those who were still taking Seroquel showed significant PTSD symptoms. (The results weren't published at clinicaltrials.gov until 2014, years after the VA *officially* stopped recommending using antipsychotics for PTSD, although its use continues essentially unabated.) Dr. Stephen Xenakis, who has done his own PTSD research, pointed out the Ham-ner studies' most glaring flaws: "AstraZeneca clearly delayed publish-ing because the data in general is weak. There are an insufficient number of subjects to show that the medication is an effective way to treat the condition." Hamner, long after antipsychotics' use for PTSD had been discredited, finally co-authored with AstraZeneca's funding a December 2016 placebo-controlled study in *The American Journal of Psychiatry* that claimed that Seroquel was "efficacious" in treating PTSD, based on research he began in 2004.

Even if Hamner's original studies were never, in fact, published when it counted, their never-ending status as forthcoming journal articles added credibility to the unfounded notion that there was some scientific justification for using Seroquel beyond just knocking out PTSD patients at night. Despite the absence of *any* independent (i.e., without drug money), controlled journal studies showing Seroquel's value for PTSD, Dr. Matthew Friedman pointed to Hamner's still-unpublished research to justify Seroquel's promise: "He presented some very interesting data that indicated that Seroquel might be better for PTSD."

Friedman and other VA researchers' casual acceptance of Seroquel and, until recently, Risperdal for use with PTSD patients might have been shaped by the funding they've received in the past from AstraZeneca and other drug companies. They strongly dispute such imputations. As *AlterNet*'s Martha Rosenberg first reported in 2010, Friedman had received an AstraZeneca honorarium and, later, served as a "Pfizer visiting professor" in 2011 at the South Carolina College of Medicine, the academic home of Hamner. When I spoke to Friedman, his ties to Pfizer weren't yet publicly known, but he dismissed the notion that any drug company funding could affect *his* views or research. As for that honorarium from AstraZeneca, he laughed it off: "That was just a luncheon symposium I hosted."

The influential Friedman continued to champion some antipsychotics, including Seroquel, as potentially useful adjunct treatments for PTSD even after the *Journal of the American Medical Association* published a damning 2011 study by the VA's own researchers which showed that antipsychotics were essentially useless for those suffering primarily from PTSD. The study was quite unlike Hamner's sketchy, unpublished early research on Seroquel or the seemingly more promising published research—largely funded by Janssen—on Risperdal's value as an adjunct PTSD treatment. This rigorous, government-funded, large-scale study on Risperdal found it caused serious side effects and was no better than a placebo for patients with PTSD or anxiety and depression symptoms. By the time this six-month randomized study of over 250 patients was published, the VA had already spent $717 million on Risperdal alone in the previous decade and $846 million for Seroquel. Roughly 20 percent of all PTSD patients at the VA were receiving these off-label, dangerous antipsychotics. As a *JAMA* editorial on this important study concluded, "The results seriously call into question the use of atypical antipsychotics in PTSD treatment. Studies are needed to identify more effective treatments."

When the study was released in 2011, Risperdal and Seroquel risks were already exposed in government liability and fraud lawsuits.

Yet none of these developments seemed to have any impact on

the policies or practices of the VA regarding the overuse of antipsychotics. The percentage—roughly 20 percent—of PTSD patients receiving antipsychotics has declined only slightly since 2011, and nearly 800,000 prescriptions for Seroquel and 430,000 for Risperdal are written annually for VA patients. In short, over $1.5 billion was spent over the previous decade by the VA for two antipsychotics never proven effective for PTSD. As noted earlier, spending for Seroquel didn't really start declining from a peak of $150 million in 2011 until the original version's generic replacements were released after it lost its patent protection in 2012, while the number of prescriptions for the widely used medication—in any version—barely slowed by 3 percent.

"After the drug companies spent fifteen years marketing this stuff, doctors are trained to use it," observes Yale researcher Dr. Robert Rosenheck, a co-author of the 2011 *JAMA* article and an investigator with the New England VA's mental health research center in New Haven. More recently, he has questioned the impact so far of the VA's new Psychotropic Drug Safety Initiative promoted by VA leaders after the Tomah scandals: "I haven't seen any data showing that these efforts are having much effect."

Rosenheck has good grounds for such skepticism. One indicator of how little the program has accomplished was the testimony of Dr. Carolyn Clancy, then the VA's interim Secretary for Health, who actually boasted to a congressional hearing in April 2015 about the success of the program launched nearly two years earlier: "We have noted a 1 percent decrease in the proportion of Veterans with PTSD and no psychosis diagnosis who received an antipsychotic medication." That's not much of a change if nearly 20 percent or more of PTSD patients are still getting the medications for unapproved uses—and a third of all veterans get psychotropic medications without having any known mental illness of any kind.

One reason risky prescribing remains nearly as high as it was before the 2011 *JAMA* study, even in the face of the increasing numbers of veterans deaths, is likely due to the lack of any high-profile alerts and enforcement by the VA over the cardiac risk of the antipsychotics. A month before the *JAMA* study was published, *The New York Times* published an article in July 2011 about a new FDA-required warning that Seroquel and Seroquel XR should be avoided with at least twelve other medicines in seven different categories—including some antibiotics and opiates—because they could cause sudden cardiac arrest. Yet busy VA clinicians have never been clearly warned about these changes by the VA, although the VA periodically sends out warnings and advisories on other drugs. Since all of the atypical antipsychotics pose cardiac risks, it's disturbing that with over 2.1 million such antipsychotic prescriptions written yearly by the agency it still hasn't bothered to unmistakably warn anyone of the potentially fatal dangers posed by the most popular one, Seroquel, when combined with other commonly prescribed medications.

The VA's medical leadership has shown little interest or concern over this striking omission. I recently asked another Yale psychiatry researcher affiliated with the VA, Dr. Ilse Wiechers, who leads the agency's psychotropic drug safety initiative, about whether the program warned about these FDA-flagged cardiac dangers. She responded: "I can't say that's the VA's position. I provide warning information to my patients and I assume it would be brought up [by other doctors] during consultations with their patients."

This failure of a program billed as a "drug safety initiative" to warn its doctors about these cardiac risks comes as a shocking surprise to experts outside the VA. "I don't understand it," says Dr. Stephen Xenakis. "It's outrageous. I'm stunned." He adds, "People are talking about reform in the VA, but with these kinds of things, it really exposes how far we have to go to change basic practices, culture and attitudes."

But these flaws in prescribing at the VA go beyond even the corrupting effect of the drug industry or the world of turf-protection and failed accountability within the agency. Rosenheck, while not criticizing the VA, points to broader factors in the culture of the pharmaceutical-subsidized mental health system at large that insulate doctors from oversight: "This is an influential industry that affects everyone's mind: 'Don't touch doctor's rights'"—a view shared by doctors, NAMI and other mental health groups and, of course, the drug industry that benefits from that messaging. "The idea is: To sell as many drugs as possible for as many illnesses as possible to increase the stockholders' value, and use our patsies in the psychiatric profession to promote our drugs," he notes.

With so many forces working against limiting irresponsible prescribing, it's not so surprising that even after the *JAMA* study was published, there was strong resistance to change within the VA and the wider field of psychiatry. Friedman, for instance, still held out hope for the value of Seroquel, and possibly other antipsychotics, with PTSD patients: "Not all atypical antipsychotics are created equal," he insisted.

In a grudging concession, he declared after the *JAMA* study that the VA would no longer recommend the use of Risperdal for PTSD patients as an adjunct treatment. Yet although the *JAMA* report was widely seen as condemning antipsychotics as a class for PTSD, Friedman said the agency wouldn't change its longstanding PTSD guidelines for Seroquel: "There is insufficient evidence to recommend for or against its use." As a result of that stance, heavy Seroquel prescribing remained essentially unimpeded. As Friedman blithely noted, "Doctors are free to prescribe medications they see as in the patient's best interest."

The failure of the VA to effectively warn its local doctors about the antipsychotics' dangers amounted to a death sentence for some patients. It led the doctors in Virginia's Tidewater area to heedlessly prescribe Seroquel and other drugs to Kelli Grese, a petite, dark-haired thirty-seven-year-old former Navy hospital corpsman who also developed psychosis—a relatively rare side effect—from Adderall given for her wrongly diagnosed ADHD, her prescription drug addiction to VA-provided Klonopin, and severe depression, all following a thirteen-year regimen of nearly thirty drugs often prescribed off-label for assorted makeshift diagnoses. She'd gone to the Hampton, Virginia, VA in the 1990s with what was originally a modest case of PTSD. But in the eight months before she died, she tried killing herself three times with the Seroquel she was repeatedly prescribed—and her final prescription was for a 120-day supply of the drug written twice in two days in late October 2010. A little more than two weeks later, on Veterans Day, she succeeded in her fourth attempt, swallowing most of the Seroquel pills given her. Shortly before a wrongful death trial was scheduled in April 2013, her twin sister Darla reluctantly settled the case for a modest $100,000 due to the financial and emotional strain. Yet the filings in the case remain one of the few public records of the agency's mishandling of psychiatric prescribing, even though the agency didn't acknowledge liability.

Kelli Grese, in truth, was pushed downhill towards her death by several physicians at different VA facilities. They couldn't be bothered to coordinate her treatments or pay attention to the side effects of the deluge of psychiatric drugs they were giving her over the years, and were abetted by nearly as inept civilian psychiatrists during her emergency hospital stays. Darla Grese points out, "She was passed on from physician to physician with no continuity. They kept writing new prescriptions, copying and pasting the old prescriptions without reading any of the complaints and concerns." (The moving story is told in full in Darla's book, *Sister Surrendered*.)

With the agency now promising to offer new and improved "integrated" and coordinated care, its failure to acknowledge its past failures with such patients as Kelli Grese and Andrew White doesn't bode well for any future reforms.

• • •

AS EVIDENCE AND LEGAL SETTLEMENTS MOUNTED ABOUT THE DANGERS OF Seroquel and its alledgedly fraudulent marketing to government health programs, the VA's continuing inaction on overprescribing took its heaviest toll on veterans struggling with both mental illness and addictions. At the Huntington VA that played a role in killing Andrew White, for instance, the latest known antipsychotic prescribing rate for PTSD patients is 23 percent, slightly higher than the VA average when the 2011 *JAMA* study demonstrated that they shouldn't be used at all for PTSD. Even more disturbing, nearly 18 percent of *all* Huntington VA patients were prescribed opiates, a rate about 300 percent higher than the national average for all adult male patients and far higher than the 7.7 percent of VA patients nationally who are using take-home opioids. (Carefully monitored opiate prescribing for patients with severe pain, of course, has a legitimate role.) Officials at the Huntington VA who provided their data said in a written statement that there are "positive trends" underway in reducing antipsychotic and opiate use, and they're following VA safety guidelines.

VA officials don't acknowledge their role in contributing to alarming opiate addiction rates among veterans through their aggressive prescribing practices. A 2012 *JAMA* study showed that veterans with mental health disorders and PTSD were three times more likely to receive opioids for pain diagnoses than other veterans. "They are essentially prescribing heroin pills; the effects of these opiates are indistinguishable from heroin and the VA jumped on this campaign to encourage highly addictive prescribing," says psychiatrist Dr. Andrew Kolodny, the co-director of Brandeis University's Opioid Policy Research Collaborative. When told about the opiate usage figure—roughly 18 percent—from the Huntington VA, all he could say, after a shocked pause, was: "Wow! That's very problematic."

"These are iatrogenic—medically-caused—addictions by the VA," Kolodny adds. "The chickens are coming home to roost."

In West Virginia and most states, the VA worsened the nation's addiction crisis—it didn't even start reporting all VA patients getting opiates to state databases until the end of 2015, a delay that allowed for more doctor-shopping and drug-dealing to civilians. The VA's Interim Undersecretary for Health, Dr. Carolyn Clancy, even admitted at a Senate hearing in March 2015 that she hadn't known that the state VAs weren't sharing data as requested. "It's shocking but not surprising," says Patrick Knue, director of the national Prescription Drug Monitoring Program (PDMP) Technical Assistance Center. The VA pharmacies were finally compelled to share prescribing records by a federal opioid abuse law passed in July 2016, but even near the end of 2016, eighteen state VA programs still weren't reporting. Independent experts say that the department is still working out compatibility problems with its software, but in a written statement, the VA claimed that its pharmacy software was "updated" to improve sharing data with state PDMPs along with the monitoring of individual facility pharmacies to ensure they share this critical information.

It seems likely that actively enforcing the mutual exchange of opiate prescribing data with state agencies simply hasn't been a high priority for the VA. Outside of sending two bland directives asking its staff to report to—and receive information from—the state databases on individuals' opiate prescriptions, with one issued as late as

March 2017, it's hard to tell from the VA's actions on this front that it's reacting to the nation's deadliest healthy scourge. In May 2016, for instance, the alarmed board chairman of the American Academy of Family Physicians wrote a letter directly to Dr. David Shulkin, then the head of the VHA, pleading for the department to impose mandatory opiate reporting on all VA programs, pointing out that the voluntary approach has failed to result in the VA "reporting necessary information to prevent the misuse and diversion of prescription drugs." More than a year later, the president of the AAFP, Dr. John Meigs, told me in a statement that the organization has still not heard back from Shulkin or anyone else at the VA. "Prescription drug monitoring programs are among the important vehicles for preventing patients from abusing opioid medications and, as such, are a cornerstone of the American Academy of Family Physicians' advocacy on dealing with this epidemic," he declared.

For the VA, not so much.

In October 2015, President Obama traveled to Charleston, West Virginia, to denounce the scourge of prescription opiate and heroin abuse, but didn't offer much in the way of funding for his proposed initiative. West Virginia has the highest rate of drug overdose deaths in the country, accounting for a third of all accidental deaths in the state. "This crisis is taking lives; it's destroying families and shattering communities all across the country," President Obama said. He didn't cite the VA's own role in spreading this wave of addiction or overmedication, or his administration's failure for years to address the rising tide of 120,000 opiate deaths under his watch—likened by Kolodny to President Reagan's inaction on AIDS.

In fact, Obama had personally honored in 2010 the then-director of the Huntington VA, Edward Seiler, over two years after Andrew White had died from Seroquel and other drugs, as one of only five VA directors given the Presidential Rank Award for federal civil servants. Seiler declared, "This is a high honor, exceeded only by the honor I have in serving America's veterans."

Stan and Shirley White were working in a different way to protect America's veterans. By April 2012, the last time I met with them in person, they still retained some hope after meeting with lame-duck

Senator Jim Webb (D-Va.) and two staff members, who had expressed concerns about antipsychotic overprescribing. Just a day earlier, the Whites learned that the Department of Defense would stop providing Seroquel in backpacks as a sleep aid for combat soldiers and removed the drug from its approved formulary list for Mideast soldiers, although authorization to prescribe it could still be obtained. The VA refused to follow the DOD's Seroquel initiative, but the retiring senator promised them that he would speak directly to the VA's chief medical officer about antipsychotic overuse. Yet years after Andrew White died and they'd begun their campaign for reform, Shirley White still needed to tell these aides: "Nothing has changed. We're hearing back from the families with soldiers who are returning that they are getting the same treatment that Andrew received." The staffers seemed sympathetic as they listened, took careful notes, and, as congressional aides always promised, they said they'd look into it.

The VA continued treatment as usual, even after the public finally took some notice a few years later in Phoenix and Tomah. In stark contrast, a radically different approach was emerging under the direction of a former Navy psychologist in rural Maryland which avoided psychiatric medications for veterans with PTSD altogether, challenging everything the VA had done for years.

CHAPTER 8

Drug-Free PTSD Recovery

By THE TIME NAVY VETERAN PAUL WALTON PLANNED TO SHOOT HIMSELF in the spring of 2012, he could see no way out. A Maryland-based electronics specialist who had worked on anti-submarine aircraft, he was in a stupefied haze, feeling lost and broken from the thirteen different opiates and psychiatric medications he'd been taking, in part because of a series of back injuries that led to a medical discharge from the Navy in 2006. That was then followed by the stresses of working for years as a military contractor, sometimes in combat zones, culminating in a breakdown during his last tour in Afghanistan in 2011 that caused Walton to be shipped back home. Yet the roots of his emotional agony and PTSD went back twenty years, long before clinicians in the military, VA or civilian world finally diagnosed his psychological traumas.

Fate saved Walton's life, in the form of Dr. Mary Neal Vieten, a Navy veteran and innovative psychologist who rejects both psychiatric medications and the medical model for wartime-caused stress disorders. As part of her tough-minded but empathetic psychotherapy offered on a sliding scale or for free, Vieten brings an alternative perspective on PTSD, along with practical stress-reduction techniques that allow veterans to truly recover without drugs. Her private therapy work has been supplemented by the week-long rehabilitation retreats she and a Maryland nonprofit disabilities organization, Melwood, offered at no cost to "warriors" from around the country about six times a year.

"Rather than serving their legitimate needs when they come back, we give them medications. I've spent my career taking them off drugs," she says. "People do not deploy to the theater of operations fit for full duty and then return mentally ill. It absolutely defies logic that they would leave sane and come back insane. They come back traumatized, and this is not mental illness. This is normal."

Even with her reframing of PTSD as "operational stress," veterans such as Walton still endure a lot of suffering. Well before he was shaken to his core by his wartime experiences and a bitter custody battle with his third ex-wife over custody of his son, he was haunted by his guilt over the rape and murder of a female subordinate while he was stationed in Guam in the early 1990s. She was a troubled young woman who was fouling up at work, and he was charged with improving her conduct and performance. She made steady progress under his direction, but on a night when they were supposed to have a friendly meal to celebrate her improvements, he got into a fight and didn't show up in time to meet her. Somehow, she ended up being fatally attacked on that same night, and he never forgave himself.

"My thought process going forward was that she was dead because of me," he says now. "I took all the blame on myself." The guilt unleashed turmoil that ravished him emotionally and physically, leaving him anxious, sleepless and angry, ready to fight anyone who got in his way—but he was too worried about wrecking his career to confide in anyone. It was especially risky to speak to a therapist in a military culture that too often scorns and drums out of the service many of those who seek help. He turned his anger inward by seeking out the most back-breaking physical labor he could find to punish himself—an environment, Walton now realizes, that injured him and left him dependent on opiates.

The VA's approach to Walton's treatment only heightened his fears to the point of despair, and ultimately led him to a church early one evening in the spring of 2012—where he planned to make his peace with God and then go home to shoot himself. There, he stumbled into a support group of churchgoers that included Robert Nielsen, an ex-veteran who had kept his eye on Walton the whole time. "I immediately connected with him," Nielsen recalls. "Without us saying a word, I could tell this man was hurting. And he had this military *persona* about him."

"Are you a veteran?" Nielsen asked him during a break. Walton confirmed it, and Nielsen said, "Dude, I can tell from the outside looking in, you're going through some major stuff. You've got PTSD. I do too, and I understand what you're going through. You've got to promise me you'll give this doctor a call. She's like no other doctor or therapist I've seen," he said—and demanded a firm vow, veteran to veteran, that he'd meet with her before he did anything else.

Walton called Vieten the next morning, and she made time to see him that day. Though overmedicated, he somehow drove himself over to her office. Even when he arrived, he was so woozy that he couldn't even come through the door at first, bouncing instead against both sides of the doorframe before stumbling into a chair to face her. She built his confidence in her therapy by citing her credentials and military service—and then cursing freely. "She cussed, she talked like a sailor, which made me feel really good because that's who I am: a sailor," he recalls. And he was especially impressed by her no-nonsense approach to the initial therapist questioning he had endured so many times before.

"How much drinking do you do?" she asked. "I'm not going to be naive: I already know you drink, so 'fess up." She was, he thought, really in his face—and, surprisingly, he welcomed it. Most critically, he recalls, "She gave me a reason to want to go back; she doesn't believe in all the medication." Ultimately, even with serious back pain, he eventually stopped taking almost all his meds, exercised more, halted his drinking and went back to college for electrical engineering, encouraged both by her and his peers in a support group she established.

He did all that in large part so he could be a better father for his son. "She kept me focused on my son; she put the carrot before the horse. She knew that was my hot button, being a good father. He's twelve now, and a lot of his being in my life is due to therapy," he says, his voice choking up briefly before he can continue. "I would not have my kid if it wasn't for Vieten," he declares.

After sessions with Vieten, Walton became a new man, learning how to confront his disabling anxieties. "I learned to recognize the onset of a panic attack and learned to meditate," he says. Still, with his years of addictions and stress not so far behind him, "Every day is a struggle," he says, but at least he now has new coping skills. Under Vieten's tutelage, he not only rid himself of his addictions, but educated his son about his condition by passing along a book for kids on dealing with a parent with PTSD, which Vieten had recommended. That made a huge difference in Walton's relationship with his son.

Walton reinforced his progress and new way of life by joining "Operation: Tohidu," the groundbreaking program launched by Vieten in 2014 at the 108-acre Melwood nonprofit retreat in southern Maryland. "Tohidu" is a Cherokee name for peace of mind, body and spirit. A quarterly, intensive ninety-eight-hour experience, the program has several vital elements that work together. It not only involves reawakening the camaraderie of military life through such outdoor challenges as high ropes balancing, horseback riding and wall climbing (all of which help these wounded warriors relax and trust each other), but includes frank group discussions and in-depth education about the root causes of their PTSD symptoms as a normal adaptation to war; this is supplemented with education about the hidden dangers of the medications they've been prescribed. "We actually have the veterans over the week live the wellness model," Vieten says. "We want the veterans to select those things that will work for them and fit into their ambitions of going back to work." Equally important, "We educate veterans on operational stress, the dangers of pharmacology and what they can do in place of pharmacology, and empower them to change their lives."

(After running eleven sessions aiding 250 veterans through May 2016 under the sponsorship of the Melwood disability organization, she left to form a new nonprofit, the Warfighter Advance, focused solely on veterans and active-duty military. It runs essentially the same program eight times a year, now called "The Advance 7-Day Training Op," at another campground near Melwood.)

For Walton, among the most exhilarating and daunting of the "experiential exercises" involved navigating on ropes between trees. Soldiers are also asked to traverse beams of wood suspended high above the ground between two poles, protected with harnesses as teammates on the ground keep the beams level by adjusting wires. As Melwood recreational program director Dora Fleisher noted, "Our idea is that if we take someone, and we get their body and mind in motion at the same time, we start to notice trends in the way we think, the way we react, and the way we problem-solve and communicate when we're under stress."

Former Army specialist Scott Barber was one of the participants seeking a new balance in his life while balancing himself during the exercises. Just a few years earlier, his heart stopped and he flatlined from all the medications, including Seroquel, that he was taking under a VA doctor's orders. When I visited the program in the winter of 2015, Barber had taken a new direction in his life after seeing Vieten, and now was starting his walk across a cable just six inches off the ground between the tall fir trees. As he alternated grabbing high and low ropes between the two trees, he was surrounded by group members who pressed their hands against him to help him steady himself. The ropes started out high, then became lower, then rose up again as Barber reached the end, a living metaphor for his military experiences. As Fleisher pointed out, "When they are up high, we ask them to consider: 'What was the high point of your military career?' As the guys are walking across the cable, they're saying it: 'It's when I got that award,' or 'When I was kicking in doors and calling in helicopters.' As you're walking, the rope starts to get low and we ask them to consider what are some of the low moments," and some cite the loss of fellow soldiers or a sense of isolation when they returned.

"Then the rope starts to get up high up again and we talk about what are the things that are going to bring you back up," Fleisher observed, such as family or faith. Two days later, they did the same exercise, but on a high ropes course way above the ground, and there weren't any spotters to keep their balance as Barber, wearing a helmet and dark winter jacket, as well as the others, made their way across the ropes to a tree with a platform. He finished by sliding a zip line, exultantly, back down to the snow-covered ground.

"The idea is to remember that when you're low, you're going to get high again," Fleisher, beaming with enthusiasm, pointed out about the ropes courses.

Later, wearing a green Melwood-issued Operation: Tohidu sweatshirt with his military rank on it, the thirty-seven-year-old SPC Barber, a formidable presence with his close-cropped hair and piercing blue eyes, declared, "The experiential learning is unbelievable. It gets everyone working together, gets you out of your own head, it really focuses you."

He's glad he is still alive to focus on anything at all. After four tours of duty in Iraq ending in 2009, the hyper-alertness that served him well in battle transmuted into nightmares, sleeplessness and a paranoid vigilance that makes any trash or item on an American road-side seem like a potential IED. "They train us to be soldiers on high alert 24/7, deployed for years and years, and we're warriors, then after that they ask us to reintegrate into the civilian population," he notes. When he said he was depressed and anxious, starting with the Army and then the VA, "They gave me a goody bag of drugs": tranquilizers, sleeping pills, Depakote, then Seroquel. "I felt like a guinea pig."

With diagnoses varying from bipolar disorder to PTSD, he was still following his doctor's orders on a Christmas Eve in 2012. He was playing Pictionary with his family when he went up to the board to draw an image and his sister suddenly noticed that his clear blue eyes had turned black—and he was bleeding out of his nose. Then he fell unconscious. The next thing he knew, paramedics were leaning over him in the ambulance and saying, "Stay with us, buddy," and apply-ing defibrillator pads to shock his heart awake. At the local hospital where he recovered for a week, the doctor reviewing his medications declared them a "recipe for death." But after he returned to the VA, they kept sending him drugs without changing their treatment plan after he nearly died. He tried tapering off on his own, but could still barely function even on relatively lower levels of meds.

Then he learned about Dr. Mary Neal Vieten.

Like Walton and Barber, most of Vieten's patients have failed elsewhere and come weaving into her office in a psychotropic-fogged haze. Many active-duty soldiers she sees keep their treatment secret from commanders so they won't be stigmatized as "nutcases" unfit for military careers, while some other veterans go through the motions of seeing conventional drug-oriented doctors and the ill-trained ther-apists at the VA in order to keep their benefits—while seeing her on the side so they can make a real recovery.

After joining the Navy as a Ph.D. psychologist in the late 1990s, she says, "When I started in the military, I had total buy-in to the medical model and the medical response to post-traumatic stress." She eventually transferred to the Naval Reserve in 2008 as a commander, and opened a private practice, though she could still be deployed. But realizing what worked for her in helping her deal with her own stressful postings, and after treating thousands of soldiers, sailors and veterans in a nearly twenty-year career, she now says, "I've come to realize that the medical model for treating trauma and for treating post-deployment issues and operational stress issues is just not valid. I haven't given a medication referral in over ten years."

Vieten first developed the model for the Tohidu program in 2003 when she was chief psychologist at a naval hospital in Puerto Rico, and needed to assist a small medical clinic at a nearby army base, Fort Buchanan, swamped by returning soldiers with assorted psychological damage, twenty-one of them with full-blown PTSD in need of immediate treatment. Using a military taps-to-reveille structure, the week-long program combined well-known, non-medication approaches to stress, wellness and recovery. In a 2004 paper in *Navy Medicine*, Vieten and her co-authors (which included Navy medic Paul Quilado, who eventually partnered with Vieten in establishing Tohidu) reported that the twenty-one enrollees saw a 20 percent reduction in symptoms in just seven days' time.

Though the Tohidu model—now The Advance—hasn't been replicated in studies by the military or VA so far, her Warfighter organization is in talks with two major research universities to formally measure outcomes. Early signs are very promising: Out of all the active-duty service members enrolled in the retreats—about 20 percent of those served by the program—fully 100 percent of them, virtually all on their way to being mustered out of the military because of their severe PTSD, have returned to active duty, with many going back to war zones. "They realized they weren't mentally ill and could work with their operational stress without needing medication," she says.

Vieten's approach to treatment earlier proved itself successful in a top-secret prison posting overseas in 2008 during the Iraq war. There, she slashed the forced psychiatric discharges of her mentally ill and PTSD-suffering guard patients to *zero*, returning them to full duty and winning a Navy commendation for her accomplishments.

"I 'normalized' and supported them and was very pro-active on prevention," she says. She helped them to understand that they were in a "crazy" environment that stressed them out, while offering, in response, caring therapy and instruction in coping skills—and she also reduced stigma by employing roving psych techs who casually counseled patients while handing out snacks to them while they were on duty. All that was in sharp contrast to her predecessor, who declared all the patients mentally ill and plied them with huge amounts of meds, then kicked them out of the military and let them fend for themselves as civilians navigating the VA maze.

Vieten doesn't believe she has a secret recipe for her successes. Instead, she sees herself as a psychotherapist in the tradition of Carl Rogers, whose humanistic, "person-centered" approach emphasizes "genuineness," joined with unconditional empathy and support that builds a true rapport between patient and therapist. Such rapport is a critical ingredient in any therapeutic improvement, almost regardless of the technique used, as confirmed by such researchers as University of Scranton psychology professor John Norcross. Vieten is just applying what good therapists should be doing, but in the culture of poorly-trained, unaccountable and swamped VA clinicians, such compassionate, individualized care is rare, worsened by the obstacle course facing veterans seeking access to treatment. "It's cheaper for the government to pay for a casket than treatment," she points out.

For Army Reserve Staff Sergeant Jacob Towner, a friend of Andrew White who saw him deteriorate and die under the VA's medication assault, two visits to the Operation: Tohidu retreats helped him grapple with his own stresses that were driving him to drink and isolating him from his family. He learned relaxation skills from yoga to breathing exercises that help steady him. The thirty-three-year-old Towner also says, "I never clicked with the people in AA, but Tohidu creates a place of so much more transparency and honesty with people who cared about you." In one group sharing exercise that encouraged frankness by having people switch seats, "I opened up to everyone in the circle." He left to call his wife in tears: "I was so relieved to get that weight off my chest: the brothers and sisters I lost in my war experience, and the loss of people after PTSD and medications," among other traumas.

Looking back, he also believes that if a program like Operation: Tohidu had been available to Andrew White, "It could have offered some new opportunity for him and helped him, but there's no guarantee." Andrew's father, Stan, told Towner about the program.

A key component of the Operation: Tohidu training is the "psychoeducation" component on a variety of psychological and treatment issues, grounded in references to scientific literature—while challenging common medical myths. At a morning training, for instance, Vieten asked the veterans during a PowerPoint presentation how many believed the "chemical imbalance" theory of mental illness. Almost everyone raised their hands. But she pointed out, "Not only is this chemical imbalance thing a theory and not a fact, but it's not even a good theory." She was also challenging what she calls the belief in a "quick hand-to-mouth answer" of psychiatric medications and diagnoses that pathologize normal human discomfort and often serve as chemical restraints.

Vieten offers a radical counterweight to the decades of drug industry marketing and deception that had victimized veterans who, like Jason Simcakoski, were all collateral damage in a deadly, greed-driven corporate campaign nearly unrivaled in modern American history. Even if her hard-line stance about the dangers of psychiatric medications, especially in the long run, put her at odds with some compassionate psychiatrists who use medications appropriately, there were good reasons for pointing to an alternative way out to undo all the damage that has been done.

These veterans had been prisoners of a system that had failed them, but they had, for now, found a way to escape. Another group of traumatized Americans—mentally ill inmates in urban jails—were not so fortunate.

CHAPTER 9

How LA County's Mental Health Officials Neglect Inmates and Ignore Violence

Before breakfast on November 8, 2014 in the women's jail in Los Angeles County, a popular inmate named Unique Moore coughed and complained she couldn't breathe. A thirty-seven-year-old African American, she had a history of diabetes, asthma and severe mental illness. Moore struggled to catch her breath on the lower bunk and desperately asked her cellmate in the top bunk, or "cellie," to call the guard for an inhaler (LA County jails do not allow inhalers in cells, as they can be used as weapons or dispensers for illegal drugs). As a lawsuit that Moore's family filed in 2016 asserted, the cellie repeatedly pressed the emergency call button inside each cell to summon help. Inside the cell in "pod" 3400 of the 2,300-woman jail in suburban Lynwood, the minutes ticked by without a response. About ten minutes into the ordeal, Moore fell down unconscious. Her cellie screamed out. But Moore couldn't be roused.

Unique Moore was one of Los Angeles County's nearly 700,000 adults with serious mental illness. Like Moore, many die far too young, and at least half receive no treatment at all. Yet each year thousands are routed into the LA County Jail, the largest single facility for holding mentally ill people in the country. The jail is a truly horrifying place, and non-violent mentally ill offenders should not have been sent there at all. Instead, their confinement made the goal of "recovery"—leading a fulfilling life while managing their illness—more elusive than ever.

On the morning of Moore's death, the guards, mostly men at that time of day, dawdled. "A lot of times when we wanted toilet paper or sanitary napkins, they ignored us," recalls Kendra Cox, who was jailed in the adjoining pod, 3300. "They probably thought it was insignificant," she says. "They were men."

But the guards for Unique's pod weren't even present. They schmoozed with colleagues in pod 3300 before their workday. Kendra alleges that, initially, they didn't answer the incessant alarm from Unique's cell, a claim that the cellmate buttressed. Kendra learned about the delayed emergency response when inmates near Unique shouted and pounded on their thick metal doors. So the inmates' yelling followed the ignored ringing of the emergency bell. In the other pod where Kendra bunked, the sounds were muffled. Yet the inmates' cries for help woke Kendra and inmates nearby.

But the shouting and pounding did not stir the guards nearby. For about twenty minutes, Kendra says, she stood near the door at her cell, looking out the small observation window and wondering where the guards were. Eventually, the guards responded. When they showed up, Unique was on the cell floor unconscious, but, they claimed in reports, still breathing. After the jail's medical staff arrived at her cell, she had gone into cardiac arrest before they could administer CPR. Then they summoned the county's Fire Department paramedics.

After she was carted away from the jail to an ambulance, word spread through the jailhouse grapevine about "Chocolate." Shortly before 8 a.m. at St. Francis Medical Center Unique Moore was declared dead.

Soon enough, it seems, yet another cover-up from the Los Angeles County Sheriff's Department (LASD) began. Based on the version of events from the LASD, the coroner reported that Moore was "routinely" checked by the jail's medical staff whenever she needed her inhaler. In Unique's case, as an LASD detective later claimed to the coroner, a deputy sped his way to the medical staff, retrieved the inhaler and returned to find that Unique had fallen to the floor, semiconscious and breathing with difficulty. The LASD insisted, "As soon as the decedent was pulled out of her cell, the decedent went into cardiac arrest." That's the LASD's story and they're sticking to it.

The LASD initially declined to comment on the incident or even concede that Unique had died. By October 2015, when I told the sheriff's department that I had obtained the coroner's report, the agency finally admitted she died, but blamed it on her drug abuse, not medical neglect.

The silence, evasions and apparent deceptions weren't surprising. After all, since December 2013, federal prosecutors have hit the sheriff's department with nearly two dozen federal criminal indictments for assault, obstruction of justice and corruption; most of the twenty-one convicted guards and administrators, including the defiant undersheriff, Paul Tanaka, have been sentenced to prison. His boss, former sheriff Lee Baca, initially faced a trial in December 2016 for allegedly lying to the FBI. It ended in a mistrial after jurors were deadlocked. Prosecutors announced in January 2017 that they planned to retry him on corruption charges. In June 2016, the stiffest sentence as of mid-March 2017—five years—was given to Tanaka, the mastermind of a scheme to block an FBI investigation into the jail's reign of violence towards inmates that he allowed to flourish. Any remaining illusions about the department's penchant for cover-ups were shattered with the conviction of the once-powerful Baca in March 2017 for obstructing a federal investigation into abuses at the jail and related charges. In May, he was sentenced to three years in prison.

Earlier, in August 2015, the LASD had finally agreed to a federally-appointed monitor to ensure that it carries out sweeping reforms across the jail system to rein in deputies' abuse of inmates and to improve care for mentally ill prisoners. The federal action followed the department's agreement in April 2015 to curb abuses documented in a class-action ACLU lawsuit stemming from decades of violence against inmates in the men's jail.

Mentally ill inmates are vulnerable across the country, but especially so in LA County and in the nation's most brutal prisons. They have been attacked at higher rates than other inmates, according to the sheriff's department's own "use of force" data and national reports by groups such as Human Rights Watch. About the same time that Tanaka was first accused by prosecutors of covering up violence in May 2015, Human Rights Watch reported on commonplace violence by guards targeting the severely mentally ill across the country, including for such minor infractions as using profanity. The report summed up, "Corrections officials at times needlessly and punitively deluge them with chemical sprays; shock them with electric stun devices; strap them to chairs and beds for days on end; break their jaws, noses, ribs; or leave them with lacerations, second-degree burns, deep bruises, and damaged internal organs." Furthermore, Human Rights Watch observed, "The violence can traumatize already vulnerable men and women, aggravating their symptoms and making future mental health treatment more difficult." (Strikingly, at least 60 percent of all jail inmates haven't been convicted of crimes, but are often too poor to post bail.)

As *The Los Angeles Times* reported, the drive to abuse mentally ill and other inmates was so great in the jail system that a rookie deputy, Joshua Sather, said he succumbed to pressure from a supervisor to beat up a misbehaving mentally ill inmate: "We're going to go in and teach this guy a lesson," his supervisor told him. A top graduate of his recruiting class, Sather soon quit the department.

Human Rights Watch cited several needless deaths in its report, illustrating that the culture of violence in the Los Angeles County Jail was not unique to California. One shocking incident involved Christopher Lopez, who died in 2013 at Pueblo, Colorado's San Carlos Correctional Facility after lying handcuffed nearly naked on the floor for hours, being repeatedly force-fed antipsychotics and suffering seizures. Meanwhile, clinicians and jailers laughed at him while chatting about vacation plans as Lopez, who had delusions that he was Jesus Christ, lay face down on the cell floor dying, according to a lawsuit his mother brought, which the Department of Corrections settled for $3 million in December 2014.

What's especially striking about official violence aimed at the mentally ill and other inmates is the resistance to making changes. For instance, the LASD didn't even start rooting out the violence and neglect until the end of 2013, after deputies were indicted, Sheriff Lee Baca retired early and the Board of Supervisors ordered the department to reform.

LA County Jail health professionals have not yet been exposed as acting as cruelly as their Colorado prison counterparts. Yet many of the same scornful attitudes have flourished for years, according to the jail's former mental health clinicians, the Department of Justice and ACLU reports. Both jail and mental health department leaders have countenanced or ignored staffers laughing at the mentally ill and ignoring inmates in physical agony. This pattern of neglect made it possible for violence against inmates, including the mentally ill, to continue unabated.

But as a former LA County Department of Mental Health jail clinician, who asked to be anonymous, points out, "The deputies and the sheriff's department are in charge." This counselor noted that the jail staff, whose ranks law enforcement officials dominate, set the tone and approach to mental health care, even though mental health services have been provided by Department of Mental Health (DMH) clinicians deployed to the jails. (Medical treatment for physical illnesses has traditionally been handled by the sheriff's department health workers, while the jail's mental health care was the responsibility of Department of Mental Health staffers.) But the culture of the jail was shaped by the brutal cruelty sanctioned by the LASD for years. That may help explain why too many mental health workers, whether at a prison in Pueblo or inside the Los Angeles County Jail, have lost their moral compass and departed from the Hippocratic Oath: "First, Do No Harm."

In the summer of 2015, the county Board of Supervisors moved to strip both the mental health and sheriff's departments of the authority to run health care in the jail, placing that responsibility with a new office in the county's Department of Health that was scheduled to assume control in late 2016. But that change won't by itself ensure that mentally ill inmates are treated appropriately or, most critically, given alternatives to incarceration.

People like Lopez and Moore should not have been in jails or prisons. Of the 356,000 severely mentally ill inmates in the nation on any given day, most have lacked reliable access to community-based services and treatment facilities, let alone high-quality care. By some estimates, ten times as many seriously mentally ill prisoners are in jails and state prisons—mostly for non-violent offenses—than in state mental hospitals. In LA County, a perfect storm of neglect, an absence of accountability and the department-wide shielding of wrongdoers led to the decades-long nightmare that brutalized inmates.

The US Justice Department in 2016 continued its criminal probe into violence, corruption and obstruction of justice at the LA County

Jail. Meanwhile, it has finalized the court-ordered consent decree announced in August 2015 to force reform of the "persistent failure" of the jail system's abysmal mental health care.

The federal oversight would come too late for Unique Moore. Kendra and other inmates often saw her, ballooning to more than two hundred pounds in part due to her meds, wandering around the open area outside the cells in a medication-induced stupor. Unique's history of serious mental illnesses included bipolar disorder and schizophrenia. Yet she was kept with the general jail population. She was also given a potentially fatal cocktail of drugs, including the antidepressant Elavil and the antipsychotic Seroquel that, according to the FDA, posed a significant risk of sudden cardiac death when prescribed together. Unique's complex medical history made her especially vulnerable. She had suffered from congestive heart failure, diabetes, asthma, anemia, chronic obstructive pulmonary disease and neuropathy, all clearly disclosed to the jail's medical staff when she was arrested for violating her probation less than a month earlier.

Unique needed careful monitoring and prompt attention in case of breathing or cardiac emergencies. But as far as Kendra could tell, few, if any, of the mentally ill inmates in the general population got medical exams. Kendra's allegations received support from a harsh assessment the Department of Justice rendered in June 2014 about the quality of care given mentally ill inmates, and the views of some current and former LA County Department of Mental Health clinicians who worked in the jail. "There was no oversight and an indifference to bad clinical care" for both medical and psychological conditions, one DMH therapist says.

But according to the LASD, Moore had received plentiful, regular health care. Its *official*, rosy version of events provided no hint of a delayed response to Unique's medical needs by the sheriff's department. Yet it suggested an alternative factor in the inmate's puzzling death: "Possibly overdosed on a narcotics substance." When I inquired again nearly a year after her death, a spokesperson for the LASD's homicide bureau told me that the medical examiner also concluded that the death was due primarily to her drug abuse history. Yet the medical examiner found no illegal drugs in her system—just prescribed medications including Seroquel, the antidepressants Elavil and Pamelor, along with Benadryl. He concluded, "The cause of death is attributed to the asthma," but he amended his initial findings after input from the LASD detectives, adding: "The mode of death is accident due to the history of drug use"—despite the absence of any illegal drugs or alcohol on the day she died.

"The state failed her," Unique's father, James Moore, believes, in part because the drug treatment programs she attended during her prison stays were undercut by the widespread availability of illegal drugs in prison.

This shoddy care has a cost. After they end up in the LA County Jail, 95 percent of mentally ill inmates have substance-abuse disorders that remain untreated. In fact, they are so unmoored from their families and communities that more than 80 percent are homeless or lack stable housing when released, as the new LA County Sheriff, Jim McDonnell, noted in testimony in February 2015 before the President's Task Force on 21st Century Policing. "Jails were not built as treatment centers or with long-term treatment in mind," McDonnell said. But that's little excuse for the apparent widespread patterns of neglect and abuse that continue in the women's jail after the men's jails have gotten so much law-enforcement and legal attention.

When Moore returned to the LA County women's jail in the fall of 2014 for the final time, it was probably one of the worst places in the country for a person with her problems to be incarcerated. In fact, DMH workers and former inmates report that female inmates' medical and psychiatric problems are often ignored for weeks. In extreme cases, female inmates pull out their own rotting teeth, according to Kristina Ronnquist, a former social worker intern in the women's jail in 2013 and 2014. Just as disturbing for some inmates, Ronnquist notes, "On the second floor [for the most seriously mentally ill], they're decompensating because of the environment. They're rubbing feces over themselves and rubbing it on the windows. And many of them are non-violent." She adds, "I had no idea any of this was going on. I was shocked and horrified."

Sheriff's deputies and detectives downplayed such complaints, similar to the way they launched a superficial inquiry into Moore's death. Although they did so within hours of her demise, the investigating officers came from the same department that allegedly threatened, terrorized and intimidated the inmates under its watch routinely. "They treated us horribly, like we were second-class citizens," Kendra says of the custody staff, noting that no inmates dared to call out the guards on the early-morning shift for their delayed response. "We didn't tell them what really happened," she says now.

But as my interviews with former inmates revealed, the sheriff's department failed to interview inmates on Unique's pod *after* they were released. Officers knew that inmates wouldn't dare snitch on them while inside. Abetted by a report to the coroner's office at odds with inmate accounts, it seems the sheriff's deputies on duty offered a version of events that put their response in the best possible light. Much of that will likely unravel in the face of the new lawsuit charging neglect, wrongful death and a violation of Moore's civil rights, supported by multiple eyewitnesses to the alleged deadly delay that cost Moore her life—and that could cost Los Angeles County millions of dollars.

• • •

BUT MOORE'S DEATH, AS WELL AS THE ABUSE, VIOLENCE AND NEGLECT that continues at the women's jail, received scant newspaper ink or TV coverage. The lion's share of media and legal scrutiny has gone to the men's jails. A citizens commission in 2012 found a "persistent pattern of unreasonable force" in the men's jails. Even before more than twenty deputies and administrators were convicted of violence and corruption-related charges, ACLU reports documented horrifying conditions at the jail. In fact, there has been two decades' worth of lawsuits, Justice Department reports and court orders highlighting abusive conditions for mentally ill inmates, mostly in the men's jail. The latest round of reforms stems from a 2011 *Los Angeles Times* investigative series that helped stoke public outrage, and the ACLU's lawsuits and reports. This public shock and anger, a belated response to decades of violence and neglect in the men's jails, is well deserved.

The seventh floor of the LA County Jail's Twin Towers building is a phantasmagoria of mental illness and human torment. In one of the sixteen single-occupant cells in this section—or pod—a naked black man, his Afro disheveled, stands behind a locked brown door howling in a deranged rage. Of the 17,000 inmates in the LA County Jail, roughly one in five suffer from a serious mental illness, such as bipolar disorder or schizophrenia. Remember, these numbers make the county jail system arguably the largest *de facto* psychiatric facility in the country. On the fifth floor, the men are jammed into dorm-like pods that include not only sixteen two-person cells, but also a common area where fourteen people are forced to sleep on bunk beds. Psychologist Sarah Hough and other department leaders contend that the county jail's seriously mentally ill inmates have access to medications and therapy, with roughly four hundred DMH staffers in the jail—including more than seventy psychiatrists and psychologists. (Hough left her leadership posts in the men's jail and, later, the women's jail by the end of 2015, but still works for DMH.)

Yet the department's role in contributing to the jail's well-documented culture of neglect and abuse has received little attention. Mental health officials defend the quality of care and seemingly ignore widespread brutality at the notorious county jail that victimizes mentally ill prisoners most of all. Yet Hough denies any mistreatment or brutality. "In the fifteen years I've been here, I've never been informed of it," from either mental health staff or any inmates, she said. (One stunned Justice Department official scoffed: "That's ludicrous on its face.")

The Pollyannaish views of Hough and other Department of Mental Health leaders contrast with ACLU reports, the successful class-action lawsuit over widespread deputy violence that the city government agreed to settle in December 2014, *and* the sweeping Department of Justice agreement designed to end inmate abuse and improve treatment of the mentally ill.

The newest round of reform efforts was triggered when the ACLU of Southern California released a report in 2011 with eyewitness accounts from a civilian chaplain and an ACLU observer of violent deputy attacks, supplemented by dozens of inmate affidavits.

After over twenty years of failing to carry out court orders and independent commissions' recommendations for change, the department, starting in December 2014, made a brand new series of promises it may or may not keep. The ACLU reformers remained hopeful real change would occur. Following the sweeping, court-enforced Justice Department settlement in August 2015, as Peter Eliasberg, the then-legal director of the ACLU of Southern California and Margaret Winter, director of the National Prison Project put it: "The reign of terror ends at LA County Jails." Yet Eliasberg remained cautious about the prospects for change in the jail: "It's better now, but it still needs a significant amount of work," he told *The Los Angeles Times*.

Change may take a while. By 2014, the Los Angeles County Sheriff's Department reported an 11 percent uptick in deputy "use of force" incidents against inmates in the jail system through September. The figure contrasts with a 36 percent rise in the women's jail in Lynwood and a 40 percent jump at the North County Correctional Facility in Castaic compared to the same period in 2013, when "reforms" began. And, as a reminder, those are their *officially* reported uses of violence—not the beatings done out of the range of cameras chronicled in ACLU reports over the years. Until about five years ago, the ACLU received roughly 4,500 complaints a year of all kinds from inmates.

In fact, the public pressure and investigations have contributed to a two-thirds decline in brutality complaints to the local ACLU since the end of 2012; those complaints are also less likely to involve broken bones and deputies piling on with savage head strikes. Yet significant problems continue: The LASD's own figures show a 167 percent annual increase to over 1,800 "use of force" jail incidents in 2016, with 314 of them resulting in injuries.

• • •

WHILE IGNORING DECADES OF VIOLENCE, DEPARTMENT OF MENTAL Health officials failed to acknowledge major problems with their care. They said they provide high-quality, regular services and screening to the mentally ill male inmates housed largely in Twin Towers and to the women in the Lynwood jail.

Indeed, the department's then-director, Marvin Southard, said the mental health staff in scandal-plagued Twin Towers delivers exemplary care. "The Department of Justice is happy with the level of service we provide mentally ill people in the jail, given the limitations of the facility," he told me in an interview shortly before the Department of Justice released a stinging report to the contrary in June 2014. The report denounced mental health care in the jail as an "unconstitutional" violation of inmate rights. Although the thirty-six-page letter acknowledged improvements in services, the Justice Department took steps to impose court oversight of the jail, which were finally put in place with the settlement in August 2015, providing a potential roadmap for reform.

But it's not clear how much the underlying culture in the jail will change. At the top, sheriff McDonnell welcomed the settlement as a "comprehensive approach to reform" that he and other leaders will "fully embrace," starting with beefed-up training, restrictions on the use of force and the hiring of hundreds of additional staffers to increase safety checks of inmates. Yet after the 2015 settlement, the department was sued again by former inmates for allegedly dumping mentally ill inmates back on the street—paving the way for a return to jail—without any hands-on transfers to new services. The county's Inspector General reported in 2016 that LASD guards used restraints to tether some near-naked, emotionally disturbed inmates to toilets, chairs and cell doors for as long as thirty-two hours, leading to two deaths in 2015, part of the twenty-one people who died in jail that year. Four jail deaths in just nine days in March 2017 then led to angry protests. "You don't magically change a culture overnight," says *Witness LA* editor Celeste Fremon.

What's clearly unresolved is the deputies' long-standing, undisguised scorn towards mentally ill inmates, and that's shown few signs of changing. Routinely, deputies refer to mentally ill inmates as "dings." In 2014, even after Department of Mental Health and sheriff's department officials claimed that they had made so much progress that federal court oversight wasn't necessary, deputies in the women's jail *still* responded to a delusionary, untreated woman standing on a table talking to herself by laughing and hooting at her, according to a former inmate, Tina Middlebrooks. In the world of the LA County Jail, the mentally ill at least are good for laughs from law-enforcement *and* clinical staffers.

The lack of decent care has been especially evident in the

women's jail in Lynwood because of the absence of meaningful outside monitoring. County officials estimate that of the roughly 1,900 inmates there now, one-quarter have a serious mental illness. (The inmate population in Lynwood dipped following a statewide referendum in 2015 reducing certain non-violent crimes to misdemeanors.) Still, only 330 health beds are set aside for them. Abuse and neglect are common, according to Kristina Ronnquist, but DMH clinicians are too scared to say anything.

Ronnquist's views were confirmed by a shocking August 2015 report by the advocacy group Dignity and Power Now (DPN), "Breaking the Silence," that chronicled the degrading experiences of several women there. The most harrowing was the story of "Nina," a forty-seven-year-old African-American woman diagnosed with bipolar disorder, schizophrenia and depression. After two weeks at the Lynwood jail, where she was allegedly denied access both to medical professionals and the medications she needed to "quiet the voices" in her head, Nina attempted suicide in September 2014 by jumping off a second-story balcony.

In addition to such neglect, untrained deputies have reportedly assaulted mentally ill inmates and even some patients who've attempted suicide for unruly conduct or slight infractions. As Ronnquist, now a volunteer with DPN, told the Board of Supervisors in May 2014, "One of my teenage clients just recently made a very serious attempt at suicide and one day later was taunted by a sheriff's deputy, who slammed her fingers in the door after she refused to move them, causing serious injury." County officials insisted they couldn't confirm her allegations after months of refusing to answer Ronnquist's follow-up inquiries. Before closing the investigation without taking action, an LASD spokesperson said in a written statement, "We remain committed to the appropriate treatment of all inmates, including the mentally ill." Yet many who have witnessed conditions there disagree.

• • •

FROM 2012 TO MID-2014, THE NUMBER OF "PREVENTABLE" SUICIDES IN THE LA County Jail system rose sharply, to fifteen. (Nationally, the suicide rate has risen steadily in jails, now the leading cause of death there.) As a result, the Justice Department moved to strengthen its ongoing monitoring of the LA County Jail's "deplorable," "vermin-infested" conditions. The federal government concluded that the poorly super-vised mentally ill prisoners "are housed in conditions that present, rather than prevent, a risk of suicide." (Recent figures show that the number of jail suicides in LA County declined to as few as one in 2015 from ten in 2013. That change was spurred in part by another wrong-ful death lawsuit, which resulted in a $1.6 million settlement in Sep-tember 2015 for transferring a hallucinating, clearly suicidal twenty-three-year-old man to an isolation cell where he hanged himself. The sheriff's department has since realized that putting suicidal and depressed patients in solitary cells is a bad idea.)

All these conditions in the LA County Jail reinforce that we're facing a nationwide crisis of mentally ill people being abused and neg-lected in the nation's jails and prisons.

Some counties, such as Miami-Dade in Florida, arrange community-based treatment programs and "supportive housing" as alternatives to jail for mentally ill offenders who commit non-violent crimes. (In contrast, Florida's state-run prison system, with a facility in the county's south end, has a sordid history of killing and torturing some mentally ill inmates.) The Florida county's programs have helped slash recidivism rates for even felony offers to as little as 6 percent. By con-trast, 75 percent of offenders with mental illness in the Los Angeles County jails commit crimes again.

If mentally ill people can somehow navigate obstacles in the county's mental health system, they are better off getting those serv-ices in the community and staying out of jail. The Department of Mental Health's seeming indifference to aiding mentally ill inmates contrasts with the achievements of the DMH in delivering consistent, high-quality services to some—but hardly all—of the 250,000 people they help each year. The agency has produced remarkable results, such as The Village program in Long Beach for the chronically homeless.

Those with life-threatening or dangerous crises usually can get an emergency response, including the help of effective outreach teams. Yet some clinics have waiting lists as long as ninety days for basic psy-chiatric care. Meanwhile, the number of complaints to the ACLU about violence in the LA County jails are still too numerous. Former inmates, their family members and reformers see a culture of neglect and violence in the jails, including Twin Towers, and seek to change it. "The treatment of mentally ill men and women in the jail is a disaster, and the fact that Southard isn't honest about it is frightening," Patrisse Cullors, director of the Coalition to End Sheriff Violence in LA Jails, said before Southard retired in November 2015. His denial of this harsh reality continues to influence the department.

So DMH officials boast about their quality jail care—including their discharge planning—unfazed by the needless deaths, homelessness and traumatized inmates signaling a broken system. "Everyone's offered after-care and we make sure their needs are met, whether it's for medication management follow-up or housing," Hough said. The new Justice Department settlement, in contrast to these claims, requires the jail to halt the dumping of disoriented mentally ill inmates to Skid Row.

Yet, even in the face of lawsuits and scandals, DMH officials remained upbeat. As Hough's then-colleague, Peter Maloney, said of the infamous Twin Towers jail, which holds most of the mentally ill inmates, "It's a better way to live," compared to other jails. In fact, he notes with pride, "The Justice Department sends mental health officials from other states to study us." Sometimes it seems that it's not the mentally ill inmates inside the LA County jails who are delusional.

As it turned out, in June 2015 the LA Board of Supervisors put an end to the DMH leaders' misguided pride *and* their role in managing jail mental health care by what amounts to a no-confidence vote. As noted earlier, they removed the authority of both DMH and LASD to run the poorly coordinated and sloppy health care in the Los Angeles County jail system. Instead, they set up a new consolidated office under the county's Department of Health, a separate agency, with a Correctional Health Director that assumed full authority in 2016.

That still wouldn't guarantee that the culture of violence and neglect harming mentally ill inmates would disappear overnight, but Eliasberg said it was an important step. In a letter to the board supporting the reform, he pointed to "the obvious unsuitability of a law enforcement agency for the provision of medical care" and the "longstanding failures of DMH to provide appropriate care to inmates with mental illness."

By removing responsibility from the DMH to run jail mental health care, the LA Board of Supervisors freed up the department to devote more resources, staff and its $2 billion budget to do things it was competent at, including delivering outreach services to troubled people in crisis that actually helped many stay out of jail; and, for the most serious and chronic mentally ill people, offering intensive, supportive team treatments that improved their lives. But until services and care were transformed for mentally ill offenders, and alternative diversion programs became commonplace, all the department's other good works would continue to be undone by the hell known as the LA County Jail.

CHAPTER 10

To Live and Die in LA: How DMH's Outreach Work Saves Lives, Stops Mass Shootings

As seen in LA County and across the country, if locking up the seriously mentally ill in jail doesn't help them or the community, then undertaking a dragnet to hunt down potentially violent, disturbed people and forcing them to take their medications doesn't hold much promise, either.

Yet a few hours after the May 2014 shooting rampage by Elliot Rodger in Isla Vista near Santa Barbara that left seven people dead, Rep. Tim Murphy (R-Pa.) seized the opportunity to draw new attention to his controversial mental health reform bill that had been stalled in Congress since 2013—in part because it emphasized forced, long-term medication and outpatient treatment. But in the wake of the Charleston church massacre in June 2015 and other tragedies, its chances looked brighter. More than a year later, mass shootings—defined as four or more people injured or killed—occurred at a rate of more than one a day, spurring a renewed interest in mental health reform. Over time, Rep. Murphy also softened the bill's outpatient commitment provision to win broader support.

His advocacy template has been set since the Newtown tragedy in December 2012. As he has so often done in recent years, Rep. Murphy, Congress's only trained psychologist, declared in the aftermath of the 2014 Isla Vista killings, "I am angered because once again, our mental health system has failed and more families have been destroyed because Washington hasn't had the courage to fix it. How many more people must lose their lives before we take action on addressing cases of serious mental illness?" A year later, even before the killings in Charleston, South Carolina, galvanized the country, Murphy reintroduced a revised version of his legislation on the anniversary of the Newtown shooting and proclaimed, "If we want to prevent the next Newtown, Tucson, Aurora, Isla Vista, Columbine or Navy Yard we have to do something comprehensive and research-based and we have to do it now."

In July 2016, after he worked to modify its most controversial elements, including mandated treatment, his sweeping mental health reform bill passed a near-unanimous vote in the House of Representatives before passing the Senate. Then it was signed into law in December as part of a broader legislative package that speeded up drug approvals by the FDA. Democrats dropped their earlier opposition to the bill for allegedly undermining patient rights. In earlier versions, it sought to use federal funds to punish or reward those states that implement involuntary Assisted Outpatient Treatment (AOT) commitment programs; in the new version, the bill simply adds funding to some existing pilot AOT programs.

Murphy's support for outpatient commitment, though, has never wavered. The nation's mental health system, he told CNN, "is more interested in protecting people's rights to be sick than their rights to be well," arguing for greatly expanded mandated, long-term treatment for the seriously mentally ill as vital for reform.

Yet Los Angeles County, it turns out, has a solution that has stopped dozens of planned school and college murders—usually without requiring the mandated long-term medication and treatment that remains a goal of Murphy's bill. But LA County's successes have been ignored in the polarized national debate over Murphy's involuntary outpatient commitment campaign that, to many frightened Americans, seems at first like a reasonable response to the threat posed by dangerous, mentally ill people.

The drive for involuntary commitment has been led by Dr. E. Fuller Torrey of the Treatment Advocacy Center. His approach has garnered uncritical attention from most media outlets, including *60 Minutes*. "You're going to have to accept Tucson and Aurora. You're going to have to accept Cho at Virginia Tech," Torrey said in 2013 after the Washington Navy Yard shootings. "These are the consequences when we allow people who need to be treated to go untreated."

But Torrey's claims of mandated treatment's magical powers to stop mass shootings aren't accepted even by those who believe that AOT combined with intensive services can have a beneficial impact. Dr. Marvin Swartz, the head of Duke University Medical School's division of Social and Community Psychiatry, says bluntly after years of studying such programs, "I don't think it makes sense to view AOT as a solution to gun violence." The state laws aim to force treatment on chronically mentally ill people who have repeatedly been hospitalized or found homeless over the years, so they don't even apply to mass shooters such as Elliot Rodger. On top of that, there are no well-accepted studies showing that mandating treatment works any better than voluntarily offering the same services. As the respected research organization, the Cochrane Collaboration, concluded in its review of mandated treatment: "It is no more likely to result in better service use, social functioning, mental state or quality of life compared with standard voluntary care." While mandated treatment won't prevent violent attacks, today's narrow, ideologically-driven debates offer few other alternatives.

With gun control dead for the foreseeable future, can the nation really have only two choices: either force meds on the untreated, chronically mentally ill who seem dangerous, or do nothing while some crazed young men plan mass slaughter? Even strong supporters of forced treatment, such as D. J. Jaffe of the Mental Illness Policy Center, quietly concede that AOT usually wouldn't be able to identify or help those young people, such as the Newtown killer, Adam Lanza, or the Aurora cinema shooter, James Holmes, who don't have long histories of hospitalizations.

But in LA County, Linda Boyd, an affable, seasoned psychiatric nurse, and the law enforcement–linked outreach teams she leads in the county's $2 billion Department of Mental Health, can't afford to wait for congressional fixes that aren't likely to prevent violent attacks. Instead, in the days after the 2014 Santa Barbara shooting, working out of her cramped tenth-floor DMH office, she and her associates reached out to the seventy-five potentially dangerous young people— along with their families and the professionals treating them—who they're regularly tracking in the nation's most sophisticated, collaborative program involving law enforcement, school officials and mental health staff. The School Threat Assessment Response Team Program (START), launched in 2007 after the Virginia Tech massacre, has already halted well over fifty planned school and campus attacks and screened more than 5,000 people, mostly students.

As Boyd explained, "We realized we needed to do something about the threats people are making, and we do whatever intervention is needed." The START team coordinates multi-agency threat assessments that include a scanning of social media, interviews with the potentially dangerous person and the key people who know him and have treated him. That's followed by usually arranging voluntary intensive services with regular at-home visits, although involuntary psychiatric "holds" are sometimes invoked initially as well.

Could all that have prevented Elliott Rodger from going on his shooting spree? "Absolutely," said J. Kevin Cameron, a leading international pioneer of multi-agency, data-based threat investigations at the Canadian Center for Threat Assessment and Trauma Response and a consultant to LA County. He was particularly appalled at the way the Santa Barbara Sheriff's deputies showed up at Rodger's home and, based on a one-time, superficial talk with him at his front door, concluded that he was "perfectly polite" and posed no danger.

"They relied on their friggin' 'feelings,'" Cameron said, "instead of relying on the data."

Based on information available from a START-style investigation, mental health workers or police would doubtlessly have had more than enough evidence to place Rodger on a "probable cause" temporary psychiatric hold. That, in turn, would have allowed police to bar him from owning weapons for five years under California law. The ability to seize weapons is a little-used power under most state laws involving seriously mentally ill people who have been committed. Some states, such as California, Connecticut and Indiana have the authority to seize weapons for between a year and five years—without requiring a formal court-ordered commitment—if people are deemed dangerous by authorities.

The big loophole, though, as a *New York Times* survey found in 2013, was that deranged people not currently acting dangerously could petition to get their guns back—and often do. The result can be tragic. Even though limited gun control laws restrict this loophole in most states, they usually aren't used.

If START-style assessment practices were in place in Santa Barbara, Cameron said, "There's no question that this particular case would have had a different trajectory." In other words, those seven young people in Isla Vista near the Santa Barbara campus would still be alive today.

Now, in the days after the Isla Vista shootings, the Los Angeles START team had to prevent potential copycat attacks and respond to new threats. (The copycat threat is no myth: A *Mother Jones* investigation found that the 1999 Columbine massacre inspired at least seventy-four plots or attacks across thirty states by November 2015.) On the first Tuesday after the murders, the LA County team learned that a high school student who was assigned a personal essay stood up in his suburban school to recite a rant about his desire to kill people in the school. School officials summoned two specially trained social workers from the START program to evaluate him. After a targeted school violence assessment, he was taken involuntarily to a local hospital for a seventy-two-hour observation period that could be extended if needed.

More typically, the START teams made sure to check up on the young people they were aiding. During a remarkable three-hour weekly meeting of the START team I attended, they reviewed the pitfalls facing four young clients they were following. (Note: The word "patient" is widely considered a pejorative.) One such client they discussed, a nearly eighteen-year-old Hispanic youth who had violent, hallucinatory fantasies about killing himself and his schoolmates, was contacted after the Isla Vista shooting and was still potentially dangerous: His psychiatrist had reported the threats to police under a "duty to warn" law that led to him being placed on an observational hold in a hospital. He also violated a restraining order barring him from any school in his town after showing up for a Halloween event on campus with a bandolier packed with real bullets. Placed on probation, he was eventually referred to intensive social work and psychiatric care from the county's "Full Service Partnership" team for youth and young adults.

The student had made considerable progress. But now he was living with a relative who doesn't believe in professional therapy, so she recently stopped taking him to sessions, Boyd learned when she contacted a DMH team clinician. "He's going to need a new home visit," Boyd said at the meeting. "He wants to engage with us, and we can help him with whatever he needs."

START's success is a challenge to the conventional thinking and political debates about mental illness and violence. In these ideologically-freighted statistical battles, it's commonly argued by academic researchers that violence by people with mental illness is extremely rare: only 4 percent of all violent acts are committed by those with a mental disorder and they're eleven times more likely to be victims than perpetrators. But those figures on violence, although understandably cited to challenge the myth that most gun violence is caused by the mentally ill, don't tell the full story. They're based on recollections culled from large surveys of mentally ill people compared with those from an annual Justice Department crime victimization survey of nearly 160,000 people.

Recent assessments of severely mentally ill people studied over time have found that they disproportionately—although rarely—commit violent acts, especially if they're not receiving any treatment. A comprehensive meta-analysis of twenty studies by Oxford psychiatry professor Seena Fazel, for instance, found that males with schizophrenia were three to five times more likely to commit violence and for women, the risk was four to thirteen times higher when compared with the general population—but most of the violence could be accounted for by the attacker's substance abuse.

Fazel joined with other leading researchers in a 2015 *Annals of Epidemiology* article that critiqued the media for promoting the stigmatizing myth that mental illness often results in violent attacks on others. In fact, the far greater risk is actually posed by suicides, which account for over half of all gun fatalities. Citing the best available epidemiological (or prevalence) reports from NIMH, they also took aim at the polarized spin on these hot-button issues: "[The data] debunked claims on both extremes of the debate about violence and mental illness—from the stigma-busting advocates on the one side who insisted that mental illness had no intrinsic significant connection to violence at all, and from the fearmongers on the other side who asserted that the mentally ill are a dangerous menace and should be locked up; both views were wrong."

Nonetheless, these and many other experts have their own blind spot: they insist, incorrectly, that it's basically impossible to predict or prevent violence beforehand. Jeffrey Swanson, a Duke University psychiatry professor who was the lead author of the paper, has argued that looking for a likely mass killer is like looking for a needle in a haystack. "You would have to detain the haystack," he told *Behavioral.net*.

As Linda Boyd scrolled through a shocking PowerPoint presentation on the warning signs the START program uses, illustrated with pictures of such notorious deranged killers as Tucson's Jared Loughner, she might have cause to disagree with those shibboleths. "What did they have in common?" she asked of the mass murderers she reviewed. "They all intersected with law enforcement, mental health and schools beforehand, but nobody ever connected the dots." After displaying the weapons stash of Adam Lanza from the Newtown massacre, she showed some of the frightening writings and drawings found in the backpacks and lockers of Los Angeles County students. Particularly troubling was the vivid calligraphy and drawings of a teenager who created a booklet called "1,000 ways to kill yourself," declaring "I just want the pain to end," with drawings of a boy hanging from a noose and a girl being cut in half with a chainsaw. Yet Boyd noted, "He's really talented, and we got him help. Now he's in an art college and he sees a future now"—one augmented by psychiatric care.

Yet despite LA County's successful approach to preventing more than fifty attacks, no national mental health organization champions START. That's apparently because the program doesn't fit neatly into either side of the intensely ideological debate over mandated outpatient commitment involving rights, safety and effective programs. If widely implemented nationwide, START would undercut Rep. Murphy's political arguments that long-term forced medication is the best deterrent to prevent the rare instances of mass violence by people with dangerously untreated mental illnesses. On the other hand, one noted advocacy group critic of Murphy's bill said she couldn't champion START because it would risk further stigmatizing people with mental illness as disproportionately violent. "We can't afford to give out a mixed message," she told me, regardless of the lives that could be saved.

At the same time, the success of the START program also challenges by example the ill-informed claims by the Santa Barbara County Sheriff's Department that there was little that they could do. And, confounding all sides of the political debate, it shows that more can be done to prevent violence beyond such oft-touted long-term solutions as more hospital beds, more medications and more outpatient clinics.

• • •

THE START TEAM, IN FACT, IS PART OF A BROAD ARRAY OF DEPARTMENT outreach services including mobile crisis teams and roughly ninety joint pairings of DMH clinicians with cops in patrol cars deployed in Los Angeles and across LA County each day. All told, the various teams help over 26,000 people a year, usually summoned through 911 and hotline calls.

Their empathetic approach to psychiatric crises generally doesn't inflict needless trauma and avoids the deadly violence that too often accompanies such encounters in other localities. But the local police departments are hardly perfect on that score. In August 2014, two apparently ill-trained, hard-line Los Angeles Police Department city policemen with the gang squad shot at close range Ezell Ford, an unarmed twenty-five-year-old man with schizophrenia. Ford died just two days after a white police officer shot and killed Michael Brown in Ferguson, Missouri. The family has filed at least $75 million in wrongful death and civil rights lawsuits against the LAPD and the city of Los Angeles. All charges of wrongdoing and racism have been denied by city officials and the two policemen, who weren't charged. Yet the city settled the lawsuit for $1.5 million in February 2017. Both the county and city police departments have paired clinician-cop patrol teams that could make such needless killings far less likely. Indeed, many local policemen have been exposed to at least some general training about people with mental illness. That doesn't mean that all policemen buy into a sensitive approach or know how to defuse a crisis.

Los Angeles County offers more than just improved crisis intervention training for police officers alone. Its unique approach to policing on this issue has sparked interest from other communities in the wake of the furor surrounding the ruthless beating death in 2011 of Kelly Thomas, a homeless man with schizophrenia, by six Fullerton, California, policemen. The acquittal in 2014 of two officers charged in his death sparked new outrage, concerns essentially confirmed by the $4.9 million settlement Fullerton paid to the dead man's father days before the opening of a 2015 civil trial against the city.

Yet plenty of improvements are also needed in the Los Angeles area as well, especially with trigger-happy LAPD officers. Between 2011 and 2015, the Los Angeles police admitted in a 2016 report, its officers shot thirty-eight people—killing twenty-one of them—and more than a third of them had an indication of mental illness.

Unfortunately for those victims and Kelly Thomas, they never got a chance to interact with caring professionals like the two Los Angeles County Sheriff's Department Mental Evaluation Team (MET) members with whom I rode along in an unmarked police car during a daytime shift. The pair—we'll call the nurse Marjorie and the deputy Gail because of their confidentiality concerns—are usually called in as mental health backup for the first police on the scene. They're also trained in START evaluations, and wouldn't have been fooled by a polite, shy Elliot Rodger. On the day of my ride-along, they're summoned when a distraught mother called 911 after her eighteen-year-old daughter with bipolar disorder exploded in a dangerous rage after her mother said she couldn't afford to buy her Proactiv acne cream. The girl had thrown her skateboard through the window. "She went nuclear," the mother tells Marjorie. "I felt scared and called the police."

Outside, Gail is gently maneuvering the handcuffed girl into the backseat of the car as they went to the hospital for a seventy-two-hour psychiatric hold. Still covered by her family's insurance, the girl, whom we'll call Maria, complains, "I'm going to have to pay for medication. It's too expensive!" Yet something remarkable occurs—Gail quietly chats with the girl about her life and learns secrets she hadn't even told her mother: the teen wasn't taking her medications because she was trying to get pregnant with her schizophrenic boyfriend. Marjorie advises her: "You have an illness, like diabetes, and you need to take your medication."

By the time they arrive at the emergency room, waiting for intake, Gail stands next to the girl in handcuffs and begins schmoozing and joking with her about makeup and styling, and eventually removes her handcuffs. As the MET team gets ready to leave while the hospital arranges for a psychiatric exam, Marjorie tells her, "Don't worry about the money, worry about feeling better. That's why you're here."

Despite such compassionate outreach, far too many policemen in California and other states simply haven't been trained properly in how to respond in a safe, responsible manner to mentally ill people who are acting in a bizarre or potentially dangerous manner. That was made clear in Los Angeles when city police in March 2015 shot a homeless, mentally ill man nicknamed "Africa"—real name Charley Kuenang, forty-three—five times during a scuffle caught on a video that went viral. Despite differing police and eyewitness versions of the tragic encounter, it appears that "Africa" was shot by police who were following up on a robbery he reportedly committed. A campaign for police reform linked this new shooting with a fatal Skid Row police tasering a few months earlier that led its victim to plunge to his death from a rooftop while fleeing arrest; they were now part of the "Black Lives Matter" movement.

The LAPD has System-wide Mental Assessment Response Teams (SMART) that operate along the lines of the county MET team run by Gail and Marjorie—but in the city, they're largely staffed by police who are assigned the jobs even if they don't want them; in the county, the positions only go to those who ask for the work. Moreover, critics say the city inexplicably won't deploy them in the neighborhood with the highest concentration of severely mentally ill people in the metropolitan area: Skid Row. The Los Angeles City police chief, Charles Beck, insists the SMART teams shouldn't get involved in such incidents, although their central mission is precisely that: to reduce the potential for violence during police encounters with people with mental illness.

Yet if you or a loved one has a serious mental illness, you don't have to be a denizen of Skid Row to be killed by police. A detailed look by *The Washington Post* at the scope of 426 deadly nationwide police shootings in the first six months of 2015 showed that a stunning quarter of all fatal shootings by police involved mentally unstable people. Some involved disputes that got out of hand, others were deliberate attempts to provoke "suicide-by-cop." On average, police shot and killed someone who was in a mental crisis *every thirty-six hours* in the first half of 2015, the *Post* noted.

More than half of these tragic encounters involve police departments that haven't provided their officers up-to-date training to deal with people with mental illness. All too often, police without proper training can feel threatened and overreact.

• • •

BUT WHAT KIND OF "TRAINING"? SURPRISINGLY, THE *WASHINGTON POST* reporting project didn't mention the most widely used training: the Crisis Intervention Team (CIT) model developed by the Memphis Police Department. Now used by nearly 3,000 communities in forty-five states, CIT incorporates safety and de-escalation training of police officers in partnership with mental health "consumers" and families to help police better understand people going through a mental health crisis. The CIT approach involves not just dry lectures, but role-playing realistic crisis situations, along with police officers apprenticing in the field with more senior members of the police intervention team.

Memphis adopted the CIT approach in 1988, led by then-Major Sam Cochran, who partnered with NAMI after a police officer killed a mentally ill man. After implementing CIT, the city's SWAT team confrontations dropped 80 percent, and injuries to police officers dropped from one in 400 to one in 2,333. "It's a program that reaches out through not only community services [such as NAMI], but training our law enforcement officers to be a first responder," Cochran told *Democracy Now*.

Now leading the University of Memphis's CIT Center, Cochran's pioneering approach is increasingly sought after in the wake of highly publicized violent encounters with police—and some lawsuits brought on behalf of mentally ill people gunned down after families called 911 for medical help.

Years earlier in Fort Lauderdale, the backing for the CIT approach came in part from the leadership of a different sort of police officer: Scott Russell, who patrolled among the homeless people in the city. Russell helped form an alliance essential to CIT's success with groups that have often been at odds with one another, including family members affected by mental illness, mental health providers and the police. "By bringing positive attention to the issue of the mentally ill," he said during the training I observed, "we're giving them a stronger voice that they desperately need." (Now a captain, Russell heads the youth and special needs services section of the Broward County Sheriff's Office, which includes that agency's CIT team.)

Fort Lauderdale was also taking action because, in the previous two years throughout South Florida, there had been a spate of deadly encounters. These included a "suicide-by-cop" a few years earlier by a crazed man waving a gun around in the street, and incidents in Miami-Dade County to the south, where a shocking *eight* mentally ill people were gunned down by police who had no specialized training. "Those are the types of incidents police come across," Russell told the CIT trainees. "You come across people who are mentally ill, who are in crisis or who aren't functioning normally. What we want to do is provide our police officers with additional skills to recognize some of those factors, to understand what's happening and also to give them some skills to de-escalate crisis situations—and to refer people to appropriate social services and mental health providers."

The officers faced a host of typical mental health crises in their role-playing exercises, most based on real incidents, with gradually escalating threats of violence. Finally, the officers practiced their responses to a crisis that has continued to periodically plague police and the veteran community to this day: an angry, deranged, armed veteran willing to kill himself or others if he can't get anyone to help. The Fort Lauderdale police sought to counsel and calm Vincent Tamburelli, a tough-looking guy with a beard, who was actually the head of a local clinic's mobile outreach team, but was now playing an angry Vietnam vet with bipolar disorder armed with a knife. He was lashed to a gate at the Oakland Park Tri-Rail station and threatening to kill people unless he got help—now.

Tamburelli played it with an eerie authenticity because he'd just been briefed by a police administrator about this real-life incident. "If I don't get help, someone's going to get hurt!" he shouted. "I need my medication, and no one will help me."

Officers Joyce Fleming and Mary Gillis approached Tamburelli gingerly as he kept his hand near his knife pocket. Fleming took the lead. After asking his name, Fleming gently instructed him, "Just put your hands by your side."

"Not yet," he responded.

But after some more smooth talk on Fleming's part, the two officers convinced Tamburelli to lie on the ground to be patted down for weapons. Then she pointed to the imaginary police car in the training conference room where he headed next, without handcuffs, as she urged him, "OK, go ahead."

Later, in reviewing her performance, Fleming won high marks from the professional therapists, although some officers in the class felt she was putting herself at risk by not handcuffing him.

The most detailed critiques of the officers' performances in different scenarios came from none other than Cochran. For instance, he assessed one officer who successfully talked down a role-player acting like a paranoid man fearful of the CIA controlling his thoughts who was barricading himself in his home. He praised the policeman for his slow-paced and courteous tone, and the empathetic way he spoke to the person in crisis about how he felt about taking his medications. "By getting that individual to talk to you, to reason with him in the here and now, it's not going to be long before that individual is going to open up the door," Cochran said.

Near the end of the training, Cochran spoke about how this work would rekindle the idealism that had brought these officers into police work. "When you ask why you became a police officer, the first sentence out of your mouth is, 'I want to help people.' But it's pretty tough being an officer, and that gets pushed to the back of our minds."

"A year from now, you'll be a different person," he concluded. "Now it's up to you to rise to the occasion."

In today's era, it's hard to remember that compassionate, dedicated police officers still exist. But they do, and in places like Fort Lauderdale or LA County or other cities where well-trained officers respond to a mental health crisis, you can see the difference they're making.

The real measure of a successful mental health system, however, isn't how quickly and empathetically police can respond to a crisis, but how the system helps mentally ill people avoid new hospitalizations, meltdowns and emergency calls in the first place. On that front, at its best, the Los Angeles County Department of Mental Health often succeeded in turning around the lives of some of the county's most chronically mentally ill people who were fortunate enough to access the agency's specialized services. Yet, despite good intentions, and in part because of the hellish failure of the LA County jails that damaged thousands of mentally ill people each year, the department's innovative treatments ultimately failed at enabling most of their clients to achieve independent, fulfilling lives.

Most clients would never find what the department proclaimed as its vision and mission: "Hope, Wellness and Recovery." And that goal remained just as elusive for the nation's troubled kids and adults who never got any high-quality services—and ended up ensnared in institutional settings often nearly as traumatizing as the Los Angeles County jails.

CHAPTER 11

Torture in Alabama

"If you're so determined to kill yourself, you should put the gun next to your head and pull the trigger."
William Knott, manager of the fundamentalist school for troubled youth near Mobile, Alabama, then handed Robert a .380 automatic pistol. The teen, who'd been kept in an isolation cell for days, naked, put the gun to his head, and pulled the trigger.

For MANY MENTALLY ILL PEOPLE AND EMOTIONALLY DISTURBED ADDICTS, such as Unique Moore, the failure to find anything approaching quality treatment in their communities as teens and young adults sets them on a downward slide towards an early death in jail, on the streets, or even in the Medicaid program itself. For others, the chaotic and dangerously incompetent local mental health system leaves them vulnerable both to the siren song of the snake-oil salesmen of the behavioral health care field—hucksters for poorly-regulated treatment facilities—and irresponsible overmedication. The key selling points for the antipsychotics that are prescribed so recklessly to young people, the elderly and veterans are that they offer a relatively quick fix for difficult mental health problems, and they can rein in troublesome behaviors. An entire multibillion-dollar residential treatment industry has flourished offering a comparable set of exaggerated claims, while profiting off of the misery and suffering of all those mishandled by their communities' outpatient programs. These inpatient-style treatment enterprises target emotionally troubled substance abusers and, especially, parents at their wit's end dealing with difficult, misbehaving kids who are struggling in school and in their lives.

Nowhere is this more apparent than in one of the most common types of private programs marketed for errant youth: the largely unregulated religious schools marked by fundamentalist beliefs and often violently harsh discipline. Inspired in part by the programs of a fiery Baptist radio preacher, the late Lester Roloff, they have been periodically exposed for whippings, beatings and alleged rapes in media outlets including CNN, *Mother Jones*, *The Daily Beast* and *The Tampa Bay Times*.

The 2012 *Tampa Bay Times* series, for example, opened with a description of a fifteen-year-old boy who was exercised to the brink of death and flown by helicopter to a hospital with kidney failure three days after entering the Gateway Christian Military boot camp in Bonifay, Florida. The school, still open today but claiming to adopt a more moderate approach, is part of the largest fundamentalist "treatment" chain for adults and youth in the world, Teen Challenge, with over eighty programs—often subsidized by taxpayer dollars through court referrals—in America, with a total of 1,100 centers in 118 countries. Regulations in the US are so loose that the controversial organization has been investigated but rarely sanctioned for such actions as allegedly using patients as unpaid workers in a reported telemarketing scam in Sanford, Florida, or hiring a convicted sex offender as co-director of its Winthrop, Maine, program. Nine states, including Florida, Alabama and Missouri, have wide-ranging "faith-based" exemptions protecting various church programs and schools from direct government oversight (while twenty-six states have no requirements for any private schools, religious or secular.) Teen Challenge has even opposed the use of twelve-step methods because references to a "higher power" in AA are, counselors tell patients, "Spitting in the face of Jesus."

National and regional leaders didn't answer my questions about these accusations, but the president, Joe Batluck, wrote me, "Teen Challenge or Adult & Teen Challenge is a US-based network of eighty-five independent religious nonprofit corporations that works with individuals struggling with chemical addiction. TC's fifty-eight-year track record is unparalleled in the field of addiction. The faith-based model has proven greatly helpful by many of the graduates."

Similar promises of miraculous changes have lured parents to send their kids to these programs for years, even to a facility in a gritty, run-down section of the predominantly African-American town of Prichard on Mobile's north side. Captain Charles Kennedy, who'd been a cop for forty-four years, didn't quite know what to expect in October 2011 when he followed up on a call from a California mother worried about her son, who was attending the local Christian school for troubled teens, Restoration Youth Academy (RYA). A few days earlier, Kennedy, then with the Prichard Police Department, had received a phone call from another California mother, Rosa Getierrez, who told him that her son had run away from the same facility, claiming maltreatment and, after holing up at a Mobile motel at her expense, returned home.

The program's executives and allied pitchmen-consultants promised parents "hope for their teenagers' future, when hope doesn't seem possible," as its website declared. "We have a highly trained staff with a heart for kids in need of guidance." And so many desperate parents were grateful for that. "I was scared I would find my son hanging from a rope or a dead from a needle," says Leslie Crawford, a Connecticut mom, about why she sent her truant, drug using son to RYA at a cost of $1,500 a month.

Kennedy was greeted at the school's forbidding metal front gates topped with razor-wire by the manager, William Knott. Kennedy thought Knott was friendly, a man with nothing to hide. He didn't know then that Knott had already been cited in two lawsuits—leading to settlements of nearly $1 million or more—for his role as chief enforcer of sadistic beatings at a now-closed Mississippi facility, Bethel Boys Academy, under his authority as "Head Drill Instructor."

Kennedy knew the concerns raised by Barry's mother and the allegations of the Getierrez boy—included in a police report faxed from California—weren't solid enough to prompt an official criminal investigation, so he tried to charm his way into places he might have needed a warrant to see. Knott provided a tour of a bare-bones classroom inside interconnected mobile homes and an adjoining cafeteria with eerily quiet, unsmiling children.

After the tour, Kennedy asked to speak alone with Barry, the son of the mother who had called him. (The names of all minors in the program have been changed to protect their privacy, unless they or their parents agreed to let their full, real names be used.) Knott agreed, but only permitted Kennedy to talk to the boy in the main office, which had three large windows and relatively thin walls, offering Kennedy and Barry almost no privacy. Barry, small for his age and clearly frightened, was brought in by Knott and placed in a chair opposite Kennedy. Knott then left the room, but hovered outside, shouting in a loud, angry voice to kids in the hallway. Kennedy saw tears welling in Barry's reddened eyes, so he reached over and pulled the boy's chair close to his, and said in a low voice, "Look at me, Barry. Don't pay any attention to what is happening out there. I am a police captain, and anything you say stays with me—no one else."

Soon the truth began tumbling out: Barry said he'd been threatened during his trip from California with a beating if he misbehaved, and once he was hustled into the compound, he was strip-searched and forced to start a brutal regimen of exercises, stark naked, in a room next to the office the two of them were now in. Kennedy later learned that this exhausting "Physical Training"—or "PT"—was common for the program's pseudo-"cadets" and included push-ups, jumping jacks and running in place.

Barry said he was also punched in the stomach, hit in the head and slapped in the face by Knott and two other drill instructors whenever he seemed to be flagging. At one point, Knott then pushed the naked boy to the ground and demanded that he do more push-ups—which Barry told Kennedy he did until he collapsed from fatigue. At that point, Barry recalled, Knott crouched down next to him, and, after yanking his head up by his hair, started pounding his skull against the floor while shouting, "You will exercise until I get tired!"

When Barry could no longer move, he was dragged by his feet into a cramped, empty isolation room and locked up for two days, wearing only a pair of boxer shorts. The door was typically opened by the staff only to allow bathroom breaks and to shove some spoiled food inside. "I asked myself why my parents spent all of their money to fly me here to put me in a place like this," Barry wrote in pencil in a sad, handwritten note he later sneaked into Kennedy's hands.

After interviewing Barry, Kennedy asked to speak to some other boys, those who'd been identified by Rosa Getierrez's son as victims of abuse. After gentle quizzing and coaxing by Kennedy, a few of them eventually revealed that they had been hit, choked and body-slammed by Knott and other staffers.

Most of the kids, however, were too scared to talk to Kennedy, but as he pursued his investigation, he found more appalling cases of degradation and physical abuse. Ryan, a thin black kid from Brooklyn, told Kennedy he had been held upside down in shackles and hit with a belt. He still bore the scars of the leg irons and handcuffs when Kennedy spoke to him during a subsequent visit to the facility. A few fellow students who dared speak to Kennedy confirmed Ryan's story of Abu Ghraib-like abuse. One boy who'd recently escaped the facility wrote a letter to Kennedy in 2012 that said, "I saw Ryan, a cadet who had escaped several times, was put in shackles in his arms and legs and went to school, breakfast, lunch, dinner, church in these shackles. I also saw Mr. Bernie [an instructor] pick up Ryan from his leg shackles and dangled him in the air."

• • •

CHARLES KENNEDY HAD ENTERED A PORTAL INTO WHAT SOME CRITICS have called "The Jesus Gulag."

The template for these schools was set by Roloff's Rebekah Home for Girls in Corpus Christi, Florida, in the 1960s, which featured vicious corporal punishment and children locked in isolation rooms where Roloff's sermons were played endlessly. He defied a state law requiring inspection of all child-care facilities, despite affidavits from sixteen girls at the Rebekah school that they were whipped with leather straps, severely paddled and handcuffed to pipes.

Roloff famously declared at a 1973 hearing following one of his arrests, "Better a pink bottom than a black soul." With dozens of ministers linking arms with him in 1979, he blocked state inspectors from entering the Rebekah Home to remove children in a stand-off that became known as "the Christian Alamo." In 1985, the state forced the closing of the home, which then moved to different states with looser oversight under an array of names, a common practice for both secular and religious "troubled teen" programs. The school briefly returned to Texas in 1998 when then-Governor George W. Bush solidified his popularity with Christian voters by deregulating faith-based programs.

The Rebekah school ultimately landed in Missouri, a haven for allegedly abusive schools, under the name New Beginnings. Not surprisingly, these leaders were accused by *Mother Jones* and in a recent Change .org petition written by survivor Racheal Anthony of abusing teens once again. "They have beaten girls with curtain rods . . . they have force-fed girls beyond vomiting," the petition declared. Spokesmen and the attorneys for the churches and schools have repeatedly denied any wrongdoing over the decades or refused to answer reporters' questions.

The stern spirit of Lester Roloff lives on in the resistance by church leaders—often abetted by local politicians—to any government oversight under the guise of separation of church and state.

These schools and programs are just part of a vast, multibillion residential treatment industry that flourishes in the United States by selling an illusory promise: a quick (and usually expensive) fix for difficult mental health problems or addictions. Yet the potential danger of abuse and neglect is a real threat for 200,000 or more youths trapped in the poorly monitored secular and religious "group care" facilities, "troubled teen" residential schools and unlicensed treatment programs. They too often profit off the misery of emotionally troubled substance abusers and parents in despair from dealing with kids they can't control.

Perhaps the largest alliance of such ultra-conservative churches is the far-flung Independent Fundamental Baptist organization with thousands of churches nationwide and numerous boarding schools that cite the Biblical importance of "breaking the will of the child."

"If you're not bruising your child," a pastor declared in a 2007 sermon captured by ABC News's *20/20*, "you're not spanking your child enough."

• • •

THE LEADERS OF RESTORATION YOUTH ACADEMY, IT TURNED OUT, TOOK that crackpot religious philosophy to its most extreme, sadistic limits. After talking to Barry and other traumatized cadets during his initial visit, Captain Kennedy tried to protect the fifty or so kids there from retaliation by acting as if nothing was amiss. Confident that the facility's staff would soon be arrested, he called Barry's mom to reassure her that her son was safe now, and that no harm would come to him as he pursued his investigation.

A few days later, Kennedy returned to RYA with a female detective to interview more boys and girls, and discovered yet another terrifying feature of life at Restoration Youth Academy: Boys with boxing gloves, usually mismatched in size, were often grabbed out of their beds in the middle of the night and forced to fight until one of them was beaten to a pulp. Kennedy stopped just such a fight in the daytime during this second visit.

Knott's casual attitude about the program's unrestrained violence was underscored when Kennedy confronted a drill instructor ("DI") about the attacks the boys watching the fight had quietly described to him. This DI, a six-foot-two, 280-pound man known as Mr. Kenny, lined up boys at shower time, where they stood naked, grasping towels, and then he walked by, randomly slapping them in the face and punching them in the stomach.

Chris Coronado, then a tough, six-foot-five fifteen-year-old Hispanic from Georgia with a history of gang-related arrests, recalls, "I knew this was something serious—it scared me. We were butt-naked and they were trying to scare you physically, treat you like a punk."

When Kennedy asked Knott and Mr. Kenny about this practice, neither denied it took place.

Kennedy knew he had a criminal case, and knew he had to stop the abuse soon, but he also knew that he lacked the hard evidence he needed to make an arrest. To make a felony arrest, he needed either the support of the DA's office, his personal observation of a crime in action or a criminal finding of abuse from the state child protection agency. For an arrest on a Class A child abuse misdemeanor, the standards weren't as strict, but he still needed either his direct observation of a criminal act, an out-of-state parent to travel to Alabama to swear out a warrant, or an eighteen-or-older survivor of the program to request that a judge approve an arrest warrant.

And so he returned yet again to RYA. During one of those visits, he glimpsed on a closed-circuit monitor the image of a naked boy, Robert, crouching in a six-by-eight isolation room with a twenty-four-hour light bulb overhead.

Kennedy asked why this cruel and not-so-unusual RYA treatment was being inflicted on this boy. Knott explained, "He's got an attitude. He's only been there for a day, and he'll be there for another day or two."

"Can't you give him some clothes?"

Knott gave a vague answer, and when Kennedy left later that day, the boy was still locked up, still naked.

Although the use of solitary confinement as punishment has been deemed torture by the UN Rapporteur on Torture, Kennedy knew that what he'd just seen wasn't illegal in Alabama. He also knew that police investigations can be compromised because these institutions bar the young people they control from unmonitored communication with family and outsiders—and most states, including Alabama, don't even protect workers who report child abuse from being fired. The result is abuse isn't reported until much after it was committed, which makes investigations and prosecutions nearly impossible.

Throughout his investigation of RYA, Captain Kennedy had been updating his police chief, Jimmy Gardner, about the potentially criminal abuses he was finding, but his chief didn't want to take action. "He telegraphed that he was not interested in making arrests, but interested in learning what I knew," Kennedy says. "He was very buddy-buddy with the mayor and Rev. Young." (Gardner says any allegations that he impeded Kennedy's investigation are "absolutely ludicrous . . . I've never done anything like that.")

When Kennedy returned to RYA two days later, Robert was still huddled in the isolation room, naked. Knott told Kennedy the boy deserved further punishment: "He told us he wanted to commit suicide." Kennedy warned Knott that he was required to notify the local child welfare department of the fourteen-year-old's precarious mental health and that he expected Robert to be released from solitary confinement immediately. He then left.

Kennedy returned again the next day to check up on Robert, who was still in the isolation room, for a fourth day, but no longer naked. He was wearing boxer shorts. Kennedy demanded to speak to him.

Robert was brought into the main office with the big glass windows and thin walls. He told Kennedy that after he had left the day before, Knott and Young took him from the isolation room and told him to shoot himself with a gun. He said Knott and the facility's owner, "Bishop" John David Young, Jr., the pastor of Solid Rock Ministries in Mobile, were frustrated by Robert's "poor" attitude and continuing depression while in solitary confinement (a leading cause of institutional suicide); and they were determined to change his behavior by any means necessary. They dragged him from the isolation room to Knott's bedroom, where Knott handed the boy the gun and encouraged him to kill himself. Robert told Kennedy he placed the barrel of the gun against his head: "I pulled it, and it went click."

When Kennedy confronted Knott and Young about this gut-wrenching, sadistic bit of theater, they didn't deny the boy's accusation. In fact, they seemed proud of their approach. Knott left the office, went back to his bedroom in the compound and returned with the gun; he placed it in Kennedy's hand, and said, "I was just teaching him a lesson."

Kennedy exploded, "This is how you treat a fourteen-year-old?"

"I knew then I was dealing with crazy people," Kennedy says now. "They were insane: you don't do that to a human being."

Kennedy knew he had to move quickly to seek felony arrests but couldn't do so without the go-ahead of the Mobile County DA, Ashley Rich. He returned to RYA in early November in a final effort to obtain confidential on-site interviews, but Knott arranged a bizarre way to thwart the investigation. Arriving after dinner, Kennedy thought he'd be allowed to interview the cadets privately in the office, but was instead led by Knott to a large shower and bathroom area where boys on their way to the shower were told, one by one, to sit across from Kennedy—while naked—to answer his questions. Even in this surreal setting, Kennedy managed to glean more damaging information from the boys.

The purpose of this stunt was explained later by one of RYA's many victims, William Vargas, who wrote, "After Captain Kennedy left, Mr. Will [Knott] told everyone to write a paper saying that Captain Kennedy wanted to see us naked, and make Captain Kennedy look like a pedophile." This missive was added to the other letters, police reports, personal observations and additional evidence

Kennedy passed to the local DA and the then-Attorney General, Luther Strange, in his futile efforts to get Knott and his sadistic staffers arrested.

After Captain Kennedy conducted those final, limited interviews in November 2011, he went to his chief, Jimmy Gardner, who gave him permission to present his findings to the DA. At that meeting, joined by DA Rich and her chief investigator, Mike Morgan, Kennedy says Gardner moved to give a briefcase to Rich with the documents Kennedy had compiled. Kennedy stopped him, and asked to check the documents before presenting them to the DA. When he inspected the briefcase, he found that half of the documents were missing, so he halted the meeting briefly and went down to his car, where he retrieved copies of all the documents intended for the DA. He then returned to give her a lengthy briefing about all he'd found at RYA—the forced fighting, the isolation cells and shackles, the beatings of naked boys.

After Kennedy made his presentation, he says Rich coolly responded, "Parents need to be more careful where they send their children." (Morgan, speaking for the DA's office, doesn't recall Rich making such a statement.)

"I was in shock," Kennedy says, "and I knew they weren't going to do anything about it."

To placate Kennedy, Rich sent Morgan to investigate. Morgan insists he conducted confidential interviews at RYA, but Kennedy says his cadet sources told him that most of Morgan's interviews were either done while being observed by Knott—or were "cherry-picked" cadets petrified to speak honestly. As a result, the DA took no action.

Karin Bazor, a former instructor for the RYA girls who quit in disgust in July 2012, says that when she approached Morgan early in 2013 with more evidence about abuses at the facility, "He looked at me like I was crazy, and said it's impossible to prosecute someone [whose program is] under a church covering."

Kennedy now gave up any illusions that local law enforcement would do anything to stop the carnage at RYA, and pinned his hopes on the DHR's Mobile-based Child Protection Services director, Beth Nelson. In a meeting with her on November 21, 2011, he laid out all he knew—the documents backing up the abuse and a long, detailed list of witnesses to contact.

Nelson, in turn, agreed to visit RYA. However, Kennedy says, again citing his sources, she made sure everything was ready for her by giving its leaders a two-day advance notice of her investigation.

Nelson found no signs of abuse at the facility, and two subsequent investigations by DHR also couldn't confirm abuse there. Even so, after Nelson conferred with DHR Commissioner Nancy Bruckner and Mike Morgan, they reached an initial decision to close down Restoration Youth Academy on November 28th. But they changed their minds after talking to Young and Knott the next day, and realized they didn't want to face the cost, liability and logistical hassles of removing the endangered kids, according to Kennedy.

Kennedy was infuriated, and called Nelson to protest. "Those are just troubled children and they got what they deserve," the child protection administrator reportedly replied, he says, and told him the agency wouldn't investigate RYA again, even if children escaped and went directly to DHR with recent bruises or wounds. "They're not fresh, so they can't be investigated," she claimed about relatively older signs of physical abuse. (Nelson, since retired, was unavailable for comment, and a DHR spokesperson said it was agency policy not to comment on any closed investigations that didn't involve a fatality.)

"There is more concern about chickens on a poultry farm in Alabama than for children!" says Kennedy.

Over the next few years, first as a police captain and then, after his 2014 retirement, as a concerned citizen, Kennedy wrote detailed letters to Alabama's attorney general, governor, DHR commissioner and other officials outlining the rampant abuse at RYA. All the while he was adding new victims to his list of people to contact.

Early in 2012, Kennedy says he got a brushoff from the Attorney General's chief investigator, Tim Fuhrman, after he'd done an onsite investigation that didn't confirm Kennedy's claims. Fuhrman apparently didn't try to contact RYA's former cadets or their families who were willing to speak about the program's horrors, a point confirmed by some victims. "Nobody ever called me or cared, except Captain Kennedy," says one parent.

On February 3, 2012, Kennedy says he got a call from Fuhrman, who told him the attorney general had determined the case wasn't worth pursuing. Fuhrman relayed AG Luther Strange's views: "These children are from out of state and their parents don't vote here and I don't want the churches mad at me."

In his July 2016 letter to me, Strange denied making such a statement: "The quote attributed to me via Chief Investigator Fuhrman is not true. A potential victim's residency has no impact on our investigation actions. The record of prosecution by this office clearly demonstrates a strong stance against the abuse of any child." He added, "The allegation that my office did a 'superficial job' is unsupported and unfounded."

Kennedy had appealed all the way up to the governor and attorney general, and nothing had happened, so he turned to the local newspaper, *The Mobile Press-Register*, as a confidential source. In March 2012, a story appeared about "questions" regarding RYA, but it focused, in the top section of the article, only on the lack of licensing for the program and its counselor, Aleshia Moffett. The article mentioned in a vague way the "rough treatment" cited by Barry's father, the traumatized boy Kennedy had interviewed during his first visit.

The issue drifted away amid the drastic layoffs at the state's major newspapers of two-thirds of their editorial staff.

In August 2012, Kennedy finally caught a break. He learned that Eric Reyes, by then eighteen, had escaped from RYA, and was not obligated to return to the school since he was now an adult. Reyes stayed with Kennedy until his father arranged to fly him home out west. Eric, who had spent eight months at RYA, was willing to fill out a police report alleging abuse against Knott. Kennedy aided him in obtaining a misdemeanor child abuse warrant that didn't require the DA's approval to be served. Eric said that in addition to witnessing the regular shackling and beating of other cadets, he had been brutally assaulted by Knott, who accused him of stealing money from another youth's wallet. When Eric disputed that claim, Knott grabbed him by the neck and pushed him against a wall, then threw him so hard against a water fountain it fell apart when Eric's head hit it, according to the police report and an eyewitness, Karin Bazor.

Eric filled out the police report on August 7, 2012, in front of Officer Robert Miles, who found it credible enough to serve an arrest warrant on Knott.

That same day, Miles got in his patrol car, heading to RYA, but his chief, Gardner, radioed him to return to police headquarters and hand over the original warrant, as opposed to returning it to the radio dispatch office for future service, according to Kennedy. (Miles could not be reached for comment.) In Kennedy's view, Gardner committed a felony that day: "He hindered the arrest of Knott and the serving of a legitimate warrant." (Kennedy says he still has the original crime report and un-served warrant; Gardner insists this incident never happened.)

In May 2013, facing the city's demand for unpaid back rent, the Prichard school moved to buildings near Rev. Young's Solid Rock Ministries church in Mobile. Kennedy didn't know where they'd gone until he spotted a white boy a few months later peeking out of a boarded-up building where the boys now slept. Kennedy kept up his writing and calls to state officials and legislators, but no one responded.

• • •

IN 2015, AN OUT-OF-STATE MOTHER PICKED UP HER DAUGHTER FROM THE RYA girl's program in Mobile. Horrified by what she saw there, she took cell phone photos of the isolation rooms and then called the on-duty juvenile division detective, Sgt. Joe Cotner, before going to the Mobile Police Department to file an abuse complaint. Cotner recalls that he was skeptical when he took that call, but after seeing the shocking photos, "We started listening to all the allegations of abuse." In March 2015, Cotner referred the complaint to the local DHR for a child abuse investigation, and the new team there—Nelson had re-tired—took the allegations seriously. A DHR-led raid a few days later rescued thirty-six children. The investigators found malnourished chil-dren, isolation rooms and the terrified kids.

Charles Kennedy hadn't known about the investigation, but he glimpsed the raid underway while he was rushing to keep an appoint-ment with a federally-funded disability rights lawyer he was prepping to file a lawsuit against the program. Driving past the ramshackle boys' home, he saw the yellow crime scene tape and the police squad cars surrounding the facility. His heart sunk: "I thought for sure some-one had been murdered." He couldn't stop to find out what happened at the moment, but as soon as he dropped off additional evidence for the attorney, he wheeled around and headed back to the home, fearing the worst. When he pulled up next to the building, he saw then-Captain John Barber, outside after viewing the torture site.

"What's happened?" Kennedy urgently asked him. "Have they killed somebody?"

"No, but I can't believe they haven't," Barber said. "His face was as white as a sheet of paper," Kennedy recalls. Barber, a veteran policeman whose brother James was the police chief, began recount-ing the unimaginable scenes of horror inside—the isolation cells, the shackles, the frightened children. Kennedy knew precisely what he was describing, the same crimes he had fought for nearly five years to stop, and told Barber, "In the trunk of my car I have two briefcases full of evidence on these people. If you want it, you got it." A short while later, Kennedy, now retired, began briefing the lead detective on the case, Cotner, aiding him in building the case against the pro-gram's leaders.

A subsequent grand jury investigation led to the arrest of Knott and the other defendants for felony child abuse in August 2015.

The trial began in January 2017, and Kennedy anxiously at-tended all four days of the proceedings. But as a potential witness, he couldn't sit inside the courtroom and instead relied on a cousin, among others, to brief him on what was happening.

On the final day, when the jury left to begin deliberations, the fatigued crusader drove home for a break. It was 5 p.m., and he was sitting on his front porch, when he got an urgent call from Leslie Crawford, the mother in Maine who had also long fought for Ala-bama law enforcement to crack down on RYA.

"Did you hear about the verdict?" she asked him excitedly.

It had only been two hours since the jury left, and Kennedy couldn't believe what he was hearing. The jury, she explained, had convicted Knott, Young and Moffett on all eleven counts of aggra-vated child abuse, the maximum charge. Kennedy was ecstatic. He asked her to repeat the verdict again to make sure he'd heard correctly.

Not only had he been personally vindicated, but the people he'd been fighting against were finally going to prison.

As he put it in an email to friends and supporters: "All of the monsters were convicted!"

• • •

ON FEBRUARY 22, 2017, KENNEDY FELT A SIMILAR SENSE OF ELATION when a Mobile judge sentenced Knott, Young and Moffett each to twenty years in prison. But his feeling of triumph and vindication is tempered by the fact they got away with it for so long. "They all knew," he says of the government agencies that ignored his pleas, "and they did nothing."

It's a pattern that continues to this day. Neither the long prison sentences nor the shuttering of the brutal facility have fundamentally changed oversight of such programs in almost all states in the country. Over the past twenty years, the Mobile effort against Knott, Young and Moffett remains one of a handful of arrests and prosecutions for physical abuse allegations at any youth treatment facility in the country. With rare exceptions unmonitored religious and secular troubled-teen facilities in Alabama and elsewhere continue to operate with impunity, generally protected by the indifference of local and state police, prosecutors and child protection agencies. "We've received thousands of police reports," but relatively few have led to prosecutions, says Angela Smith, the founder and national coordinator of the Seattle-based Human Earth Animal Liberation advocacy group, better known as HEAL.

Now seventy-three, Kennedy is trying to close other facilities. Most recently, he's briefed the district attorney's office in Baldwin County, Alabama, about troubling abuse allegations at a facility in rural Seminole called Blessed Hope Boys Academy, which is run by pastor Gary Wiggins. In September 2015, an openly gay teenager, Lucas Greenfield, who had been imprisoned at RYA before the March raid was then shipped to Blessed Hope by his mother after he returned to his hometown; in a September 12, 2015 police report, and in conversations with Kennedy, the teen charged that Wiggins had assaulted him, declaring beforehand, "I'm going to get the demon out of you and make you straight." In December 2016, DHR officials and county police raided the place in response to escapees' complaints of solitary confinement and hours-long exercise sessions, leading twenty-two students to be sent back home. Thus far, however, Kennedy's pleas for prosecution have been ignored. "Once again, Alabama law enforcement has failed to protect children," he says. (Wiggins said of the charges: "It's lies, all lies," before hanging up.)

Since the convictions, law enforcement and other public officials such as Morgan and Strange have begun trying to discredit Kennedy, using his final interview with the boys against him. While Kennedy says Knott forced the boys to take off their clothes—and the evidence from Vargas and others supports him—Knott told state and local investigators otherwise. Some officials such as Morgan and Strange now claim that's in part why they failed to act—even though they've long been aware such charges are bogus, Kennedy says. "We had questions about the way Kennedy conducted his investigation," Morgan told me, citing the naked interviews.

Morgan added, slyly, "I don't want to imply he did anything improper."

Kennedy's response: "This is not true."

Kennedy is equally outraged that former state Attorney General Luther Strange has been appointed a US senator to replace Jeff Sessions, the new US Attorney General. "He [Strange] threw the children under the bus so he could grease the way for his political ambitions," Kennedy says. "All these politicians have lined their pockets with the blood of children."

• • •

THE REFUSAL TO ACT BY NEARLY EVERYONE IN AUTHORITY IN ALABAMA took its toll on the children imprisoned in the school, and its horrific legacy lives on long after the program was shut down. Erin Rodriguez, now eighteen, was a pill-popping runaway in suburban Atlanta before she was sent to RYA. "They would whip me," she says. "They stripped me to my underwear and bra and took out a belt and hit me until I bled."

At Prichard, she was also placed in an isolation room for a month after an escape attempt. "I was crying and angry every day, and I was in shackles and handcuffs." She pounded on the wood door, shouting to be released, but was only given brief bathroom breaks about twice a day, and, a few times a week, the chance to take a shower. "I felt like a dog," she recalls, lying on the hard concrete floor with nails sticking up here and there, trying to avoid the bugs crawling all around. "It was nasty."

She tried to tell her father about the whippings and beatings and isolation rooms when she went back home on brief leaves, but he didn't believe her and kept sending her back. She was there when the police and child protection workers swept in to take her and the other fourteen girls held in the all-girls facility, augmenting the raid that took away twenty-one boys from the home across from Rev. Young's church about the same time. Erin says it felt like a SWAT team rescue operation. "They were shouting, 'Where are the girls? Where are the girls?'" she recalls. "I was so happy to be going home to Atlanta." She continues to have nightmares about what happened to her.

There is plenty of talk these days among experts about "trauma-informed care" for young people whose brains are especially vulnerable to severe trauma as children and adolescents, but there is almost no guidance offered about how individuals—like these RYA survivors—can go about obtaining such specialized care.

(There's no definitive list, but good places to start are the certified Trauma-Focused Cognitive Behavioral Therapy clinicians found at https://tfcbt.org/members/; the outpatient clinics that are part of the National Child Traumatic Stress Network at www.nctsnet.org/about-us; and the licensed professionals certified by the group promoting an alternative, evidence-based practice for trauma known as Eye Movement Desensitization and Reprocessing (EMDR) therapy at www.emdria.org/search/newsearch.asp.)

Dr. J. Douglas Bremner, the Emory University psychiatry professor who specializes in PTSD, has outlined self-help stress reduction techniques and a guide to proven professional care in his indispensable book, *You Can't Just Snap Out of It*. He points out that only about 15 percent of people who experience traumatic events actually develop long-term PTSD, but, he says, "Half of those patients experience short-term symptoms, but they will eventually grow out of it." Yet in the end, many of the young people who went through the program remain severely damaged. And neither the long prison sentences handed Knott and his accomplices nor the shuttering of their brutal facilities have fundamentally changed oversight of such programs virtually anywhere in the country.

Yet, surprisingly, in fundamentalist-dominated Alabama, there's finally some hope because of a new law in the state to regulate all private residential teen programs under DHR. Kids are required to be allowed unlimited communication with outsiders, while local police where the programs are located have been granted the unfettered right to inspect the sites in response to abuse allegations and bring charges if needed without relying on the children's guardians or parents. It's the strongest law in the country, and with the support of the state's religious groups, it passed the legislature unanimously in May. Its success was due in part to the exposure of the crimes of RYA leaders, with added attention brought to Kennedy's reform crusade by an investigative feature in March 2017 on ABC's *20/20* and, possibly, my article on the RYA sadists in *Newsweek*. But that law doesn't help those people who've already been brutalized.

After being released into the custody of his grandparents in a small Texas town, Robert, the bipolar teen given a gun to shoot himself by Knott, continued to unravel. In the late fall of 2016, the traumatized, suicidal youth was found by police sitting on his mother's grave with a gun and some drugs, then arrested and sent to jail by the officers. The police and juvenile court judge ignored pleas from Captain Kennedy that he needed mental health treatment instead, as he had argued after his first drug arrest in 2015. After the first arrest, with his family too poor to afford bail, he wrote to Captain Kennedy, "Each day I'm subjected to 'ISO' [isolation], I grow more and more depressed. The flashbacks are becoming realer, so real in fact I've woken up in a cold sweat gasping for air as though I was being strangled, which was sometimes a daily event in RYA." (As of this writing, he's been suffering from untreated mood swings while in jail more than ninety days, even if he's not kept in solitary confinement.)

In another town, Eric's father, Joe, is just left with the memory of all the money he wasted—nearly $15,000 on school fees alone—and a son, now twenty-two, continuing to deteriorate after coming back home to California.

Eric shouldn't have ended up in RYA in the first place after he mutated into a depressed, drug-abusing teen. There were few mental health professionals available in the Coachella Valley, where the Reyes family lived. One evening, Joe heard strange noises coming from sixteen-year-old Eric's bedroom, and entered to find him hanging from a rope slung over the top post of a bunk bed. He rushed forward to hold up his body to prevent strangulation, then called 911. Eric was sent to an under-staffed area hospital for a few weeks, then he was kicked out without any treatment plan, medications or referrals, still deeply depressed. Joe turned to RYA after finding it online.

These days, he is not always sure where Eric is: Sometimes he sleeps out in the streets, sometimes he drifts back to the house. "I am very upset. I can't do anything for him," Reyes says, unable to speak for a while, choking up with tears about the son he tried to help. "He's not doing good at all. It's taking forever to recover, and all he has are bad memories."

The traumas such young people face is why Kennedy continues to fight against abuse.

"One of my greatest satisfactions is knowing that these children who suffered so much at their hands know that justice has been served in some way," he says, but "you can't return the youth that was stolen from them, you can't restore the mental and physical damage that was done."

Yet for one forty-five-year-old woman, Jodi Hobbs, the president of Survivors of Institutional Abuse, the ongoing failures in Alabama and other states have a deeper, personal meaning. She has sought for over a decade to provide services to victims and prevent future abuse, in part to help others avoid the trauma she experienced as a seventeen-year-old girl in the Victory Christian Academy, shut down amid allegations of physical and sexual abuse in 1991. She worked with *The Tampa Bay Times* in publicizing and then helping close the founder's new facility nearly twenty-five years later in Florida. She's moved on with her life, becoming the mother of five and having a successful tech consulting career, while helping win passage last year of a California law extending at least nominal oversight to religious programs. But when she learned about RYA's isolation rooms and violence, it brought her back to her own time that broke her spirit in her academy's "Get Right" confinement rooms. "When I saw what happened at Restoration Youth Academy," she says, "it breaks my heart, I feel so defeated as a survivor."

Despite recent successes, like the convictions of Knott and the new California law, she doesn't see real change in enforcement happening until a broader shift in public and family attitudes takes place. "These are throwaway children," she observes. "They are looked at as dollar signs, not as individuals."

CHAPTER 12

Profits and Losses from Residential Treatment: The Story of Bain Capital and CRC Health

THE APPARENT NEGLECT AND TORTURE ENDURED BY ERIN RODRIGUEZ and Eric Reyes and the other teens in an Alabama religious facility were, sadly enough, hardly unique. This sort of victimization did not result solely from a fanatical application of fundamentalist beliefs, but also arose from something even more common: exploiting desperation for profit.

When Dana Blum, a recent widow living in Portland, Oregon, made the fateful decision to send her son Brendan to Youth Care, a residential program for troubled teens located in the suburbs of Salt Lake City, it seemed like a beacon of hope. "Our treatment center," Youth Care's website proclaimed, "is an excellent vessel for adolescents to begin turning their lives around with the help of our highly trained and dedicated professionals."

Brendan, a fourteen-year-old boy with Asperger's syndrome, had been extremely aggressive for years; he was even arrested a few times after attacking members of his family. Local therapists hadn't helped, and six months after her husband died, Dana was frantically casting about for solutions. A consultation with UCLA's neuropsychiatric unit convinced her that Youth Care's therapeutic and educational program would finally make a difference.

Four months into his stay there, Brendan had earned a reputation as a temper-prone student who tried to shirk his obligations. So on the afternoon of June 27 when he complained to medical staff that he felt very sick, as if something was "crawling around" in his stomach, his concerns were dismissed. After 11 p.m., he woke up, complaining of stomach pain, and defecated in his pants. The on-duty monitors took him to the Purple Room, a makeshift isolation room used to segregate misbehaving students. There, he suffered a long night of agony, howling in pain and repeatedly vomiting and soiling himself. According to court transcripts and police reports, the two poorly paid monitors on duty did little more than offer him water, Sprite and Pepto-Bismol. They never telephoned the on-call nurse and waited until nearly 2 a.m. to contact the on-call supervisor, only to leave a voicemail. There was little else they felt they could do—Youth Care's protocol on emergency services meant they were too low on the totem pole to call 911 themselves.

"They didn't trust our judgment in emergency situations," explains Josh Randall, a former Youth Care residential monitor, who wasn't on duty that night. "If you're working for $9.50 an hour on the graveyard shift, you don't want to buck the system." At any rate, the monitors had little expertise in how to respond—it was an entry-level job requiring only a GED, plus a CPR and safety course overseen by Youth Care itself.

When the morning staff arrived at 7 a.m., they discovered Brendan facedown on the floor of the Purple Room, his body already stiff with rigor mortis. The state's chief medical examiner later determined that Blum had died of a twisted bowel "infarction," which requires emergency surgical intervention.

"It made me very angry that they couldn't provide better emergency services for my son," Dana Blum told the online magazine *Momlogic* in 2009. "I feel like he was murdered." In fact, no court has ever found Aspen Education, the corporate division overseeing Youth Care, or its staffers and subsidiaries, guilty of murder or other crimes. Blum, with the help of insurance and school district aid, paid Youth Care $15,000 a month in 2007 for Brendan's care. Now she can't speak publicly about the case as part of a wrongful death settlement she reached in 2011 with Youth Care of Utah and its parent company, CRC's Aspen Education.

The failure at Youth Care was not due simply to the carelessness of a few workers—a point underscored when a Utah court found that the threshold needed to pursue criminal negligence charges against the two monitors in 2008 wasn't met and the charges were dismissed. And it wasn't the only example of alleged negligence or abuse at treatment centers for adult addicts and "troubled teens" that were owned by Aspen's parent company, CRC Health Group, according to a review of government reports, court filings and official complaints by parents and employees, along with interviews with former clients and staff.

In late 2014, CRC Health was sold for $1.3 billion to Acadia Healthcare, a chain of addiction and mental health facilities. That amounted to a modest profit for Bain Capital, which bought the firm in 2006. But that acquisition doesn't necessarily mean a shift in the CRC facilities' corporate culture: The CEO of CRC Health Group, Jerry Rhodes, an executive with CRC since 2003, remained in charge as it joined Acadia. That could be seen as a potentially ominous sign for those aggrieved staff members, patients, surviving family members and young people all too familiar with those sorts of operations.

To be fair, Acadia, under the leadership of CEO Joey Jacobs since 2011, has faced relatively few of the public lawsuits, investigations and complaints about neglect and deaths that have dogged the other major behavioral health companies. These include Jacobs's own Psychiatric Solutions, Inc. (PSI), once the largest provider of inpatient psychiatric services, which he sold to the larger, scandal-plagued Universal Health Services chain in 2010 for $2 billion. Jacobs has long disputed allegations of neglect, sexual violence and wrongful death at PSI facilities following a *ProPublica* series that started in 2008.

So it didn't really seem to matter to investors that CRC or its Aspen Education division was marked by several wrongful death lawsuits; a $9 million settlement in 2014 with the Justice Department for allegedly defrauding Medicaid by providing substandard care; and at least ten potentially preventable patient deaths so far since being acquired by Bain in 2006. These deaths included four patients in less than two years at its premier drug-treatment facility, Sierra Tucson in Arizona, known for treating celebrities such as Ringo Starr and Rush Limbaugh.

All told, since CRC acquired the high-end, $50,000-a-month treatment center in 2005, six people have died in the facility as of this writing, most recently in August 2015.

Sierra Tucson has been considered a world-class treatment facility, especially proud of its expertise in dealing with "dually-diagnosed" patients with mental illness and substance abuse. Its website proclaims, "If you or a loved one is battling a chemical dependency concern and the debilitating symptoms of a mental health condition, look no further than Sierra Tucson's Addiction and Co-Occurring Disorder Program."

Despite that promise, January 2015 began with the death of one such patient when a fifty-five-year-old Pennsylvania man, Richard Lecce, who was supposed to be on suicide watch, hanged himself with a belt in his room. He was found "unconscious but still breathing" in his room by staffers who had spent the previous two hours looking for him, witnesses told investigators for the Pinal County Medical Examiner's Office. A few weeks later, Sierra Tucson's CEO, William Anderson, said the staff was "extremely saddened," but asserted, "Suicide prevention is a key focus." In December 2015, Lecce's family filed a wrongful death lawsuit, citing the program's monitoring failures in the death of the deeply depressed engineer whose family cashed in $64,800 in savings to pay for his uninsured care. Sierra Tucson's CEO William Anderson told the *Arizona Daily Star* that he couldn't comment because the issue was being litigated.

Unfortunately, Sierra Tucson's staff and leadership—consistent with the general practice of CRC over the years—don't seem to learn from their mistakes, and virtually never apologize or admit wrongdoing. With toothless state oversight so commonplace, why should they? For instance, when the facility reached a June 2015 settlement with the state to improve monitoring and pay a $7,500 fine following Lecce's January 2015 suicide, its lawyers said the agreement wasn't "an admission of violation, wrongdoing or liability." Yet it was just a few months later, on August 27, 2015, that a fifty-nine-year-old California man hanged himself in his bathroom closet with shoelaces— despite the facility's previous promises to track patient movements. Even so, in October 2015, state health officials *still* didn't crack down: they ended the facility's probationary period, loosened oversight and accepted yet another fine for $27,000.

As usual, Sierra Tucson's leadership followed the same script they have used ever since a suicidal patient's corpse was found on the grounds in 2011. In their October 2015 agreement with the state, Sierra Tucson officials vowed yet again to make improvements in screening and monitoring patients. But the problems continued: The facility was also required to pay another $4,000 in July 2016 for its repeated deficiencies, some involving failed health monitoring, in its fifteen-bed psychiatric care unit. Anderson issued a statement after this penalty: "The safety and well-being of our residents is our utmost priority," while noting the facility's full cooperation with state regulators to "understand guidelines" affecting the program.

Yet by the end of 2015, the year of the last reported fatality, there had been so many allegedly needless deaths due to the same sorts of staff mishaps that it was hard to keep them all straight. It would take an entire book to chronicle all the mistakes in full, but it's worth offering a summary review of the deaths so far. (Some of the wrongful death lawsuits and state health reports can be viewed online at this book's companion website, mentalhealthinc.net, and at Tucson.com.) With perhaps one exception, virtually all of them follow a similar pattern: It begins with a suicidal or disoriented patient signaling to the staff his interest in killing himself or exhibiting other signs of severe distress. Then after the patient commits suicide, the similarities continue through the state's death investigation, which usually ends with a modest fine and Sierra Tucson agreeing to make improvements. Then sometime later, another patient dies and the cycle starts all over again.

At some point in these deadly repeat performances, families usually get around to filing their wrongful death lawsuits—and executives dutifully decline to comment while litigation is pending or after they reach confidential settlements. Of course, the size of the regulatory fines, the precise method of death and the promised reforms vary in specifics, but the general framework remains the same. Reviewing the highlights puts this string of deaths in a broader context:

- In March 2007, a few years after CRC bought Sierra Tucson, a thirty-four-year-old patient, Toby Blanck, drowned in the facility's swimming pool but nearby staff didn't respond. As recounted in the *Tucson Sentinel* and in online memorials to him, he favored long stretches of underwater swimming but blacked out. Citing a confidential source, the *Sentinel* reported that staffers may have believed he was pretending to drown as he had reportedly done in the past. The family's wrongful death lawsuit against the facility was settled out of court in 2013.

- In August 2011, shortly after admitting a deeply depressed patient, California physician Dr. Edward Litwak, the staff assessed him as being at "high risk" of suicide, but he was nonetheless transferred to the center's poorly monitored residential section. He was soon reported missing, but it took the staff *two weeks* to find his body on the grounds near the horse stables. A wrongful death lawsuit against the facility was settled for undisclosed terms in September 2014.

- In January 2014, a fifty-nine-year-old patient from Phoenix with a history of depression and anxiety hanged himself with a shoelace attached to a showerhead, as *The Arizona Daily Star* first reported. The day before the incident, a staff counselor overheard the distressed man telling his wife on the phone of his plans to kill himself. His alarmed wife immediately called the staff to inquire about removing him, yet they convinced her to let him stay, while failing to note the incident in his chart or to increase monitoring of him. Though the state fined the facility $2,000 for its apparent neglect, the facility didn't admit liability and Sierra Tucson avoided further damages by apparently settling with the family even before a lawsuit was filed.

- In April 2014, a disoriented, depressed twenty-year-old patient confided to a nurse, "I want to die," even as his doctor later assessed him at "low risk" of suicide. A few days later, he was found face down on the floor of his room. He died two days later from what an autopsy determined was lethal drug toxicity. It's still not clear whether his death was accidental or a suicide, but his mother filed a wrongful death lawsuit in April 2016, blaming Sierra Tucson's lax procedures. The state penalty imposed on Sierra Tucson for the tragedy: a $250 fine and an order to train staff again on suicide monitoring protocols.

- On January 2, 2015, staff members seemingly chose to ignore the lessons from those required suicide prevention trainings imposed after the earlier suicides. As a result, they allowed the new middle-aged patient from Pennsylvania, Richard Lecce, to wander around unobserved for hours before he hanged himself. Sierra Tucson entered into a new state enforcement agreement in May 2014 to improve suicide risk assessment, hold more prevention trainings and upgrade monitoring of drug interactions.

- In August 2015, a fifty-nine-year-old California man hanged himself in his bathroom closet with his shoelaces tied together. Sierra Tucson officials promised again later in the year to make reforms.

• • •

So in 2016, when Sierra Tucson officials paid their most recent fine—for deficiencies in their psychiatric inpatient unit—they followed the same time-tested response virtually all CRC facilities have employed for over a decade: they didn't acknowledge any culpability. Once again, no one in authority at CRC appeared to be held accountable for anything that went wrong.

Welcome to the world of loosely monitored for-profit behavioral health care in which profits and cost-cutting priorities can easily trump patient safety. By January 2015, after the Acadia deal was signed, the leadership of CRC Health appeared ready to turn the page and put all those messy lawsuits and deaths behind them—until two more Sierra Tucson patients killed themselves before the summer of 2015 was over. Akin to VA officials rarely facing punishment for wrongdoing, when there was no culture of accountability and enforcement in Sierra Tucson and other CRC programs, patients' lives were seemingly also endangered.

CRC originally purchased Sierra Tucson in 2005 for $130 million as its "crown jewel" shortly before plans to sell CRC to Bain were announced. "Then the business side started controlling admissions," says a former employee, who worked at Sierra Tucson before and after the CRC acquisition. "It doesn't take a brain scientist to realize that if you reduce staff [in key programs] and add sicker patients, there's going to be trouble." By 2009, even before Litwak's 2011 death, the state health department fined the facility for having insufficient staff to prevent high-risk patients from wandering off.

Nevertheless, any fines, deaths or wrongful death lawsuits across the CRC chain didn't prove to be much of a problem for potential buyers of CRC by 2014, when Bain looked to sell the company. Bain was following its customary practice of increasing an acquisition's revenues and then reselling after five to seven years. The CRC firm was considered an appealing asset in the burgeoning $220 billion behavioral health field, which includes government clinics, nonprofit hospitals and for-profit treatment centers. Dana Blum and other grieving family members, however, were likely not cheered by this upbeat financial news.

• • •

IN LOOKING INTO CRC IN 2012 FOR *SALON*, I FOUND PREVIOUSLY UNRE-ported allegations of abuse and neglect in at least ten CRC residential drug and teen care facilities across the country, including three I visited undercover in Utah and California in 2012. When I looked again at CRC in 2015 and 2016, the same types of dangers seemingly continued unabated, emblematic of broader failings in the residential treatment field. These include facilities owned by corporate leaders such as the UHS hospital chain; small locally owned sites such as the Tierra Blanca ranch for troubled teens in New Mexico, whose owners faced lawsuits for alleged fraud, "torture" and wrongful death until the claims were quietly settled in 2016, but they continue to strongly dispute the allegation; and, of course, the unfettered, brutal religious programs such as Restoration Youth Academy. I was surprised to learn that some facilities I had covered earlier, such as Sierra Tucson, had apparently become even less safe after the scandals erupted. With the rare exceptions of the publicity aimed at a few CRC facilities in Arizona, Utah and Tennessee, the incidents I found have largely escaped national notice or even sustained local attention because the programs are, thanks to lax state regulations, largely unaccountable.

Court documents and ex-staffers also charged that such incidents reflect, in part, a broader corporate culture at CRC Health Group, still a leading national chain of treatment centers even though it's operating as a division of Acadia. A series of lawsuits alleging wrongful death and abuse, augmented by the criticism of former staff and clients, have portrayed CRC as prizing profits—and the avoidance of outside scrutiny—over the health and safety of its clients. (Back in 2012, I sent specific questions on these basic charges to CRC and its original owner, Bain Capital. CRC would answer only general questions; Bain did not reply. Acadia executives didn't reply to my recent requests for comment.) But the Acadia company, despite its over $1 billion in revenue, conceded in its 2015 financial statement that its rosy predictions for CRC and other divisions faced some risk: "The occurrence of patient incidents could adversely affect the price of our common stock and result in incremental regulatory burdens and governmental investigations."

And CRC's corporate culture, in turn, still reflected in large measure the no-holds-barred attitudes and financial imperatives of its owner for eight years, Bain Capital, the private equity firm co-founded by Mitt Romney. (The Romney campaign in 2012 did not reply to written questions about Romney's continuing investment revenues from CRC after he left Bain Capital.) As early as 2007, Romney also personally faced public scrutiny over his ties to reportedly abusive teen programs: Two of his leading GOP fundraisers, Mel Sembler and Robert Lichfield, founded and ran controversial chains of troubled-teen facilities, Straight, Inc., and the World Wide Association of Specialty Programs and Schools (WWASPS). Those scandal-marked programs and their spin-off facilities have variously faced allegations and lawsuits over horrific abuse, false imprisonment or neglect they have strongly denied. *Time* magazine's Maia Szalavitz, the author of the first major book on these programs, *Help at Any Cost*, wrote a scathing article about Romney and these influential donors for *Reason* magazine headlined: "Romney, Torture and Teens."

• • •

WHEN BAIN PURCHASED CRC IN 2006, IT LOOKED LIKE AN INVESTMENT masterstroke. The CRC company, founded in the mid-'90s with a single California treatment facility, the Camp Recovery Center, had quickly grown into the largest chain of for-profit drug and alcohol treatment services in the country, with $230 million in annual revenue. Under Bain's guidance, its revenue nearly doubled, to more than $450 million by the time it was sold in 2014. CRC now serves over 30,000 clients daily—mostly opiate addicts—at more than 140 facilities across twenty-five states. Of course, when CRC was sold to Acadia, certain Bain investors made out well, including presumably Mitt Romney, when the company received 6.3 million shares of Acadia stock valued at almost $2 billion. Bain's original purchase of CRC, a leveraged buyout, had also saddled CRC with massive debt of well over $600 million.

The 2006 CRC acquisition immediately made Bain owner of the largest collection of addiction treatment facilities—both inpatient and outpatient—in the nation. And by receiving millions of shares of Acadia stock in 2015, Bain Capital is still heavily invested in the behavioral health care field. In a report in April 2015 on the health-care market for private equity investors, Bain Capital remained optimistic about the profit potential of the US behavioral health segment, citing continuing loose regulation and the expansion of the health-care market under the Affordable Care Act.

Even after the sale to Acadia, the story of Bain Capital's handling of CRC Health remains an object lesson in how the drive to maximize revenues can place vulnerable people at risk. According to company executives and independent analysts, hands-on oversight of subsidiary companies was a hallmark of both Bain and CRC, so any major problems in their facilities should have been known to officials in charge of CRC.

These factors are still at work in the maltreatment, needless deaths and fraud alleged in lawsuits, media accounts and government investigations aimed at today's giant in this field, the UHS chain. With nearly two hundred behavioral health care facilities—including troubled-teen and addiction programs—in the United States, joined by a few dozen general acute care hospitals, it rakes in over $9 billion in revenue annually, over half of it from Medicaid and Medicare. It is by far the nation's leading provider of inpatient mental health and addiction services, with 20 percent of the market. The company's Chief Financial Officer, Steve Filton, even admitted to investors in 2013 that weak oversight of UHS and other behavioral care providers is a key to the field's financial success: "It tends to get, I don't want to say no attention, but a fairly minimal amount of attention from [government and private] payers, which I think is generally a good thing." (For nearly thirty years, spokespeople for the company have denied corporate wrongdoing in the deaths or suicides of patients at their facilities, going as far back as two teenagers who died while being restrained at UHS facilities in Pennsylvania and North Carolina in the late 1990s. Occasionally, states have stopped sending kids to UHS centers.)

Bain was flexible in using its private equity strategies to squeeze more money out of CRC Health. Unlike some Bain Capital acquisitions, which have led to massive layoffs, Bain's approach with CRC was to boost revenues by gobbling up other treatment centers, raising fees and expanding its client base through slick, aggressive marketing, while keeping staffing and other costs relatively low. But that rapid pace of acquisition couldn't be sustained in the mostly small-scale drug treatment industry alone. So Bain Capital and CRC set their sights on an entirely new treatment arena: the multibillion-dollar "troubled teen" industry, a burgeoning field of mostly locally owned residential schools; Residential Treatment Centers (RTCs) offering mental health and drug treatment services; and wilderness programs. As mentioned earlier they all served, nationwide, at least 200,000 kids facing addiction and emotional or behavioral problems, according to GAO estimates and other reports.

One of CRC's first acquisitions under Bain ownership was the Aspen Education Group. Founded in 1998 with about six schools, Aspen Education had expanded to thirty troubled-teen and weight-loss programs by 2006, including Youth Care of Utah. With Bain's backing, CRC purchased Aspen for nearly $300 million in the fall of 2006.

Less than a year later, Brendan Blum was dead.

• • •

AT THE TIME OF THE CRC ACQUISITION, ASPEN ALREADY HAD A HISTORY of abuse allegations, including at least three lawsuits, and two known patient deaths, one by suicide. Featured on *Dr. Phil*, Aspen grew out of schools inspired by the "tough-love" behavior-modification approach of the discredited Synanon program, which was eventually exposed as a dangerous cult.

Aspen, in some ways, sought to present itself as the more professional and somewhat kinder version of Mel Sembler's Straight, Inc., but one that would still use tough-love techniques to dramatically improve kids' lives. The spartan, harsh conditions, ostensibly designed to toughen the spirit of wayward youth, also saved money and boosted profits.

In October 2006, just nine months before Brendan Blum died and as Bain's deal to purchase Aspen Education was being finalized, CRC received an alarming assessment of Aspen's quality. Following some phone conversations, family therapist Elisabeth Feldman walked into CRC's Cupertino, California, headquarters to see Dr. Thomas Brady, a psychiatrist then serving as CRC's chief medical officer, in order to confront him about a host of issues at Youth Care. She had stumbled upon the problems while trying to help her son's former girlfriend, a teenage girl who had suffered what Feldman called "gross mistreatment" at Youth Care. Of particular concern to Feldman was a three-month delay before Youth Care hired a psychiatrist to assess the young woman's deep depression and a failure to treat her Lyme disease. Feldman's ultimately unsuccessful crusade to get the woman released had led her to seek the services of a Salt Lake City lawyer, Thomas Burton, who had earlier settled two lawsuits against Aspen Education for fraud, neglect and abuse.

Feldman had been part of Brady's professional referral network for years, but this visit wasn't congenial. Feldman presented Brady with a one-hundred-page sheaf of legal and corporate documents about Aspen Education programs—including her affidavit describing "brutish punishment and isolation" at Youth Care—in order to support her charges of abusive treatment and neglect. These claims included reportedly covering up the alleged sexual assault of a female student by an Aspen employee at Turn-About Ranch in Utah—the girl was later duct-taped and restrained by staff, a former employee, Toni Thayer, told Feldman. Thayer had written complaints about abusive staff conduct to management, state regulators and the Garfield County sheriff in 2004—but no sanctions followed.

According to Feldman, who has passed away since I interviewed her, Brady said he wasn't aware of any problems at Youth Care or Aspen Education and sought to mollify her about Bain's pending purchase of Aspen: "I have to trust that Bain did their due diligence," she recalled him saying. Brady confirmed, by email, that he spoke on the phone and met with Feldman, but said he has "no recollection" of making those remarks. And he insists that the documents she brought didn't support her claims of mistreatment. Even so, he says he took her concerns seriously and that CRC and Aspen conducted a thorough review. "I came to the conclusion," he said, "there was no merit to the accusations." He remained as CRC's medical director until May 2009, and said that although he encountered a few "untoward event" cases at Aspen during his time there, he saw no "pattern" of unsafe care.

At any rate, Bain's purchase of Aspen Education went ahead smoothly. When, months later, Feldman learned about Blum's death, she was horrified to realize her warnings had had no effect. "For Bain and the big guys, nobody cared," she said. "It was all about the money."

• • •

BRENDAN BLUM'S DEATH WAS THE FIRST PUBLICLY REPORTED DEATH DUE to apparent neglect in CRC's twelve-year history. But in the years since Bain Capital acquired the company in 2006 and, later, when Acadia took over, there have been at least ten more seemingly preventable deaths of patients at CRC's residential programs. Starting with the initial Bain takeover, critics and former employees charge that corporate attitudes have too often emphasized cutting costs and limiting public scrutiny at the expense of safety and quality of care. These tendencies appear to have produced risky, potentially life-threatening practices—only a handful of which have drawn public attention. Despite several lawsuits settled confidentially, CRC has been a significant player in the scandal-prone, decentralized field of teen residential treatment that has by some measures about 4,000 scattered facilities; the firm has roughly twenty therapeutic schools, drug treatment programs and wilderness sites catering to youth (not all of them using "tough love" techniques) out of its roughly 145 facilities nationwide.

These days, it's not at all clear that anything has changed in the philosophy of CRC after its sale to Acadia Healthcare. Jerry Rhodes, CRC's then-CEO, boasted at the time of the 2014 sale: "Together we will grow and excel by providing industry-leading patient care at a time of profound need in behavioral health care." In truth, the CRC that Acadia purchased was hardly a model of across-the-board quality care. After too many lives were damaged and some lost forever, it became, if you looked closely behind the shimmering facade of caring it presented, a cautionary model of something else altogether: what can go wrong when the profit motive enters the sensitive arena of helping people with mental health and addiction problems turn their lives around.

CHAPTER 13

Recipe for Disaster?: Residential Treatment Programs for Addicts and Kids

By February 2015, when Acadia finalized its takeover of CRC from Bain Capital, the decades of failed regulation that made the residential treatment field so appealing to corporations had proved to have an unwelcome downside. Now Acadia was responsible for cleaning up the legal mess CRC left behind with some of its wrongful death lawsuits while Acadia's executives also had to fight off new pending and potential legal claims.

A spate of rehab incidents well before Acadia acquired CRC suggests a corporate culture at CRC that often downplayed safety and quality of care. In 2010, at least two drug treatment patients died while being treated at the overcrowded New Life Lodge in Burns, Tennessee, according to wrongful death lawsuits and an investigative series in *The Tennessean*. A third patient died shortly after being discharged while allegedly overmedicated, according to yet another wrongful death lawsuit. According to the account in *The Tennessean*, one of the patients, a twenty-nine-year-old mother named Lindsey Poteet, came down with pneumonia and was drifting into unconsciousness when she was driven in a private van to a Nashville hospital thirty miles away. The journey was undertaken on orders of the facility's medical director, although another hospital lay just eight miles down the road. Poteet stopped breathing en route and died the next day in Nashville. This wrongful death lawsuit was settled by mediation for an undisclosed sum in December 2013.

After *The Tennessean* series first reported on these incidents, the state's Department of Mental Health froze all new admissions to the facility. (It was finally allowed to admit a smaller number of new patients in early April 2012, but Medicaid and Medicare still won't pay for patients there.)

One former patient, Malea Fox, who had befriended Poteet at New Life, told me that she called state Medicaid (also known as Tenn-Care), the facility's primary funder, to complain that the facility was far too overcrowded for personalized care. "All they [New Life] care about is making money," she told me.

There's a continuing mystery about Lindsey Poteet's death that haunts her mother and investigators: Why did the center staff drive her past the hospital emergency room down the road to a hospital nearly an hour away?

This puzzled everyone looking at the case, except, I later discovered, the workers at a comparably dangerous and woodsy CRC drug facility in California's Santa Cruz County, Camp Recovery. They weren't surprised, and told me that most likely the New Life staff and administrators didn't want to draw further attention to their allegedly life-threatening, slipshod care by repeatedly calling ambulances to take their sick or dying patients to the nearest emergency room. At Camp Recovery they, too, were instructed to avoid calling 911 or police in emergencies if at all possible. Trevor Bottoroff, a former Camp Recovery counselor, told me about the program: "I remember witnessing a lot of discussions among staff about whether they should call 911—but that couldn't happen unless the executive director gave permission."

In a field rife with neglect and poor quality care enabled by indifferent government oversight, CRC's New Life facility stood out because it was particularly bad. The Department of Justice won a $9.25 million settlement in 2014 against CRC for submitting false claims to Medicaid because care there was allegedly "substandard." It's hard to overstate just how rare such a legal initiative is because poor quality care is so commonplace. As ably documented in Anne Fletcher's definitive *Inside Rehab*, most, but hardly all, drug treatment facilities are mediocre, sometimes harmful and overwhelmingly ineffective, in part because they usually don't offer state-of-the-art treatments. In a statement announcing the settlement, Assistant Attorney General for the Justice Department's Civil Division Stuart F. Delery declared, "We will not tolerate health care providers who prioritize profit margins over the needs of their patients."

The Justice Department ultimately accused New Life of engaging in a variety of deceptive and harmful practices in a civil complaint, including billing Medicaid for substance abuse therapy services that weren't provided. CRC, once again, avoided admitting any wrong-doing. Like Camp Recovery, New Life remains one of the CRC companies that are still part of Acadia, now doing business as Mirror Lake Recovery Center.

In the spirit of Aspen Education and CRC, Acadia's new leadership also took a "No retreat, no surrender" approach to handling controversy. In Acadia's 8-K filing with the SEC in May 2015, it announced it would fight the remaining wrongful death cases against New Life seeking a total of $27.5 million in damages from the facility, brought on behalf of two other patients who died, Patrick Bryant and Savon Kinney.

In a conference call with investors, analysts and business reporters in April 2015 about their booming quarterly results, Acadia and CRC executives also hailed CRC's robust revenue performance and quality. There were no reporters' questions about lawsuits, Department of Justice fines or needless deaths that took place in the past and might again in the future in the pursuit of higher profit margins. All that counted for both the executives of Acadia and the reporters covering them was that the company was making money, seemingly fueled by what Jerry Rhodes, CRC's then-CEO, had boasted was "industry-leading patient care."

• • •

IN REALITY, HERE'S WHAT THAT INDUSTRY-LEADING CARE LOOKED LIKE close-up.

In 2009, the state of Oregon forced the closing of two teen programs run by Aspen Education. State investigators found nine cases of abuse and neglect at Mount Bachelor Academy in central Oregon, including incidents of "sexualized role play," in which young patients were allegedly forced to give lap dances during therapy sessions. After Mount Bachelor and its director initially filed a potentially costly counter-claim against the state, the state's Department of Human Services softened the language of the report; CRC claimed the allegations were false (while also fighting $48 million in abuse lawsuits over the school's practices.) Even so, DHS "stands by our findings," a spokesperson said of the 2009 report.

By January 2015, fifty-one former students privately settled three separate lawsuits asking for millions in damages against Mount Bachelor (which closed in 2009), Aspen Education and CRC for alleged sexual abuse and maltreatment. As usual, there was no finding of wrongdoing and no public damages required of CRC—an approach that, critics note, the Catholic Church also used successfully to keep the lid on abuse allegations for decades.

In 2009, the same year that Oregon investigators found abuse and neglect at the CRC-owned Mount Bachelor, its SageWalk Wilderness School proved deadly for a student in another part of the state. In Redmond, sixteen-year-old Sergey Blashchishen died of heatstroke on his very first school hike on a sweltering August day, outfitted with an eighty-pound backpack and scorned by staff as he staggered and fell to the ground exhausted. They contended he was faking his symptoms and didn't call 911 until his pulse had stopped. The county sheriff recommended homicide charges but none were ever filed by the prosecutor; the state ordered the school shut down and a lawsuit brought against the school by Sergey's mother was settled for an undisclosed amount.

These sorts of complaints generally bring a standard, canned reply from CRC. To CRC officials, the lawsuits, criminal investigations and state sanctions all come in response to isolated events, aren't "systemic," and shouldn't reflect on the dedication and quality of a large company now serving over 30,000 trouble-prone teens and substance abusers each day. The company declined to respond to my written questions outlining allegations made by alumni, parents and former employees about questionable practices at specific programs, citing a legal requirement to protect patient confidentiality. But a public relations consultant, Robert Weiner, who worked closely with CRC and its most prominent board member at the time, Gen. Barry McCaffrey, President Bill Clinton's drug czar, did respond in general terms in a phone interview: "The people you cited can whine all they want, but that's just a bunch of specifics we can't talk about compared to 40,000 people a day we're making better lives for," he said, citing the higher enrollment figures in 2012.

"In a human-run company there will be human errors in some cases," Weiner added. "But in other cases, it's garbage," discounting the accusations.

Over the years, CRC officials have disputed criticisms aimed at the company because of the reported deaths, citing positive surveys of parents and clients, and certification by regulators and accrediting agencies. And in a conference call in 2011 for investors, the CRC CEO before Rhodes, Andrew Eckert, discounted the controversies over New Life in Tennessee as merely "unwelcomed bumps in the road." In fact, later in the call he claimed that "CRC is in the process of staking its ground as the definitive leader in clinical excellence."

• • •

SUCH CLAIMS OF EXCELLENCE DO NOT SEEM TO HAVE PIERCED THE CANOPY of the Santa Cruz redwoods, home to Camp Recovery, the first drug treatment facility CRC purchased in the mid-'90s and still a part of the Acadia portfolio. According to former employees, safety and quality both eroded once Bain purchased the facility in 2006. Meanwhile, state agencies periodically reported—but did nothing—about increasingly troublesome findings of violence, neglect and drug dealing after 2006, while prices tripled to as much as $18,000 a month. The governing view, according to a former Camp Recovery counselor, Tom Corral, was to accept even the sickest and most mentally disturbed patients: "You've got to keep them at all costs."

Camp Recovery is registered with the state as a nonmedical facility, and so patients needing intensive medical or psychiatric care should be referred elsewhere. But such restrictions soon collapsed, say former staffers, in a drive for profits. "Certified nurses were reprimanded when we complained to the intake office," says one former nurse. "When I didn't want to admit a person who was falling down drunk, they wrote me up."

The administrative resistance to calling 911 was so pronounced that when one overmedicated, mentally disturbed patient fled the facility in hysterics one summer day in 2008, she was left to lie on the road outside the gate, screaming for help before collapsing into convulsions. One camp executive told staff on duty at the time, "Leave her alone. We don't want to make a scene," according to Bottoroff and other former staffers. It was left to neighbors to call 911. Nevertheless, the camp still made more emergency calls than any comparable facility in the Santa Cruz area, according to addiction and ER doctors who reviewed 911 log data I obtained—perhaps a measure of just how ill many of the patients are at this facility, which isn't even licensed to provide medical care.

Camp Recovery's culture of secrecy was especially pronounced when it came to alleged instances of statutory rape of underage kids by adult patients, teen assaults on staff or fellow patients, and on-site drug use among the adolescents in treatment, former staffers say.

In September 2012, all these concerns about failed oversight allowing facilities like CRC's Camp Recovery to run amok were confirmed by a scathing report issued by the California Senate Rules Committee, "Rogue Rehabs: State failed to police drug and alcohol homes, with deadly results." The health division originally in charge of the programs was shut down, but its successor agency, the Department of Health Care Services (DHCS) allowed felon-run treatment centers engaging in fraudulent billing to flourish, according to a 2014 state audit and a joint 2013 CNN–Center for Investigative Reporting investigative series. Two years after the story broke, prosecutors were arranging plea deals in eleven criminal cases, but few seemed likely to go to prison.

It also remained unclear if the DHCS division promising tighter oversight would make much of a difference. Camp Recovery was still in business and the California rehab field doesn't seem to have fundamentally changed. Early in 2016, one of California's largest insurers, Health Net, launched its own sweeping anti-fraud investigation of California addiction treatment centers for paying kickbacks to win patient referrals, and for fraudulent billing.

• • •

IN MANY WAYS, CRC'S FACILITIES ACROSS THE COUNTRY HAVE GENERALLY faced far fewer sanctions and scrutiny than those rogue rehab centers in California. (Camp Recovery was mildly chastised by state investigators for offering unlicensed psychiatric evaluations and medications.) That's because the complaints against the CRC programs have rarely led to consequences for either the company's drug treatment or youth programs, let alone their executives. The troubled-teen industry, in particular, is a regulatory Wild West, with some states lacking any licensing system at all for these residential programs. Even some states that do license, such as Utah, appear unable to guarantee patient safety: about a dozen young people are known to have died due to neglect—countless more due to suicides during their confinement or shortly afterward—since 1990 while attending Utah residential and wilderness programs.

As Greg Kutz, a GAO investigator, said in congressional testimony about the industry in general before the House committee, "It seems that the only way staff could be convinced that these kids were not faking it was when they stopped breathing or had no pulse."

This mindset has contributed to the deaths and injuries of dozens, if not hundreds, of young people. But because the exact same indifference, ignorance and brutality have been exhibited so many times since then, it shouldn't come as a surprise now. But the horror is indeed magnified because these attitudes are still commonly held throughout the troubled-teen industry today.

Out of all the federal and state inaction came a chance to grow a thriving business for CRC. Where some see neglect and dangerously lax regulation, others see investment opportunities. In California, although fraud by inpatient rehab clinics has finally garnered statewide attention, the regulation of outpatient drug treatment facilities still appears especially ineffective. Yet what's not widely known is that the now-closed California Department of Alcohol and Drug Programs (ADP), for example, had never investigated the deaths of nearly two hundred patients over five years at CRC's dozen or so outpatient methadone clinics in the state. Remarkably, those deaths, followed by over three hundred fatalities annually in all of the state-approved methadone programs, *still* remain unexplored by the broader state health department that took over ADP's role, the DHCS. (A spokesperson for the department declined to answer questions or offer any examples of any government response to the wave of methadone clinic deaths.)

Mostly likely, addiction experts say, the clients' rampant substance abuse is the culprit, not sloppy practices at CRC or other clinics, but that supposition has not been rigorously tested. In fact, in 2011 Pennsylvania regulators cited two of CRC's methadone clinics for failing to properly screen patients for drugs or narcotics use, a potentially deadly oversight.

In subsequent years, more problems with CRC's methadone clinics—many of whose patients suffered from serious mental illnesses as well—were revealed whenever state agencies bothered to look. There are over eighty methadone clinics nationwide owned by CRC, and the upsurge in opiate addiction is surely good for business. Yet by 2013 and even earlier, according to *Bloomberg News* and other media outlets, law enforcement officials and state regulators in Virginia, West Virginia, Indiana, Maryland and other states uncovered a disturbing trend: CRC clinics were allegedly involved in loosely regulated take-home methadone practices that may have played a role in deaths and illegal drug-dealing. In response, a spokesperson for CRC said it had many safeguards against misuse, including screening people for take-home privileges and the use of lockboxes for their home supplies of the drug.

Yet there's little sign that CRC subsequently actually took a tough-minded, fresh look at their methadone clinics' practices. And in states like California, patient protections were eased up further: California regulators and law enforcement agencies haven't sought to look closely at why so many CRC methadone patients are dying, let alone explore the trends in illegal methadone use nearby where CRC clinics are located. At the same time, as reported by the World Health Organization and the Institute of Medicine, methadone, along with the drug Suboxone, has real treatment value *when properly distributed and monitored*: it can significantly reduce illegal drug use, and this "medication-assisted treatment" also lowers overdose mortality by 75 percent, as noted in Maia Szalavitz's recent book, *Unbroken Brain*. Due to what amounts to criminally negligent regulation in California, however, "The programs have experienced the reality that there are no consequences if anyone dies," says a knowledgeable former California rehab regulator about the state's drug programs. These include CRC's methadone clinics, which have become the chain's cash cow.

• • •

THE LOOSE OVERSIGHT SEEMS TO HAVE BEEN CRITICAL IN ENABLING CRC to flourish. It's hard to imagine, in particular, that without the scandalously weak monitoring of the teen treatment industry, CRC's Aspen division would have been able to continue its harshly regimented, unproven behavior-modification methods and dicey emergency protocols.

This apparent lack of oversight in the teen industry, combined with a widespread view by providers that their charges are manipulative troublemakers, has allowed a toxic culture of psychological abuse and medical neglect to prevail, according to parents, alumni and federal officials. That culture was visible even at Aspen Education's most upscale residential programs, such as Island View in suburban Syracuse, Utah. One former student there, Colleen Davidson, now twenty-four, who graduated from the program in 2009, recalls her alarm when she coughed up blood one morning as she stood at the bathroom sink. She says she was never allowed to see a doctor because, by the time the nurse wandered by a few hours later, another student had rinsed the blood from the sink. "They assume you're lying," she says.

For months, CRC denied me press access to any of its facilities, so I visited Island View in 2012, posing as a father of a troubled girl. During that visit, director Laura Burt confirmed this skeptical stance towards potential medical emergencies. She said the nursing staff would see my (fictitious) daughter immediately in case of a medical crisis but would monitor her if they suspected fakery: "We're not going to rush her to the hospital if she's just saying that and there is nothing that says it."

These incidents seem to illuminate an institutional culture that allowed Sergey Blashchishen to die in 2009 before ever receiving emergency medical aid. As one government investigator told me about the field instructors at SageWalk, where Blashchishen died, "They were highly trained, but the culture overrode that." The SageWalk Field Instructor Manual—like other Aspen manuals that were vetted by CRC, according to a former CRC official—requires staff to go through a rigid "chain of command" before emergency help can be summoned.

CRC spokespeople, including Weiner, insisted that safety is a top priority and there are no major problems. They pointed to a recent initiative by CRC to ensure that all its teen programs are certified by two leading accrediting agencies, the Commission on Accreditation of Rehabilitation Facilities (CARF) and a body known as the Joint Commission, a sixty-year-old industry-funded nonprofit that accredits thousands of health-care programs in the United States.

This offers scant comfort, given that members of Congress harshly criticized the Joint Commission in the wake of revelations of medical negligence at Walter Reed and other Joint Commission–accredited hospitals. Moreover, many facilities in one of the most notorious chains in the teen treatment field, Mel Sembler's Straight Inc., were approved by accrediting agencies, including the Joint Commission, until they shut down in the wake of lawsuits and state action. Some maintained their high ratings even after Straight Inc. and several of its spin-offs were hit by state investigations and as many as ninety lawsuits alleging abuse.

• • •

DESPITE THE ACCUMULATING LAWSUITS, STATE INVESTIGATIONS AND EVEN criminal inquiries, neither Bain Capital nor Acadia forced any major shake-ups in the culture or leadership of CRC when the company was acquired. Aspen co-founder Elliot Sainer and CRC CEO Barry Karlin remained in their executive posts until they retired in 2007 and 2010, respectively. Trina Packard, the executive in charge at Youth Care when Brendan Blum died, remains in her post.

Rather than instituting reforms, CRC seems to have responded to the series of lawsuits, in part, by requiring parents to sign elaborate contracts that feature sweeping "hold harmless" clauses even in the case of death.

Aspen Education, now down to just four treatment facilities, uses what the teen treatment industry calls a "levels" model that grants more privileges and freedoms as students follow the rules, but imposes varying degrees of humiliation and harsh sanctions on those who slip up or disobey. Punishments were more often psychological than physical at Aspen programs. According to former students, emotionally brutal isolation punishments and peer-driven encounter "therapies" were commonly employed to break down resistance, especially at Island View. These concerns about Island View's prisonlike environment were also raised in two lawsuits filed in early 2014 by ex-students. Both lawsuits were ultimately dismissed on technical grounds, one for being filed after the statute of limitation.

As is all too common in the troubled-teen field, Seroquel and other antipsychotics were part of the behavioral control arsenal used on teens at Island View, according to a disturbing investigative article in *The Huffington Post* in August 2016. Regardless of FDA rules, the teenagers at Island View were swamped with off-label antipsychotics. Emily Graeber, then a fifteen-year-old who ran away from Island View and was sent back by her parents, received the maximum dosage of Seroquel approved for adults: 800 mg. "I feel like they kept us sedated for ease of control so people wouldn't have as many outbursts," Graeber, now twenty-three, told *The Huffington Post*, a charge denied in the article by a former Island View administrator.

Shortly after the 2014 lawsuits were filed, Aspen Education closed down Island View, but it reopened with a new name, Elevations, under a new company, Family Help and Wellness, headed by a former Aspen Education executive—and with the same tough-love philosophy. Nearly 80 percent of its employees are the same. Apparently, not much has changed at Elevations in terms of Aspen-style practices, according to the *Huffington Post* investigation. In addition to the ongoing use of off-label antipsychotics, the article by Sebastian Murdock revealed, "Staff are still isolating and physically restraining children. At least one has attempted suicide. Others have tried to run away." (A spokesperson for Elevations denied in *The Huffington Post* any cruel or improper treatment of kids, claimed all therapies are accepted by the state, and said that the four-by-four isolation cells cited by Murdock were just "time-out rooms" because the doors were unlocked.)

Yet if the same therapeutic approaches that operated at Island View have continued at Elevations, kids may be in further danger. The confrontational sessions at Island View were so terrifying that girls resorted to desperate measures to avoid attending, according to Colleen Davidson. She recalls that some girls choked themselves to induce fainting; one rubbed feces in her own eyes to cause an infection.

"They break you down, but they don't really build you back up," she says of the Island View approach, still widely emulated in other teen programs. "I have nightmares from it, and the memories are really awful."

• • •

CRC DECLINED TO ADDRESS ANY PROGRAM-SPECIFIC ALLEGATIONS WHEN I researched the company in 2012, and spokespeople for the new owner, Acadia, have since declined to reply to any of my phoned questions.

Short of rigorous evidence that their programs work, CRC's PR machine offered up testimonials from pleased parents and CRC-funded surveys of parents and students that report positive outcomes. CRC's spokesperson at the time, Kristen Hayes, put me in touch with one of these parents, the mother of a self-destructive, drug-abusing fifteen-year-old son whom she sent to Island View, the Aspen program Colleen Davidson attended, after other treatments had failed. "I didn't want to stand around and wait for my child to die," she said bluntly. Enrolling him in Aspen, she said, was the turning point. "I wish all kids were as lucky as my son," she observed.

And what can't be washed away by good PR can always be described as an unavoidable tragedy. At Youth Care of Utah, admissions counselor Claire Roberts offered up this sort of soft-focus gloss when she told me about the death of Brendan Blum. "It was very traumatizing for us," she said. Then she added philosophically, "These things happen."

Surprisingly, by 2016, there were small, hopeful signs of change. These include a new state oversight law in Washington lobbied for by HEAL. Most significantly, in September 2016 California passed a law—then among the toughest in the country—requiring the licensing and monitoring of troubled-teen sites, including religious schools. The California law passed largely because of a brilliant, media-savvy alliance between an older generation of victims who were members of the Survivors of Institutional Abuse (SIA), and the politically influential Los Angeles LGBT Center, which was outraged by the troubled-teen industry's efforts to harm gay teens while claiming to "cure" their sexual or gender identity. But it was not certain that these new laws would be any better enforced than regulation of drug treatment programs in California or youth programs in Utah. Still, Jodi Hobbs, the president of SIA, while praising the California law, struck a forceful note after it passed. "It's not enough," she said. "Until we finally pass federal legislation to regulate this rogue industry in every state, the lives and well-being of youth remain at risk." SIA estimates that over the years as many as three hundred kids have died in these programs or killed themselves afterward.

Indeed, the states, once called the "laboratories of democracy," have proved to be in this regard experiments in failure and death. In most states, government inaction that allows the death, neglect, abuse and rape of young people to continue remained the rule, not the exception. Perhaps no state in the country, with the possible exception of Utah, illustrated just how dangerous all these factors could be as much as Florida. There, government and law enforcement agencies often looked the other way as literally hundreds of emotionally troubled kids were abused, raped and killed.

CHAPTER 14

Florida: Free-Fire Zone for Killing, Abusing and Raping Kids?

Shortly after 8:30 p.m. on March 3, 2011, sixteen-year-old Susan Jackson returned to the Vanguard School in Lake Wales, Florida, after a trip to Starbucks with a classmate. The girls' dorm monitor, Kami Land, had driven them in her car to the coffee shop and then dropped them off near Boyd Hall, their dorm at the center of campus. They were supposed to be in bed soon.

Curfew at the private Florida boarding school for kids with learning disabilities was 10 p.m. In Susan's case, however, the campus had imposed a 9:30 p.m. curfew on her in January 2011, after she had been hospitalized after smoking methamphetamine-laced marijuana that she and a friend had bought off-campus.

Instead of heading to her room, however, Susan walked away from the main cluster of buildings and towards the gym, the athletic field and the woods that ringed a lake on the south end of campus, which is just south of Orlando. During the day, students played tennis, soccer, golf and paintball on the grounds or canoed on the pristine water. At night, however, the campus's remote areas became popular spots for students looking to hook up or do drugs.

Therefore, they were off-limits to Susan unless a staff member accompanied her. When Susan failed to return by her curfew, a security guard went looking for her. He eventually found her—distraught, frightened and disoriented—behind the school's greenhouse near the woods.

"She was upset and very scared," recalled Ellen, a student who lived across the hall from Susan. "Her hair was messed up. She had mascara on her face, and it was obvious that she had been crying."

"I asked her, I said, 'Are you OK?' And she said, 'I was raped.'"

The details gradually emerged that night and the next day. (For confidentiality reasons, I'm withholding the real names of all juveniles in this chapter.) Two male students I'll call William and David had tricked Susan into walking with them into the woods on school grounds, the sixteen-year-old girl reported. Then they forced her to her knees and made her give one of them, William, oral sex. The night of the alleged attack, after she had returned to her dorm's kitchen, Susan told her dorm monitor, Kami Land, what had happened.

Nobody working at the school—or in local law enforcement or at the state Department of Children and Families (DCF)—adequately followed up on claims by Susan or several other victims of similar alleged crimes at Vanguard. For instance, Det. Mary Jerome of the Lake Wales Police Department allowed the school's president to help in questioning the suspects and suggesting alibis, which is not an accepted practice. And cops closed the case the same day the rape was reported without obtaining any evidence supporting the suspects' alibis, according to legal and police documents filed in the case.

Perhaps just as alarming, I reviewed a twenty-one-page list of 911 calls from the Vanguard School to the county's emergency call center between November 2010 and September 2014, plus a list of the far fewer service calls and even fewer arrests by Lake Wales cops. They indicate dozens of phoned-in emergencies, including at least a dozen assault cases and other violent disturbances—and some attempted suicides.

It also seems incidents are sometimes neither reported nor logged. For instance, on January 17, 2013, according to former teacher Gail Bonnichsen, a teenage girl was allegedly assaulted on the grounds by a student who jammed his hand inside her, causing vaginal bleeding. But staff on duty that night brushed aside the girl's concerns and didn't call police or seek medical help—until the girl told Bonnichsen about it late the next day. Bonnichsen claims she called a DCF abuse hotline and two local police departments, but the agencies never responded. "Nothing was done about it, and nobody gave a crap," Bonnichsen says.

Vanguard caters primarily to children and teens with learning disabilities who may also have developmental problems. But over time, it has increasingly become a haven—or "dumping ground," as one disgruntled parent calls it—generally for affluent disturbed and violent youths. Even so, Vanguard's website promises that its "safe, supportive environment facilitates physical, social, and emotional growth of all students" and that its "dormitories are a home-away-from-home for [its] residential students."

In a 2011 reply to a lawsuit filed by Susan's family, the school's attorneys denied negligence. Despite repeated email and phone inquiries from me, school officials declined to answer any broader questions about student safety and the alleged failure to properly report crimes. Polk County-based attorney Richard Straughn, who represents the school, wrote me, "The health, safety, and well-being of students are top priorities at the Vanguard School . . . Part of our commitment includes complete respect for the confidentiality and privacy rights of our students and families."

The allegations of trouble at Vanguard embody a pattern of regulatory failure common across the entire field of troubled and disabled teen programs. Private schools and residential programs for youngsters, as noted in earlier chapters, not only house kids with learning disabilities but also with emotional, behavioral and addiction problems. Vanguard, though, doesn't employ the notorious tough-love approach common in many other teen residential programs. Vanguard isn't the worst program in the country, but in the absence of any state or federal agency reliably tracking deaths and abuse, there is no way of knowing which residential program is in fact the most deadly.

Yet the law enforcement and regulatory lapses that made Vanguard such an apparently dangerous place for its most vulnerable students are worth understanding because, in some ways, they are so commonplace. The accused roughnecks and torturers at Restoration Youth Academy who eventually were arrested are in some ways extreme outliers. Vanguard was led by well-educated professionals, some with advanced degrees, who used their influence, and the school's economic importance to the community, to protect themselves from scrutiny. In addition, the local police department's response to allegations of assault and rapes at Vanguard is far more representative of those hundreds of police departments that generally ignore violence

at residential programs until someone is killed. There was no dedicated Captain Kennedy on the Lake Wales police force doing his best
to protect children and prosecute wrongdoers.

"I am not surprised by what happened with the Vanguard
School situation in Florida," Angela Smith of HEAL observes, "It is
not unusual for regulatory and law enforcement agencies to ignore
abuse complaints." She adds, "Sometimes the complaints are ignored
because the people are disabled and being disabled to some apparently
means having a credibility issue." By taking a close look at how an
indifferent police department operates—while state regulators look
the other way—we can better understand why genuine accountability
is so rare. In this anything-goes field, Florida's monitoring stands out
as among the very worst in the country.

Fortunately, there have been no deaths at the Vanguard School,
but it's fitting that perhaps one of the most notorious cases in this
field took place in Florida: the beating death by guards of a black
fourteen-year-old boy, Martin Lee Anderson, that began when he
stopped exercising at a Bay County Sherriff's Office juvenile boot
camp in 2006. Seven guards and a nurse were charged with
manslaughter, but they were acquitted by a jury of their rural Florida
peers. The controversy led to the closing of state-run boot camps, but
the state's juvenile justice department still contracts with reportedly
abusive programs.

What all of these programs share is a lack of accountability.
Few, if any, states do a strong job of monitoring. Trade groups such
as the National Association of Therapeutic Schools and Programs
(NATSAP) have successfully defeated both federal and state efforts to
impose greater oversight. Robert Friedman, an emeritus professor of
the Department of Child and Family Studies at the University of South
Florida and founder of the reform group ASTART for Teens, observes,
"You not only need good licensing law and policy, you need good
monitoring and frequent review—and the states do not have adequate
staff to do the reviews."

On top of all that, advocacy groups remain loose, mostly under-
funded networks of volunteers lacking real clout. Courts are generally
no remedy either, with parents slow to admit they've been duped and

lawyers reluctant to take on anything except wrongful-death lawsuits.

Florida is especially notorious for its lax oversight of vulnerable children. Private schools are barely monitored. Outside of an easily obtained business license, they don't get the oversight normally given to public schools or even state-sanctioned residential group homes that receive government funding. Some examples of the toll in children's deaths and abuse in Florida:

In January 2014, University of South Florida researchers announced the findings from a makeshift graveyard at the notorious state-run Arthur G. Dozier School for Boys in Marianna, Florida, which closed in 2011 after a long history of abuse and scandal. At least ninety-six children died at the reform school between 1914 and 1973.

In 2012, *The Tampa Bay Times*, as mentioned earlier in the book, exposed widespread patterns of brutality at unmonitored Christian academies, some operating outside the state's minimal private accrediting requirements. That prompted a preliminary state review and a tepid government response, but didn't lead the state to examine unlicensed secular schools such as Vanguard.

Most strikingly, DCF allowed nearly five hundred children—mostly five and under—to die under its watch in a six-year period, killed mostly by parents or other family members, as *The Miami Herald* reported in a horrifying 2014 series. The agency scrambled to cover up the real causes of most of the children's deaths and continued to do so even after the newspaper broke the scandal. Limited new reform legislation was introduced and the Secretary of DCF resigned following the onslaught of negative publicity.

As with the abuses and deaths at the VA, New Life Lodge and countless other scandalous health-care programs, nothing was done until media attention focused on all these needless deaths. Those Florida child-killing atrocities were made possible by the same pattern of apparent bureaucratic neglect and indifference—although not leading to any deaths—that seem to be at work on a smaller scale in the weak response of officials to alleged incidents of sexual and physical assaults at the private Vanguard School for learning-disabled kids.

. . .

Dangerous conditions at first glance seem unlikely at the bucolic Vanguard School, a self-proclaimed "international learning community" that boasts a state-ranked basketball team and claims 95 percent of graduates attend college. Most of all, however, it promises desperate parents a safe and supportive environment for students with dyslexia, attention-deficit disorder and Asperger's syndrome, who also often have emotional disturbances. The cost: up to $44,000 a year in tuition.

Before attending Vanguard, Susan Jackson was a pretty, doe-eyed girl whose affluent parents from a Mid-Atlantic suburb had been scrambling to find a program that would allow her to succeed. She had been diagnosed with an autism-related disability known as a "nonverbal learning disorder (NLD)," which made her particularly trusting, unable to read social cues or facial expressions and easily swayed. When she arrived at the school in September 2010, her parents hoped she'd fit in better and make greater academic progress than she had at her previous specialized private school.

Her parents also expected that the Vanguard School would do a good job protecting their daughter. However, rather than calling the police or a doctor immediately about her alleged rape in 2011, dorm monitor Kami Land contacted her immediate supervisor, Felix Lugo, the assistant director of residential life, on the phone. She then sent an email at 1:08 a.m. to top officials at the school, including then-Vanguard president Cathy Wooley-Brown, telling them what had happened. The incident report was labeled as having "high" importance.

After a drive from her home nearly an hour away, Wooley-Brown didn't call police until she spoke to staff members and the boys the next morning—perhaps with an eye to keeping all their alibis consistent. Later that morning, before police arrived to investigate Susan's rape report, Wooley-Brown took extra steps to keep the full story quiet, according to her dorm-mate Ellen's deposition. When Wooley-Brown took Ellen to the infirmary on a golf cart to rest, the exhausted high-schooler confided in her that she'd been told that one of the boys had previously raped another female student. The victim herself had told Ellen.

Wooley-Brown then allegedly looked Ellen in the face and said, "You don't need to get involved in drama like this," Ellen said in a deposition. "And I think that is horrible. That is wrong for her to have said that." That earlier alleged rape by the same suspect was never reported to police. Indeed, police records show Ellen was never interviewed by police in Susan's case.

In sworn interviews led by Detective Mary Jerome in the president's office at Vanguard later that morning, the boys, prodded by Wooley-Brown's alibi-oriented questions during the "interrogation," offered an alternate version of events from the previous night: Susan was looking to trade sexual favors for drugs.

"She said, 'I want to have sex with you if you give me some drugs.' I said, 'No.' I walked away," William said in his interview, according to police records.

Detective Mary Jerome allowed the president of Vanguard to sit in and ask supportive questions of the suspects throughout the so-called interrogation. She treated her with unbecoming deference and essentially as a fellow interrogator who could jump in when Wooley-Brown chose—rather than as an administrator with a vested interest in squelching any scandals at her school. Wooley-Brown questioned them in a way that aimed to establish a timeline of events that showed they were in their dorms when Susan said she was raped—and essentially reminded William to tell the detective his tale about Susan's purported offer of sex for drugs.

At the end of the questioning, Wooley-Brown and Detective Jerome implicitly reminded the suspects to tell the version of events that the school president wanted to hear. Detective Jerome urged William to "tell the truth."

Wooley-Brown added: "Are you telling the truth today?"

William answered, "Oh yes, ma'am."

The police report transcripts don't tell us what sort of body language, facial expressions or tone of voice Wooley-Brown may have used to better convey to witnesses and suspects the meaning and subtext of her questions. It's reasonable to suspect that the school president's presence was an intimidating one for the students whose academic careers she held in her hands, so it was in the mutual interests of both the suspects and administrators that it appear as if no rape had happened.

Then Det. Jerome closed the case the same day the rape was reported, accepting Wooley-Brown's unverified claims that the school had videotape proving the boys were in their dorm rooms when Susan said they had raped her. Wooley-Brown never produced the videotape during either the criminal investigation or the lawsuit that followed. Detective Jerome's closing of the case was approved by a captain, James Foy, who himself had pleaded "no contest" to having sex with a fifteen-year-old girl while working at another police department. He was fired in January 2012 after a county prosecutor said he would no longer accept the captain's testimony as credible.

Indeed, there was no verifiable evidence supporting the suspects' alibis, a review of Jerome's report and other depositions in the civil lawsuit reveals. And Susan's timeline of events clashed with that of the school staff and the suspects.

During the course of the civil lawsuit, though, the contradictions were eventually settled in Susan's favor. The family's attorney produced a time stamp—that Jerome had never obtained—from the front gate showing that Susan had arrived back at the school around 8:30 p.m. as she had claimed, not at 9 p.m. as the dorm supervisor Land, Wooley-Brown and all the suspects had alleged. Retired Detective Kirk Griffith, a former top investigator with the innovative Sexual Assault Unit of the Dallas Police Department, reviewed the case for me. "A lot was lacking in some of the things needed for verification," he says, taking particular notice of Wooley-Brown's presence at the interrogation. "The supposed interrogation of suspects was not a true interrogation."

In the fall of 2011, Susan's family sued the school for negligence. By August 2013, as the civil lawsuit moved ahead, Detective Jerome reportedly disavowed the findings and accuracy of her original report, according to a knowledgeable source familiar with her criminal investigation.

The suit was settled in October 2013 for an undisclosed sum. President Cathy Wooley-Brown faced no public consequences for her actions, nor has she answered questions about the Vanguard School outside of the deposition she gave in Susan's lawsuit. She left the school in January 2015 to form her own educational consulting firm.

• • •

THE FAILURE TO TAKE SUSAN JACKSON'S RAPE ALLEGATION SERIOUSLY contributed to an environment at Vanguard that allowed subsequent attacks to victimize other students without consequences. For example, on January 18, 2013, Gail Bonnichsen, then a teacher at Vanguard, listened with horror, she says, as a student she mentored described a sexual assault on Vanguard's football field. A student musician with long fingernails, the girl said, had scraped her vaginal walls. Bonnichsen says she discovered that school staff had the night before brushed aside the girl's claim because she was known to be promiscuous. "She needed medical care," Bonnichsen observes. She says she contacted her own gynecologist, who treated the girl.

At 7:22 on the night she learned of the attack—she recorded the time—Bonnichsen says she called the DCF abuse hotline. Then, referred by DCF, she phoned the county sheriff's office—and later spoke to the police department nearest her hometown. But DCF and three Polk County police departments, including Lake Wales, deny they were ever notified about the alleged rape at the Vanguard School. On top of that, Bonnichsen contends that Vanguard's principal, Derri Park, even chastised her for reporting the alleged attack to DCF's child abuse hotline, although the call was supposed to remain confidential. "I told her I did what I was charged to do: 'This is abuse and I had to report it,'" Bonnichsen declares. (Park, who still works at the school, didn't respond to my phone and email inquiries.)

Bonnichsen left the school in summer 2013 after working there only two years, and was reprimanded by supervisors again for reporting to authorities such incidents as a knife attack on one of her students. In her view, the school's general approach to violence is "a cover-up," worsened by the apparent failure of law enforcement to respond. "I hope you understand how sad this makes me. I tried to do the right thing," she says.

• • •

AIDED BY SUCH APPARENT COVER-UPS, REFORM EFFORTS IN THIS FIELD— or in any campaign to protect Florida's most vulnerable children—face a steep uphill climb. The state's news media, including *The Miami Herald*, have long chronicled DCF's failures to protect kids from neglect, abuse and death. Most of the secretaries of the scandal-plagued DCF and its predecessor, Health and Rehabilitative Services (HRS), have resigned under fire since the 1990s.

There have been myriad legislative fixes and vows of reform, yet not much has changed over time. Even with the passage of laws in the 2014 state legislature designed to create more transparency and strengthen abuse investigations, DCF's historically toxic culture of neglect, secrecy and incompetence seems unmoved.

But some advocates, such as Broward County attorney Howard Talenfeld, have made a major difference, both through the courts and effective lobbying. Founder of Florida's Children First, a group dedicated to protecting children under state care, Talenfeld successfully pressed for a change in DCF's law requiring the agency to investigate teen-on-teen rapes up through age eighteen of the victims. But that change applies only to youth under state care or custody, not to students at private schools such as Vanguard. "Nobody tracks which kids are sexually aggressive between twelve and eighteen," he says. "This is a big issue."

And, as usual, there's still no federal response to any kind of abuse in residential treatment. Although the House of Representatives passed an oversight measure in 2008, the "Stop Child Abuse in Residential Programs for Teens" bill never made it through the Senate. The hopes for any national legislation have faded along with the retirement of the leading advocate for federal oversight—Rep. George Miller—and the reluctance of Congress to pass tough new regulation of any industry.

Even for Susan Jackson, the trauma is far from over. The day after the reported sexual assault in March 2011, the parents of the then-sixteen-year-old flew to Florida and pulled her from the school. "Susan and her family have been shattered by this," says a Vanguard parent who knows them well but asked not to be identified.

Susan confided in a counselor at her new school that she didn't tell anyone at Vanguard at the time about alleged multiple sexual encounters with a Vanguard staff "monitor," apparently because of the fear, trauma and shame she felt then. Thoughts about the monitor's alleged sexual exploitation recurred following new nightmares over Vanguard: "I don't know, I just blocked it out," she explained to her Utah therapist when asked why she hadn't complained about it earlier.

Lake Wales police detectives identified another underage Vanguard girl allegedly exploited by the same man, adding credibility to her claims. But they couldn't complete an investigation because neither girl's parents wanted to put their daughters through an arduous, potentially traumatizing criminal probe with an uncertain outcome. (The alleged perpetrator was never charged and denied any misconduct.)

Indeed, troubling memories of her time at Vanguard continued to plague her. A school counselor's report in March 2012 detailed her psychological state: "Flashbacks/nightmares began that were associated with the sexual assault situation that had occurred with two boys at the school."

These days, the Vanguard School seems to have sidestepped the scandal. A new president, Harold Maready, has taken over from Wooley-Brown, but, so far, he remains mum about the allegations against the school and the lawsuit. There has been no local publicity about the lawsuit or the two police investigations involving Susan or the numerous emergency calls to the county dispatch center about crimes and attempted suicides—even after I wrote a long-delayed article on the school for the South Florida *New Times* chain in November 2014. Because there has been no public acknowledgment that school officials did anything wrong, there has also been no indication that there have been fundamental changes at the school.

When I approached the front gate of the Vanguard School in the fall of 2013 near the end of my week of reporting in Lake Wales, and asked for Cathy Wooley-Brown, I was told, "She's not available to come to the phone."

The silence protecting the Vanguard School in Lake Wales, it seems, still continues.

CHAPTER 15

Karen's Story and the Mental Health System That Never Was: Saving Families, Young People from Lifelong Madness

WITH ALMOST ANY OTHER DISEASE THAT RAVAGES SO MANY PEOPLE, you would think the government would take it seriously by now. The National Institute of Mental Health has estimated that the country's neglect of mental illness costs the country not only in preventable deaths and blighted lives but also $444 billion a year in lost earnings, federal disability costs and about $200 billion in direct health-care costs, not counting the spending on incarceration.

"The system is perfectly perverse," says seventy-four-year-old Dr. William McFarlane, the former director of the Center for Psychiatric Research at the Maine Medical Center, a professor at Tufts University medical school and a leader in developing effective treatments. Medicaid, the primary payer for public mental health services, spends freely on costly psychotropics for people who don't need them and on programs that don't work, such as "day treatment" outpatient care that usually mimics old-fashioned state hospitals. But it skimps on or denies funding for proven programs that go beyond a standard medical model to make a difference in people's lives. McFarlane has created two pioneering evidence-based practices that harness the potentially positive impact of families on people with serious mental illness to reduce relapses by up to 400 percent and even *first* psychotic episodes to as little as 6 percent, thus preventing lifelong disability and endless years of schizophrenia.

Yet such effective programs are rarely implemented by local, state or federal health-care agencies. This not-so-benign neglect continues despite the way McFarlane's and other well-documented programs save lives, are supported by decades of research, dramatically cut costs and have won endorsements from the influential SAMHSA.

"It's sad that the American mental health field is still using [therapy] methodologies developed in the '50s and '60s. The results are abysmal," he points out. "Insurance companies pay for a fifteen-minute med check but not much else, making hospitalizations almost inevitable. They cost an ungodly amount of money and the profit margins are huge."

"The public mental health clinics just give the typical outpatient therapies 'supportive therapy' that doesn't work, and when they fail, as they usually do, it doesn't cost them if the patients go into the hospital," he continues. "And then the hospitals make a ton of money off them. If the clinics actually implemented them, they wouldn't see a dime in savings." And why should they care personally about long-run savings to the larger system? Some executives at top-paying Medicaid-funded nonprofits earned as much as $10 million a year—while the then-CEO of New York's Institute for Community Living, Peter Campanelli, pulled in as much as $2.8 million annually in 2011 for his program providing housing and other services to the mentally ill. So there wasn't much extra incentive to work harder training people to provide intensive, time-consuming programs.

As for the federal-state Medicaid programs that pay for most of it, those officials are too mired in turf battles, opposition from health-care providers resisting change and bureaucratic inertia to take action. As McFarlane and others see it, for the lead federal agency, the Centers for Medicare & Medicaid Services, "It's perfectly obvious that CMS hasn't done anything to support evidence-based practices." He says federal officials didn't even stir themselves to start raising awareness about them "until they were all caught flat-footed by the massacres [by crazed gunmen like Adam Lanza and James Eagan Holmes]," while still doing substantively little to apply them.

Yet "evidence-based practices" still became a mantra that federal mental health leaders would invoke from time to time for PR purposes, but few clinic directors today are paying any attention.

• • •

TAKE A LOOK AT AN UNLIKELY REVOLUTION IN THERAPY THAT WAS TAKING place a while ago inside a mental health clinic in a small town in south

Maine, a snapshot in time from the early days of the SAMHSA-supported programs for people with serious mental illness. Its success ultimately helped lay the groundwork for something previously unimaginable: preventing some people from developing schizophrenia at all.

About twenty people—patients with schizophrenia and their families—are sitting in a circle of folding chairs, shooting the breeze about the Red Sox and their holiday weekends. On the walls of the classroom, there are a few heart-shaped collages with homilies reflecting the spirit of the group, such as "Stick with me through thick and thin." The families have often been struggling to do just that for years, and now, after seeing their loved ones go in and out of hospitals, they've finally turned to this new multifamily "psychoeducation" group for information about the illness, mutual support, encouragement to take medications and other help. The group may be new—only five months old at the time—but it's a treatment model that's been proving itself in controlled studies for over thirty years. Yet only in the 1990s did it begin to spread and win recognition as perhaps the most effective family-based treatment—generally combined with carefully monitored medications—ever devised for any mental illness, reducing relapses to as low as 10 percent annually.

This multifamily group (MFG) in Maine is being gently guided by two "facilitators," clinical social workers Dawn Hardy and Marilyn Wanyo, but there's no hiding the pain in the room. Tonight, Wanyo, a tall, low-key counselor who sees several of the patients privately at the clinic, soon steers the talk to the schizophrenia that has brought them together. "How have you been handling the illness in the last two weeks?" Wanyo asks. For now, Karen, an earnest thirty-five-year-old woman hospitalized twice in recent years, is remaining quiet, but will later tell the group how she has a calmer relationship with her parents and is looking to return to at least part-time work.

As Wanyo passes a pencil as a signal for speaking to Mike, a short-haired former dockworker in his forties, who begins the "sharing" portion of the meeting, it becomes clear how intractable, but hardly hopeless, this illness remains for many—even as recovery remains a real possibility for all those given effective care. (The names of "Mike" and other patients have been changed to protect confidentiality.) His head is tilted down as he mumbles something about starting new medications, and then says what's really on his mind: "I was thinking about hearing voices and having bad thoughts; a lot of them are true." He adds, "The Devil's on my case." Karen nods in agreement, understanding well how her feelings about evil and the Devil had distorted her life.

"This sounds really important," Wanyo says, calmly turning to his parents for their views, unruffled by the patient's ongoing delusions. His mother offers a more reassuring perspective: "He doesn't seem as drugged as he's usually been," she says, while noting that he's been experiencing medical side effects from new blood pressure medicine that he's also been taking. "It all comes down to that I'm over the hill," he jokes as the rest laugh; it seems like a throwaway line, but it's actually a small breakthrough for him: he hasn't participated much or shown any humor in previous sessions. (Wanyo, comparing his current status to the progress he made with her in individual therapy, later observes, "The patient is so much better.") As each new person speaks, the sharing illustrates both the variations in the illness and the common bond between them.

Later in the session, Wanyo and the group will devise solutions to a patient's problem through a process of group brainstorming, with the therapist having just one of many equal voices worth hearing.

For both clients and families, the family psychoeducation group means something special to them: a way to both learn about the illness and ease the isolation it imposes on them. In interviews later, its value becomes clearer. To Karen, "It was kind of scary at first being in a group, but it's good knowing that there are other people suffering from the same problem who you can identify with." And both she and her mother underscore the value of the treatment's psychoeducation component; it not only explains the biological roots of the illness, freeing the family from blame, but also offers pointers to families on creating a calm, low-stress environment designed to defuse the often intense, hypercritical or overemotional family response to patients that's known as "expressed emotion." While avoiding the phrase "expressed emotion" or warnings to families about how it can lead to more relapses—and thus avoiding even more blame of families—the psychoeducation program does offer pointers on creating a calmer, less pressured environment.

These findings and strategies led McFarlane to start wondering if the same insights could help younger people with a genetic history of schizophrenia and who had troubling early warning signs—including feeling "presences" or hearing nearby voices—from developing full-blown schizophrenia altogether. He was encouraged by major research in Finland that found that children born to mothers with "schizophrenic-spectrum" illnesses raised as adoptees in intrusive, critical families were an astounding 800 percent more likely to develop schizophrenia—at a 13 percent rate across age groups. That's compared to similarly genetically high-risk children raised in well-adjusted families, who developed schizophrenia at a 1.5 percent rate. "Their genetic background predicted nothing," he says when accounting for the differences in families.

Back in Maine, McFarlane and members of the family group found that a new muted atmosphere in families fosters recovery and helps avoid relapses. "I think my parents understand me better, and aren't so apt to criticize me," says Karen, who was living with them after she had to give up her own nail salon business a few years earlier. Her mother admitted at the time, "I didn't understand the illness."

This shortcoming is remedied in part by the psychoeducation workshop that comes early in the program—reinforced throughout the course of treatment—which teaches the family that schizophrenia is a biologically based illness that's continually affected by the social environment. "It's a 'biosocial' illness," says McFarlane, who created and studied the program for over two decades by that point. He points out that independent research shows that families that manifested high "expressed emotion" did not see schizophrenia as an actual illness amenable to treatment. As McFarlane notes, "They tended to feel guilty; they tended to work hard to correct the situation with everything from excessive attention to anger and criticism, especially when their efforts and concern failed to achieve improvement. High expressed emotion families were in a very real sense victims of lack of information. A principal cause for that kind of agony was professionals' failure to inform, support and guide the family."

That's an apt, high-toned description of the sort of hell Karen and her family went through. But thanks to the multifamily group, Karen and her parents—her mother, Martha and her father, Dan—had a better understanding of the illness and treated her in new, gentler, empathetic ways. After years of turmoil and madness and tears, it's a hard-won understanding they would have welcomed earlier in their lives, but they didn't get it until the summer of 2002.

Karen always was a tense, troubled child in some ways, but no one thought she'd ever end up raving in a mental hospital about being the Devil. Growing up in a blue-collar Massachusetts city, her family's hard work and savings permitted them to lead somewhat more affluent lives than some of their friends. Karen was one of three children of a hard-working schoolteacher (Dan) and an office administrator (Martha); she was a nervous, insecure kid without many friends. As a teen, she recalls that she "didn't like school," but doesn't elaborate on that; there were few if any signs to forecast the breakdown that hit her when she was thirty. She had little in the way of outside hobbies or interests, but she was far from being crazy. Tensions mounted between mother and daughter when her parents finally retired in their mid-fifties, in 1991, in the house the father had largely built himself over several summers in Maine (while keeping another home in Florida). In Maine, home all the time now, her mother felt Karen's touchy personality was making it difficult for Martha's sons and grandkids to visit her, and, Martha told me, Karen was jealous of attention shown to others. For instance, when Martha's grandson was born on the same day as Karen's birthday, she began crying, complaining, "I can't even have a birthday by myself." Karen, in turn, remembers visiting her brother and new nephew for a subsequent birthday party and being resentful that "they didn't care one way or another" about her birthday. The father was resentful of what he saw as Karen's spendthrift ways—an issue that at the time caused some problems between the two.

Over the next few years, Martha gradually began to feel that her control of the house was slipping away to her daughter, who still lived at home. Meanwhile, Karen's business, which she launched in 1991 when she was twenty-five, grew more successful (though she never earned more than about $35,000 a year). Eventually, Martha felt, "It wasn't my house anymore," and she and her husband moved out to an apartment owned by a son in another part of town. Karen was left alone, and it's likely the troubles began there, adding stress to what most scientists believe is an innate biological vulnerability.

At first, Karen enjoyed the new freedom she had, sprucing up the place, repainting the walls white, bringing in new rugs, and getting rid of some of her parents' items. But the town was, Martha said, a cold and unfriendly place, and Karen would call, sometimes late at night, about being lonely. In the wintertime, when her parents were away in Florida, she really had only one friend, who was often busy with a husband. Karen was either working or staying by herself in the house, and so the isolation mounted.

About this time, Karen became more religious, attending a Catholic lay Bible study group, sometimes quoting the Bible to her mother when they had arguments. She even went on a religious retreat, developing an unrequited crush on one of the priests there. Karen was impressed by the devotion of one of the kitchen workers, humbly peeling corn. Neither incident seemed like that much at the time, but when she visited the retreat again in the days before her subsequent breakdown a year or so later, they took on an outsized importance in her fevered mind. "Things were building, you could see it in her eyes that she was getting worse," her father, Dan, said. But before that first breakdown in the summer of 1996, she seemed suddenly eager to make changes in her life and began planning a fun, life-affirming experience: a trip to Europe with some younger students at the college where she was taking night courses in business. She closed the shop for a month, paid all her bills ahead and prepared for an exciting new journey.

But it became the first leg of a journey into madness. Then thirty, she felt estranged from the young college kids on the trip, and bizarre new worries began to occupy her mind. Her flight to Italy was on a TWA flight, and on the way over she began ruminating on the possibility that she had caused the crash of another TWA flight to Paris a week earlier. She kept the thought to herself, although she didn't even think it was crazy, and remembers a lot of that stressful time: "Everything was piling up on me, and I had a lot of guilt." Over what? She's not specific about it, nor was there any rational reason for that feeling, but she notes that in the prayer group she'd begun going to, "There was a lot of talk about the Devil, and somewhere along the line, I became more interested in the Devil than in God." She didn't become a Satanist or anything like that, but after she returned from her trip to Europe, she gradually became convinced that she herself was the Devil.

The paranoia and delusions became more intense during and after a brief visit to the Catholic retreat. According to her mother, Karen left the retreat in Massachusetts feeling intensely guilty about her crush on the priest. And when that humble kitchen worker greeted her by saying, "Long time no see," Karen recalls, "It freaked me, wicked." She barely knew the person, and there was something about his greeting that struck Karen as eerie, too intimate and, perhaps, part of a conspiracy. On the long trip back to Maine by herself, she wept the whole way, and strongly felt that "I didn't know where I was supposed to be." It was a feeling of being "out of sync" with life and at a crossroads facing choices she couldn't quite define.

She showed up at her family's apartment, upsetting her mother with all her crazed talk about sin. "She started talking about the Devil, that she was bad and evil," Martha recalled. At night, Karen couldn't sleep, and they'd stay in the same bed, Martha holding her hand as Karen wept. "I didn't know what to do," Martha said. "I thought she was putting on an act; I thought she was being a spoiled brat." Martha felt Karen was trying to manipulate them with a "guilt trip" so that the two parents wouldn't go back to Florida. After a few days of Karen "not making any sense," Martha recalls, she asked a friend who was a registered nurse to meet with her daughter, and after a few hours of talking, the nurse recommended that she should be taken to an in-patient mental health facility then known as the Pavilion in Portsmouth, New Hampshire.

Once there, she was given medication, but she was discharged after about a week without being given a fair trial to see if the drugs could have much impact. During this hospital visit, she was diagnosed as having bipolar illness, and it wasn't until after a subsequent hospitalization in Maine two years later that she was told she had a form of schizoaffective disorder, or depression with psychotic symptoms.

In any case, after a few days in the Portsmouth hospital in 1996, the psychiatrist there recommended that she receive shock treatments, a decision both her mother and daughter eventually felt was too hasty, and Karen continued to return on an outpatient basis for the treatments, a total of six times.

Karen also recalls the group therapy sessions at the hospital, and how they differed from the multifamily group she went to in Maine. "Your family was with you in Maine, and because it's a long-term group, we got to know each other. In the hospital people came and went," she says.

In the two years after her shock treatments, she would go on and off her medicines, worrying her family. But for a while, her delusional symptoms were kept under some control by the passage of time, periodic use of medications and the sheer effort of Karen's will: "I had to keep talking to myself and say, 'I don't think I'm evil.'" But she had trouble getting along with customers at work, sometimes throwing someone out in anger, and she couldn't get along, either, with the women in a "Women Alone" support group she joined at the suggestion of her mother. Part of the problem was Karen's belief that they were engaged in an evil conspiracy to somehow use her in some nefarious spiritual way. After a blowup with two of the women in the group, she got so angry with them that she scrawled "BITCH" and "I HATE YOU" on their cars with lipstick. The next day she wrote a letter to the leader withdrawing from the group and asking for her money back—and then made plans to hang herself.

She bought herself a rope and called her mother at home in Florida, announcing her intention to kill herself. Her mother frantically called Karen's psychiatrist but didn't receive any response, despite repeated calls. So she called her son in another part of the Maine town and a next-door neighbor, asking them to go over and look in on her. Karen's brother went over reluctantly, telling his mother blandly, "If she's going to do it, she's going to do it." The neighbors, an elderly couple, dropped in briefly but didn't offer much help or comfort. Karen drove herself to Counseling Services of Southern Maine's emergency center, which referred her to a nearby hospital's psychiatric unit. There, she was surrounded by what she felt were some screaming madwomen and was distressed when hospital staff made her take off her jewelry, an apparent preventive measure against suicide. At the hospital, the psychiatrist urged her, "You've got to take responsibility." She notes, "When he told me to take responsibility, I thought he meant I had to take responsibility for my family"—not exactly the message someone in her condition wanted to hear. She also focused her mind on a bird outside the doctor's office, and when she saw the doctor the next day wearing a tie with a picture of that bird, she knew it was part of a plot against her.

She only stayed for a few days: "I just pretended to get better to get out of there."

She continued to work, with increasing dosages of antidepressant medication and a mood stabilizer, but her work lost any meaning for her, and she kept getting into arguments with her customers. Her parents came back to Maine early because she wasn't getting any better and they now knew she shouldn't be alone. "I felt she'd be better with us," Martha said. The parents sold the Maine house in 1998—staying instead in the apartment when visiting—and Karen found a buyer for her business, almost giving it away for under $15,000. She continued to suffer from some milder, occasional delusions, but back in Florida and during her returns to Maine, her doctor recommended increased exercise, and she also got more socially involved, even joining a bowling league.

So when Marilyn Wanyo, her counselor during her summer visits to Maine, started a multifamily group in May 2002, she was somewhat open to participating, even though their summer return meant that they joined the group a few weeks late. Initially, she didn't like it and was wary, but later came to enjoy going. "I finally felt connected with people," she says. She also welcomed the opportunity to learn about others' problems and help them as well. Karen says, "I could identify with their pain as far as dealing with the illness on a daily basis." She adds, "Their dilemmas are not the same, but basically by taking care of each other, we're making sure you're taking medication and finding ways to console family members." Problem-solving exercises, in particular, helped underscore their common ground: "It was nice when they talked about their situation, and you have the same situations," she says.

She blossomed a bit by helping others, too. "She offered some good suggestions," her father said of her participation in the problem-solving exercises. Moreover, her mother said, "By looking at everyone else's problems, it brought her out of herself. With that disease, all they think of is themselves." Karen, for instance, made a suggestion to one of the women in the group about checking with her doctor to find a counteracting medication to leg-shakes induced by the antipsychotic medication the woman was taking (Karen knew about the drug because a friend had a similar problem); the woman followed Karen's advice, and her doctor indeed suggested such a drug. "People learned from you," Karen says.

In addition, compared to other groups she's been in at various times (including some for overeating and depression), "They weren't judgmental, and the people were very patient," Karen says. Her parents noticed that once Karen started to like the group, her mood improved, and as her willingness to return to the job she quit indicates, she was willing to take steps to repair ruptured relationships that she wouldn't have taken before.

As for her parents, "the group did wonders for us," Martha said when I met her. It offered some comfort, as well as insights into the illness. The psychoeducation component also inspired her to alter her behavior towards her daughter. "I made changes because I understood the illness," she added.

When she was living with her family in Florida for most of the year, Karen wasn't able to find the kind of support she found in Maine. To her, the primary benefit of the Maine group has been "the connections to people," and she's not sure she'll find that kind of connection again in Florida, where multifamily psychoeducation groups are rare, if they exist at all.

• • •

IN THE YEARS SINCE I FIRST SPOKE TO KAREN, SHE VISITED NEARBY CLINICS in her county for conventional psychiatric care, went on and off various medications, and periodically ended up back in the hospital, lonelier and more isolated than ever. Some years later, she suffered a hard blow when her parents died, and she moved back to Maine by herself.

Suspicious and fearful, apparently still struggling with her illness, she didn't want to talk about what was going on in her life now. With both her parents dead, she was no longer eligible to participate in a multifamily psychoeducation program, even if she wanted to do so.

In January 2015, SAMHSA hailed "Recovery Month," spreading the message that mental health services can enable people with mental illness to "live a healthy and rewarding life." But by failing to actually spread the ongoing use of something perhaps even more valuable—programs that work—the agency's sweeping promises don't touch the lives of people like Karen who still need help.

McFarlane knew that there were many more people like Karen he and his programs could reach, even *before* they developed schizophrenia. He learned from the successes of the multifamily education model and sought to apply it more broadly, incorporating most of the elements of the best evidence-based treatments, such as supported employment teams, to improve work and school performance. The science of spotting early warning signs was well-developed by the time he took his program into the Portland, Maine, community in 2000; then with over $17 million in funding from the Robert Wood Johnson Foundation, he and his associates at the Portland Identification and Early Referral Program (PIER) launched it in six cities in 2006, from Glen Oaks, New York, to Sacramento, California. All six sites worked to "proactively" educate thousands of community members, health professionals and educators about the early signs of severe mental illness, then identified at-risk young people and got them into treatment. The program's promising results reduced psychotic breaks within two years among high-risk patients to as low as 6 percent, compared to nearly 30 percent of high-risk young people who don't get such treatment.

"If you want to identify someone at risk, then you would be talking with and educating the people who spend a lot of time with adolescents," McFarlane observes. As part of researching the outreach program, this became the psychosis-prevention version of a community-wide diet, exercise or anti-smoking campaign.

It seemed like an admirable goal, and real people would be helped, but the underlying approach soon became an inadvertent part of an intellectual firefight over a proposed diagnostic code in the then upcoming American Psychiatric Association's DSM-5 diagnostic manual. The proposed diagnosis of "psychosis risk syndrome" or "attenuated psychosis syndrome" was seen by its critics as a stalking horse for the overmedicating of kids. The opponents were led by Dr. Allen Frances, the former chairman of Duke University's psychiatry department who led the committee that produced the previous diagnostic manual. "The results could be a disastrous misdiagnosis, stigma and exposure to unnecessary and harmful antipsychotic meds," he said. "Preventing psychosis would be a great idea if we could really do it, but there is no reason to think we can."

In the media firestorm that followed these sorts of attacks in 2012, the APA announced it was dropping the diagnosis (although a variation was buried elsewhere in the manual when it was published in May 2013). Dr. Allen Frances became something of a mainstream hero to those who saw psychiatry as invariably endangering people with needless, greed-driven medications. No matter that McFarlane only approved small, short-term doses of Abilify as a rare, last resort in his program, and he wasn't publicly drawn into this raging debate, but his research programs then underway in six cities were entirely ignored in the media controversy. Looking back, McFarlane sums up Frances's views with one word: "Poppycock." He points out that Frances ignored a vast research literature on how psychosis could develop at any point over two decades in a young person's life from age twelve onwards, let alone the research he and a dozen other clinicians have done worldwide, showing that prevention of this most frightening and disorienting of all mental illnesses was indeed possible. Yet in some ways, Frances had good reason to object to the pre-psychosis diagnosis being used because, if applied by most harried conventional clinics and psychiatrists who often dole out antipsychotic meds like candy, the dangerous prescribing he feared could well have spread to this new diagnostic category of patients.

Frances's warnings about this controversial diagnosis, despite his ethically questionable research for J&J decades ago, are well worth noting. In a statement he emailed me, he argued, "The larger problem is the misuse of a diagnosis once it gets into the DSM. We already have massive overuse of antipsychotics in kids for questionable indications—and 'pre-psychosis' could make this worse. Researchers always see benefits of their pet projects, but don't appreciate risks when applied sloppily in the real world."

Even with these dangers, a proven program thwarting schizophrenia before its onset wasn't something that could neatly fit into the usual ideological framework that pitted proponents and opponents of psychiatric medications against each other. When it comes to something as dangerous, elusive and complex as schizophrenia, it needed to be challenged by a program with nearly as many interwoven elements as the illness itself. Lives were at stake; over 10 percent of people with schizophrenia kill themselves; and those with untreated schizophrenia are three or more times as likely to commit violence than the average citizen, even though they are 1,000 percent more likely to become victims of violence. Either/or answers were not a solution, and like so much else that works in the mental health field, McFarlane's early intervention successes would refute ideologues on all sides of the debates over psychiatry and medications. But as with most of the other evidence-based programs that actually help people recover by managing their illness, finding work or living independently, narrow-minded government agencies would often prove to be an obstacle to mentally ill people seeking meaningful and stable lives.

CHAPTER 16

Why Can't We Just Do What Works?

Before he became the director of the Dartmouth Psychiatric Research Center and pioneered a work program that has transformed the lives of thousands of mentally ill people, psychiatrist Dr. Robert Drake was a graduate student in psychology in the 1970s who visited patients confined in mental hospitals and shoddy group homes. He saw them sitting around in listless boredom, doped up on the reigning antipsychotics Haldol and Thorazine, mired in lives without hope. "It was clear to me that people didn't need to be in institutions for a long period of time. They just needed basic supports in the community," he says. "That's what we needed to do then and it's still true. But we have been bombarded with polypharmacy that hasn't changed course or helped people make an adjustment to live in the community."

"They need good housing, they need a job, friends, social supports and they need families who know how to help them," Drake adds. Though his views may sound like common sense or simple human decency, very few have access to most of those basics. A little over half the nation's ten million adults and six million children with serious mental illnesses and emotional disturbances—including those adults suffering from schizophrenia and bipolar disorder—receive any kind of treatment in the course of a year. Yet less than 2 percent of adults in treatment are involved in the proven "psychosocial" programs such as Independent Placement and Support (IPS), the supported employment approach co-developed by Drake that can make their lives meaningful and help reduce relapses that lead to hospitalizations, jailings or suicides. About 85 percent of seriously mentally ill people don't work at all, even though most have expressed a wish to do so—a higher rate of unemployment than with any other disability. A 2014 report by NAMI showed that unemployment rates were as high as nearly 93 percent in Maine for those in the public mental health system, and even in progressive California rates were at 90 percent.

In that context, the results of supported employment are especially astounding: More than two-thirds of people with serious mental illnesses not only land actual jobs but often keep them for years. The core practices and philosophy of IPS involve using a "job coach" embedded with a clinical team to provide guidance and to seek out employers with the goal of rapidly getting clients hired for truly competitive jobs. No one is excluded, regardless of how severe their mental illness or their addictions. The client's goals are paramount, while staff ensures they retain all their benefits and don't face cutoffs by earning too much. All this is at odds with the still-dominant approach of conventional vocational rehab, if that's offered at all. Most seriously mentally ill people are seen as too sick to work outside of "sheltered workshops" or doing menial tasks inside a mental health program—and they supposedly need months, if not years, of "pre-job" practice before they're ready for work in the real world.

In contrast, Anne Peyer, the vocational services director of Cornerstone Montgomery, a full-service mental health program in Silver Spring, Maryland, observes, "We strongly believe that anyone who wants to work, can. It is a matter of finding the right job." Their results prove the point: 69 percent of their six hundred youth and adult clients work.

One of Peyer's clients is James, a bright man in his fifties, who had his first psychotic breakdown in the 1980s while enrolled as a medical student. James welcomes the independence and confidence work has brought him. With ten years at a health-care supply business in an administrative post, he says, "You feel like you matter to society and that you're contributing. Every day, you have something to get up for and you get to know people: that's really healthy for you." And of course, there's the paycheck: up to $25,000 a year in a thirty-two-hour-a-week job, thanks to promotions, while still retaining Medicaid and remaining on Social Security disability rolls, although payments are lowered as his income rises.

That's a very different experience from when James was beset by the demons of schizophrenia and the strong belief, while volunteering in a nursing home as a student, that he was communicating telepathically with the patients. He stopped working, eventually dropped out of school and was so introverted he could barely talk to other people. After being hospitalized several times, James took part in day-treatment programs while suffering severe side effects (including muscle rigidity) from the older generation of antipsychotics. He was helped, despite its potential risks, by taking the then-new antipsychotic Clozaril in 2000, and felt the drug's value for him was worth the weekly blood tests to check his white blood cell count. Clozaril helped him act on renewed stirrings of ambition and enroll in a community college for an associates degree in computer programming. "I always had goals," he says. After another hospitalization, though, he was referred to Cornerstone Montgomery. There, counselors asked him questions he'd rarely heard before: "What do you want to do, and where do you want to go in your life?" Still not feeling quite himself, he searched for an administrative job and, by January 2005, landed a clerical position he's held ever since. One sign of the job's impact on him: "For a good ten years, I had trouble waking up. Once I got the job and showed up on time, I wasn't exhausted." Today he holds a more senior administrative job.

Cornerstone Montgomery values the program so much that each client has two counselors to work with: one to handle job-specific issues, the other to offer help with other life problems. For James, the job coach has intervened a few times with bosses at work over the years, by, for example, asking for a supervisor to cut him a little slack over his work pace when some of his symptoms worsened. It's up to each client to decide whether to disclose to employers that they have a mental illness history, but the health-care firm where James worked knew he worked with the program and scouted him after he was referred for an interview.

It was James's first real job since dropping out of University of Pennsylvania medical school many years earlier. His therapist, who spoke to me with his permission, told me, "For someone with schizophrenia to go to work every day, it's really difficult. It was very helpful for him and gave him more confidence. He's done amazingly well: he's gotten bonuses for never being late and he has a strong work ethic."

James hasn't escaped his illness, but he manages it—the real definition of recovery. After a brief hospitalization a few years ago, he still finds himself bothered periodically by obsessive thoughts. But with the help of the Cornerstone Montgomery staff, he returned to work. "I feel competent," he says. "I feel like a good worker." A reclusive, quiet man, he also has something he's never really had before: a few close friends.

Indeed, when people like James see themselves as steady workers, rather than as patients in the mental health system, their employment also dramatically contributes to positive outcomes in other areas of their life. Over a ten-year period, the costs these clients incur for outpatient treatment and repeat hospitalizations are a stunning *$166,000* less per person than for those enrolled in conventional treatment programs, according to a study co-authored by Drake in the journal *Psychiatric Services*. A year of supported employment services only costs an added $4,000 or so for each client, Drake notes.

"The best mental health treatment in the world is a *job*," Drake once told me, in a moment of enthusiastic hyperbole, at a conference several years ago; of course, as James illustrates, supported employment is offered along with other services, including counseling and if needed, medication. But the ability to find and hold a competitive job is viewed by most experts as a central measurement of recovery and personal fulfillment. Now with two dozen controlled studies worldwide over two decades and the program adopted in portions of approximately twenty states and endorsed by leading European countries, all part of a collaborative network based at the Rockville Institute near Dartmouth, there is clearly interest among the savvier, more dedicated mental health administrators in putting it into practice. But to do so, US agencies and clinics have to overcome an obstacle course of byzantine government disincentives and a hodgepodge of funding sources, barriers that combine to keep people with mental illness permanently impoverished and hopeless for life. Drake and others have partially blamed the billions wasted on medications that often don't work—government funds that could have been used to hire and train more clinicians and counselors to offer personalized care and cost-effective programs like supported employment.

"It's all based on false advertising," he argues. "We spend billions on ineffective medications, and we won't spend a few million to get people back to work and off of the Social Security rolls. Does that make any sense?"

For mental health programs that just want to help people live independently, it's a funding and logistical nightmare. Administrators must struggle with obtaining funding from a myriad of different federal and state agencies. Medicaid generally won't pay for employment support and contradictory, arcane rules make it difficult to cobble resources together. In contrast, it's always easy for health-care providers to tap into centralized funding sources, either Medicaid or Medicare, to pay again and again for dangerous antipsychotics that can, at their worst, kill people—but no federal agency will coordinate funding for programs that can restore dignity, well-being and purpose to people with a serious mental illness. Drake offers a clear, obvious answer for addressing supported employment, but it isn't part of the congressional discussion on mental health reform: "Fund treatment and rehabilitation as an integrated and bundled package through Medicaid," he wrote in 2014. "This solution recognizes that [supported employment] is good treatment, helps people to recover their lives outside of dependence on the mental health system, and reduces costs over the long run."

A few states, such as Illinois and New Hampshire, have wisely begun paying more to clinics implementing supported employment. In these cases, though, it's not clear if they would have done that on their own: Class-action disability rights lawsuits brought by, among others, each state's federally-funded state disability rights legal center under the Americans with Disabilities Act (ADA) have forced some states to adopt evidence-based psychosocial practices. These enable the seriously mentally ill to flourish in their communities, rather than languish in institutional settings or receive third-rate, drug-oriented clinic care—the national norm. As a result of the 2014 settlement in New Hampshire, supported employment is part of a broad package of mandated reforms that serves as a blueprint of effective programs, including Assertive Community Team outreach work and "supported housing": subsidized apartments combined with access to an array of services that let the seriously mentally ill live independently.

Drake is glad to see more states use supported employment and such allied approaches, but he's angered at the continuing resistance of most state and federal agencies to providing effective care. "Medicaid hasn't given much attention to mental health reform, just to cutting costs," he says. "We're funding vested interests to suck profits out of the system, rather than helping the patient."

Despite all the roadblocks faced by supported employment and related psychosocial programs, such as McFarlane's family-based psychosis treatments, Drake and other proponents remain determined to see proven programs spread more widely. It has been fashionable for political leaders and advocacy groups in Washington to call for the adoption of evidence-based practices and early intervention programs as part of Rep. Tim Murphy's mental health reform package. But few of the champions of these programs understand how the federal government has handled—or mishandled—such initiatives before and how it continues to undermine them today.

• • •

THESE CAMPAIGNS WERE LAUNCHED YEARS AGO WITHOUT MUCH TO SHOW for it. Drake headed the Evidence-Based Toolkit Implementation Project, a groundbreaking, ambitious program launched in 2001 under the direction of HHS's feckless SAMHSA, which was first supposed to promote best practices through guidebooks (or "toolkits") for clinics, agencies and family members. That effort, in turn, was followed by carrying out the practices in a pilot program. The agency, though, after endless rounds of internal discussions and required approvals, didn't make the toolkits available until about 2008, by which time the supported employment guidebooks (still in online form) and accompanying DVDs were periodically out of stock. Those belated publications were issued well after the second, clinical implementation stage of the project in eight states was already completed in 2005, and their results were published in 2007. Other agency publications were canceled altogether after the one communications office staffer working part-time on preparing all of SAMSHA materials just gave up, a knowledgeable agency source says. A former SAMSHA official familiar with the toolkit program and other agency publication projects admits, "Millions of dollars were wasted and the delays took much longer than anyone expected." A staffer at a local clinic involved with the project, who had waited in vain for the toolkits says, "SAMSHA officials were totally incompetent and bungled everything," while some in the agency blamed the Dartmouth Research Center for turning in instructional materials that weren't reader-friendly.

During that fiasco, Drake's center, starting about mid-2002, developed their own materials that their staff and contracted technical assistance experts could use in the field, training more than fifty clinics in eight states in a two-year span to adopt five under-used methods, including supported employment and family psychoeducation. Given limited funds, the project simply sought to measure whether clinicians and providers could show "fidelity" to the practices as they were supposed to be implemented because outcomes had already been established in years of well-designed studies on the methods. On that front, at least, there were some major successes: A 2007 *Psychiatric Services* study showed that more than half the sites could follow these models in practice, with supported employment among the most faithfully implemented of these proven approaches, while they had more trouble carrying out the "dual-diagnosis" programs that treat both mental illness and substance abuse. The clinics got specialized assistance, plus salesmanship on the cost-effectiveness of the programs from Drake and his state allies—but, surprisingly, not extra funds for putting the practices in place.

Later, Dr. Gregory McHugo, a research professor of psychiatry at Dartmouth and a co-author of the 2007 study, wasn't sure those gains would continue. "They were doing things on a shoestring," he observed. "The feds just don't provide enough money for this. You have to put incentives in place to make [clinicians] do the right thing. People in the field respond to incentives and go where the money is."

Unfortunately, because there's relatively little money in the mental health system, there's even greater reluctance to adopt new approaches. By 2014, two years after the shootings at Sandy Hook Elementary School spurred an increase in state mental health funding, funding slowed again. State programs had slashed over $4 billion from their mental health budgets over a three-year period ending in 2012. "This damage is a long way from being repaired," NAMI reported.

With limited funds, federal and state programs are especially reluctant to adopt the pre-psychosis risk program for young people developed by McFarlane, despite its proven effectiveness. The six-city, Robert Wood Johnson–funded community outreach study published in 2014 in *The Schizophrenia Bulletin* found that those with serious pre-psychotic symptoms were three times as likely to remain in school or be working than those who didn't participate in the early prevention program. Most strikingly, people taking the program were as much as five times less likely to develop psychosis than those with those same early symptoms. All told, using McFarlane's model or comparable pre-psychosis interventions, fifteen studies worldwide have shown the positive impact of this combination of family-based intensive services, individual counseling and working in partnership with the client to achieve their goals—with low, brief doses of medication as a last resort.

The PIER model that became the basis of the broader six-city study cut the number of people hospitalized for first psychotic breaks by 26 percent in the *entire city* of Portland, Maine. "If we don't do anything before they're hospitalized, we'll have another generation of people with the illness [schizophrenia] having a 12 to 15 percent suicide rate," McFarlane points out.

But that is precisely what could happen because NIMH is potentially putting some people at risk by downplaying the value of *any* pre-psychosis programs, claiming the evidence just isn't in—and advising state governments that they shouldn't spend any of the federal "set-aside" grants on them. Despite some in-depth, laudatory coverage of these programs, the media accounts paid little attention to the fact that this proven treatment modality available now—intensive pre-psychosis supports—was being denied federal funding in communities, although NIMH has commissioned some long-range studies in this field. (The media accounts sometimes conflated NIMH's post-psychotic break programs, known by the acronym RAISE, with McFarlane's *pre-psychosis* work that employs similar psychosocial strategies with different, but complementary aims.)

The McFarlane model faced powerful enemies. The NAMI advocacy group strongly opposed allowing states to use federal funds for the program, claiming that it was following the research guidance of NIMH. Congress rejected requests in 2014 for expanded permission to use the funds on pre-psychosis programs from the National Association of State Mental Health Program Directors (NASMHPD), whose leaders recognize the cost-effectiveness of preventing the suicides, homelessness and hospitalizations resulting from psychotic breaks. Nevertheless, in 2015 and 2016, at the urging of NAMI and NIMH, congressional budget bills banned spending any early-prevention set-aside funds—from the $520 million in total "block grants" to the states—on pre-psychosis programs. Stuart Gordon, the state program directors' policy director, says of the opposition of NAMI and federal officials to such spending, "It's really odd that major mental health organizations should oppose a prevention intervention." In a mental health system struggling for funds, however, the emphasis on primarily helping early on those who have recently been hospitalized for a psychotic break makes a certain economic and public health sense, even if more people could be helped before becoming psychotic.

Federal officials haven't yet commissioned research on Open Dialogue, a promising crisis-intervention response to young people experiencing early psychotic episodes. Open Dialogue was studied in a recent small pilot project in Massachusetts. It shares some of the cooperative, flexible spirit of McFarlane's PIER psychosis prevention approach, but goes well beyond RAISE and other post-break psychosis programs in downplaying the role of psychiatric medications. It has been championed by critics of conventional psychiatry because of the astounding reported results popularized in Robert Whitaker's influential 2010 book *Anatomy of an Epidemic*, although it hasn't been replicated in randomized controlled studies, as with RAISE and the overseas research on PIER-style programs. A five-year observational study of forty-two young participants in Open Dialogue in rural Finland, where it was first developed, found that 86 percent of those diagnosed with psychosis were now working or in school, 14 percent were disabled and only 17 percent were still being prescribed antipsychotics.

"When I first saw those results I thought there's no way this could be true, it's implausible," says Dr. Chris Gordon. He ended up developing an Open Dialogue pilot project as medical director of the Advocates community mental health program in Framingham,

Massachusetts, working with a team of University of Massachusetts and Boston University researchers. After visiting Tornio, Finland, and meeting with the chief academic researcher there, he concluded, "The reported outcomes are exactly as they said. This isn't a flim-flam." The approach is as much a philosophy as a specific method: it involves a pair of therapists approaching the person in crisis and their families at home and working in collaboration with them on how they can provide help. Open Dialogue doesn't rely on diagnostic labels the clinicians view as stigmatizing, or, in many cases, medications. "We meet the person where they are and engage with the person in crisis with a wide open mind," says Gordon.

Partnering with Dr. Douglas Ziedonis, the chairman of the UMass psychiatry department, and his research colleagues at Boston University, they published in *Psychiatric Services* in July 2016 the results of a small fourteen-person study: it showed that nine of the young men and women enrolled in the program were still in school or working. Yet even in this empathetic, low-medication, cooperative approach, medications and hospitalizations were used. During the course of the year, four of the people needed to be hospitalized, two of them involuntarily, a 28 percent one-year relapse rate that's roughly equivalent to conventional treatment. And while some of the people, ages fourteen to thirty-five, went off their meds or began taking medication, by year's end, 50 percent of the participants were taking antipsychotics. The real importance of the program, Gordon argues, is this: "It's empowering people to do better in their lives through shared decision-making and enhancing their connections to their support network." But it's not likely to be widely adopted in the US without rigorous controlled studies backing it. But thanks to a *New York Times* article on the program and other alternatives in August 2016, it's now on the map for policy-makers and may eventually draw NIMH's interest.

Despite the brief flash of publicity for McFarlane's pre-psychosis programs and, more recently, Open Dialogue, most of the media attention has focused on RAISE, the well-researched Recovery After Initial Schizophrenia Episode program. That's a related but different early psychosis program, led by NIMH, that emphasizes the value of low-dose medications and combined psychosocial services for those experiencing "first-break" or early psychotic episodes. Announced with a flourish in September 2015 with the publication of a two-year study in the *American Journal of Psychiatry*, RAISE showed significant but modest improvements in symptoms, school and work functioning of those enrolled in the program *after* psychotic breaks, but no difference in hospitalization rates—a critical barometer of recovery that has been dramatically cut by the McFarlane model and other pre-psychosis treatments. McFarlane critiqued the high repeat breakdown rates of RAISE: "That's nothing to boast about." (In an email, NIMH officials explained away a troubling repeat hospitalization rate of 34 percent for both conventional and RAISE treatments by contending that by comparison the community care treatment was actually quite good.)

Still, RAISE deployed an array of services similar to the McFarlane model and Open Dialogue, although RAISE generally placed a greater emphasis on using antipsychotics, but in low doses and in consultation with the young clients. Also, like McFarlane's approach, it offered family support programs and one-on-one talk therapy. What drew so much media attention was that RAISE, like McFarlane's work, not only eschewed high doses of antipsychotics and other psychotropic drugs but collaborated with patients when a medication plan was needed—a far cry from the drugging onslaught that played a major role in the deaths of Gabriel Meyers and Andrew White.

One beneficiary of RAISE is Belle, a twenty-three-year-old student in Portland, Oregon, now studying to be an occupational therapist. As a teen, her early depression and anxiety eventually blossomed into a full-blown psychotic episode at nineteen after her psychiatrist crudely diagnosed her as having ADHD, then plied her with a stimulant and the antidepressant Effexor. The combination of medications, Belle believes, pushed her into a downward spiral when she began hearing voices, staying up sleepless for days and becoming paranoid. In response, the doctor just added some new medications, including Zoloft and Adderall, the amphetamine that, as with Kelli Grese, has possible psychosis side effects. "She blew past the risks," Belle says. Despite hospital stays, she didn't really improve after she got a mix of mood stabilizers and antipsychotics that kept changing. Before she was discharged a final time, a nurse referred her to Oregon's Early Assessment and Support Alliance (EASA), a program that is among the leaders in the nation in developing both pre-psychosis and "First Episode" psychotic break approaches.

In Belle's case, she was enrolled in a program similar to RAISE and was immediately struck by the empathy, concern and attention to her goals that the treatment staff offered her. She had failed all her previous classes and lost most of her friends from her bizarre behavior. So when they asked her, "What do you want to do?" she told them that she wanted to return to school and taper off her medications. She weaned herself off of most of her meds (but still stays on a mood stabilizer), graduated college after enrolling again part-time and started working as well. "My functioning improved and I learned to empathize with myself," she says. Their caring approach also inspired her career goal as an occupational therapist.

To Tamara Sale, director of care for EASA, both of the early psychosis approaches complement each other and have value. But she points out, "NIMH has put so much emphasis on the RAISE project because there's all this investment behind it"—over $20 million.

Sale has found that the pre-psychosis program, shaped by her group's involvement in the Robert Wood Johnson six-city study, has important benefits that can't be overlooked in the rush to support and promote the RAISE model. Once a person develops schizophrenia, as opposed to preliminary hallucinatory symptoms, she points out, "They are at extremely high risk of adverse events such as legal involvement, accidental death or involuntary hospitalization."

NIMH, though, dismisses McFarlane's work (and virtually all pre-psychosis research in this field) as poorly designed, purportedly because they don't meet the "gold standard" of a randomized clinical trial with exactly matched control and experimental groups. These arcane statistical issues may appear dry, but they're worth knowing if the federal government has in fact decided to cut off all funds for using the pre-psychosis model in the field, thus depriving people of needed care. An NIMH spokesperson said in a statement, "Set-aside funds should be reserved for interventions shown to improve outcomes in First-Episode Psychosis." Yet there are at least a dozen worldwide, rigorously controlled studies with an experimental and a "control" group—but none in the United States—that show that the use of pre-psychosis psychosocial interventions can cut the risk of a psychotic breakdown by 50 percent. That's what the medical literature shows, according to studies sent to me by the world's pioneering expert in this field, Australian researcher Dr. Patrick McGorry, executive director of Australia's National Centre of Excellence in Youth Mental Health. McGorry, himself a recipient of a $6 million NIMH grant to study non-drug treatments on this population, says, "I guess their attitude is if it didn't happen in America, it doesn't count."

McGorry and McFarlane share a philosophy of focusing more on the early stages of mental illness, rather than waiting for advanced or fatal outcomes. That approach helped save the mind and possibly the life of Tiffany Martinez, who got involved in the McFarlane program when she was in college when the program was still based primarily in Portland, Maine. She got help early that allowed her to bring under control the scary symptoms of shadowy figures and strange voices haunting her—and move on with her life. Today, at twenty-eight, she works as a psychiatric nurse practitioner helping others struggling with mental illness. "They really took their time with me," she says gratefully of the staff of the Portland Identification and Early Referral (PIER) program she learned about in college.

Unfortunately, when Tiffany tried to gradually go off her psychiatric medications with the advice of the PIER staff, some of her crazed and depressed thinking returned. Eventually, aided by cognitive behavioral therapy that helped her challenge those thoughts, she graduated college in 2008 and weaned herself off all psychiatric medications. "I believe in mental wellness," she says, staying active and healthy by lifting weights, getting enough sleep and having a steady routine that includes caring for her two dogs.

She argues, "There are early symptoms of psychosis and manifestations you can't ignore. If you can get someone trained to assess you, you're better off getting the specific help you need."

CHAPTER 17

Putting People Before Big Pharma: Overcoming the Barriers to Recovery

"RECOVERY" FROM SERIOUS MENTAL ILLNESS IS REAL: THE ABILITY TO manage otherwise disabling conditions and to live a meaningful, independent and fulfilling life involving work, relationships, a stable home and ties to the community should be available to all. It's still hard for many people to believe that skilled early intervention or even a supportive family environment can potentially help some people from developing full-blown schizophrenia, bipolar disorder and other devastating mental illnesses. But it's worth recalling that even the likelihood of a genetic predisposition underlying these "biosocial" illnesses doesn't doom people for life—and serves to underscore the importance of traumatic life events and social conditions in shaping mental illness. Unfortunately, because 75 percent of psychiatric illnesses develop by age twenty-four, and two-thirds of children with mental health problems receive no treatment at all, millions of people grow up struggling with disabling mental illnesses.

Hard as they are to find, there are still valuable programs and caring professionals at work who can make an enormous difference in the lives of people with serious mental illnesses. The barriers to accessing such effective programs and compassionate clinicians are in some ways worsened by the arguments over the appropriate use—if any—of antipsychotics and other psychotropic drugs. In reading the disturbing stories about drug industry corruption and needless deaths in this book and in the occasional investigative series, one might be tempted to conclude they should never be used because the dangers are too great—a view held by psychologist Mary Vieten and Dr. Peter Breggin, among others.

Unfortunately, the debate over the appropriate use of antipsychotic medications has become deeply polarized. As we've seen, while proponents such as Dr. E. Fuller Torrey score political points by calling for forced medication of seriously mentally ill people deemed too dangerous or unstable, critics, led by the influential journalist and author Robert Whitaker, have forcefully argued against involuntary treatment and contend that antipsychotics are widely over-used. They've marshaled studies that show there is limited evidence of efficacy even for those for whom the drugs were first developed: people with schizophrenia, as the history of pharmaceutical fraud so amply reveals. Whitaker's once-heretical argument, based on decades of scientific research, that the long-term use of antipsychotics usually worsens outcomes for people with schizophrenia has prompted some—but not most—influential mainstream researchers to question such conventional uses. Even Dr. Thomas Insel, for instance, wrote in *JAMA Psychiatry*, "Antipsychotic medication, which seemed so important in the early phase of psychosis, appeared to worsen prospects for recovery over the long-term."

What's too often downplayed in the either/or debate over antipsychotics is the notion that these medications—if judiciously prescribed and coupled with proven therapies, caring therapists and social supports—can be quite helpful for those ravaged by the symptoms of schizophrenia, at least in the short run and in relatively low doses. The harsh reality, though, is that few people disabled by the most severe and persistent forms of mental illnesses such as schizophrenia, bipolar disorder and major depression—a little over 4 percent of the population—will ever get the targeted, empathetic help shown in programs such as The Village in Long Beach, even though they too often face the long-running calamities of homelessness, repeat incarceration and hospitalizations. Meanwhile, millions more are needlessly exposed to antipsychotics they don't need and that pose real dangers to their health and possibly their lives, but neither influential reform organizations nor government agencies are doing much about it.

The commonly marketed notion of an imbalance of chemicals, as noted in the introduction, has largely been discredited by recent research. While there is no single definitive biological marker that's yet been found for depression or other mental illnesses, there are enough indicators showing that biology doubtlessly plays a key, if not yet precisely determined or quantified, role in mental illness. These include studies of identical twins; neural imaging studies highlighting malfunctioning brain activity; and research into abnormal brain development. That research has helped to spur a new federal "brain initiative" by NIMH, but that's not likely to offer answers anytime soon, especially since real-world clinical research accounts for only 10 percent of the institute's budget.

In the meantime, clinicians and consumers hope for the best with the tools at hand. Psychiatrists in the field simply can't wait decades for new research to offer definitive solutions, or for the longstanding battles over the role of biology in mental illness to be finally resolved. Rigid debates about medication and diagnoses don't help psychiatrists such as Dr. Mark Ragins, founding medical director of Mental Health America's "The Village," a successful program for the long-term mentally ill homeless in Long Beach. "This feels philosophical, an inside baseball debate that's quite removed from the everyday lives of people with schizophrenia," he says. "They've got concerns like: How do I get enough money to have a place to live? How do I find a primary care doctor and get him to take me seriously? How do I stop a policeman from shooting me?"

He agrees, though, with many of the common critiques of conventional, rushed, pill-dispensing psychiatry. He shares with fellow critics of psychiatry the horror at the legacy of abusive and forced care for people with schizophrenia: "There is no other non-contagious illness in history where people are quarantined for life; or that you put ice picks into people's brains and chop them up." Even so, he demurs: "I admire the critics' efforts to decrease all these negative things, but by putting psychiatrists, medications and hospitals in with all these medical things in one pile, they've made it difficult for me to be a compassionate psychiatrist who uses medications in prescribing," he says. "They're not acknowledging the humanity of relieving that suffering."

For instance, he describes the case of a disheveled man in his forties who was first found by The Village's outreach staff on the street after being discharged from the hospital yet again. He was silent, sunburned, disoriented and angry, glaring up at the worker offering help, with a history of as many as eighty jailings and hospitalizations over twenty years. He never took medication on his own and never could get it together to get disability payments—and once beat up his mother so severely that she ended up deaf. "His family was terrorized," Ragins notes. The man cycled between jails and hospitals and the streets of Long Beach.

The Village social workers knew he'd never come for a formal medical appointment, but they invited him to lunch to meet Ragins in the cafeteria. He could barely talk or even eat a sandwich: "He was like a wild animal," Ragins recalls. Even so, the outreach workers arranged for him to stay at a sober living facility whose kind-hearted manager tolerated his odd behavior. Ragins learned from the hospital that the man had briefly improved on an antipsychotic, Risperdal, which does have serious side effects. But Ragins still prescribed it, and it helped the client make progress while he reconnected with his once-estranged sister, who came by each day to bring him a meal. A Village case manager eventually started taking him and a few other clients to go bowling, and while at first he still couldn't manage to tie his own shoes, he did get up and bowl some impressive strikes, a sign that he was starting to engage with others. A few months later, Ragins says, "Now he is coherent, taking his medication regularly, and he has lunch with us. He can have a conversation, he's clean and he walks." Unfortunately, Ragins notes, "He has gained thirty-five pounds."

Ragins spotlights the dilemma he's facing as a psychiatrist: "When you talk about when to prescribe meds, here's a guy whose entire life has changed: he can have a conversation, his family's back, his mother is no longer in danger, he's living someplace, he's connected with people—but he's got a dangerous side effect of gaining weight."

"I can talk to his sister about giving him less burritos, but it comes down to: Do I lower the dosage and allow him to get sicker?" he says. "But his life has been changed, so we have to ask: What are we balancing it against?" Ragins is trying to bring a balanced way of assessing this thorny issue: "If the person is not going to be able to live in the community and be tolerated, the person *is* going to be incarcerated either in hospitals or jails. If the person is going to be rejected and homeless repeatedly, it's not necessarily the height of [compassionate] philosophy to say, 'Good, let them be without meds.'"

Informed by such a caring perspective, there's little question that Ragins, his staff of clinicians and the teams of "personal service coordinators" available for 24/7 assistance have made a striking difference in people's lives. Guided by a "whatever it takes" philosophy, The Village helped pioneer intensive, cost-effective services in California designed to reduce chronic homelessness, arrests and repeat hospitalizations, which inspired a statewide referendum leading to a specially-funded Mental Health Services Act in 2004. California spends about $1.5 billion annually on innovative and intensive services statewide. Its revenues derive, amazingly, from a tax on millionaires.

Most psychiatrists have yet to adopt the nuanced, thoughtful approach to prescribing and treatment that Ragins and the Village staff represent. Moreover, their successes don't rest on just one talented physician but on a spirit of compassion and dedication that is set at the top of the organization. What's striking is that they don't focus on degrees and credentials in their hiring of caseworkers, or "personal services coordinators," and other staff who make up their "Full Service Partnership" teams, but on their warmth, friendliness, openmindedness and caring—the qualities people in a psychiatric crisis need.

For Brad (who didn't want his full name used), those attitudes made all the difference. He spent years in and out of treatment and jail, but when his final possession reminding him of his humanity—his bicycle—was stolen, something inside him turned on and he resolved to work seriously with the Village staff to turn his life around. "I realized that someone could kill me and no one would even notice," he says. As a result of the regular outreach work on the streets The Village does, he got involved in treatment and discovered that he was bipolar. He became sober, now lives in a halfway house, has reunited with his family, works part-time and is no longer gripped by the suicidal depths of his bipolar disorder or alcoholism. But it's his connection with his caseworkers and other clinicians at The Village that helps keep him on course: "Everyone on that team is all there for you," he says.

These days, The Village program has helped slash re-hospitalizations and re-arrests by rates ranging from over 80 percent up to 96 percent, and, through direct housing programs and other assistance, to cut homelessness by over half, according to Mental Health America of Los Angeles. During a visit there in 2014, I saw how Ragins carried out his mission to offer individualized, helpful care. He seeks to promote recovery (in short, managing mental illness successfully), hope and respect for individual rights by collaborating with his clients over their own goals, medications and personal views of their symptoms. It's in the same spirit as McFarlane's psychosis prevention work and the Open Dialogue model.

Ragins's approach brings the sort of personalized attention to his clients that a broad spectrum of psychiatry's critics, including psychiatrist Dr. Daniel Carlat in his book *Unhinged*, decry is generally missing from psychiatry today. Ragins spends enough time with clients to learn what factors in their background and lives, including any history of abuse or rape, have contributed to their current crises— and tailors his treatments towards their preferences and personal objectives. For example, he commonly asks those who are hearing voices, "Are they a blessing or a curse?" Then he fashions his prescribing to fit their needs, including lowering dosages in a way that allows those who find their hallucinatory experiences comforting to hold on to them to some degree.

That apparently seems to be a response in part to the burgeoning Hearing Voices Movement, popularized by British founder Eleanor Longden in her TED talk with nearly four million views. As *The New York Times* recently reported, there's a growing alliance called the Hearing Voices Network for people seeking a non-medical approach through support groups, drop-in centers and peer-run respite centers for people in crisis. Part of the interest in these alternatives is due to the problematic side effects of antipsychotics, which cause as many as two-thirds of the people using them to stop within eighteen months. Yet what's gotten less attention is that Longden and other "peer" leaders in the movement also accept the role of medications as often helpful if collaboratively prescribed.

For his part, Ragins, to demonstrate the importance of fully understanding his clients' points of view, holds up his hand and tells the story of a patient who once held out his hand in front of Ragins's face, and asked the doctor, "What do you see?" Ragins proceeded to describe the inside of the palm and assorted lifelines, but the patient soon interrupted him, offering a metaphor, "Until you can see the knuckles and hair on the back of my hands the way I see it, you won't really understand me."

Ragins regrets, in some ways, that the broader community doesn't offer a more loving, tolerant response to madness. "We have to deal with the way the society and treaters are at present," he says. He contends that the current debate over psychiatric medications posits a false choice: "It's not meds *or* individualization—it's meds *with* individualization." Even so, only about 75 percent of the roughly five hundred people being served at The Village are currently on medications, and the therapists accept that clients can stop taking their medications after shared decision-making and being fully informed about the consequences—with the door remaining open for help if they get in trouble again. This reflects the cornerstone of The Village's success: building and maintaining strong relationships with their clients. (Ragins recently left The Village to work as a consultant for other mental health programs and to write a book.)

Yet as a rare last resort for the most extremely violent or endangered clients seen at The Village, even the liberal-minded staffers there sometimes seek involuntary commitment. These people could be placed in treatment facilities although there are relatively few available beds or, under a hotly-disputed new Los Angeles County law, in expanded court-monitored AOT programs. But Village staffers generally avoid the mandatory commitment strategies touted by hard-line advocates such as Dr. E. Fuller Torrey and Rep. Tim Murphy. This philosophy of voluntarily engaging severely mentally ill people in treatment is applied county-wide by other providers when they use the AOT program that could lead to involuntary commitment, with nearly 90 percent of those reached willingly by AOT consenting to accept services.

The best of the Los Angeles County's Department of Mental Health programs, as at The Village, can have a powerful and uplifting impact. But since there is little long-term follow-up and no commitment to helping people obtain competitive jobs, even the most dedicated staff can't help the people they serve live truly independent lives. That reality is barely masked by the department's co-option of the emerging mental health consumer movement under the guise of offering volunteer opportunities in clinics and awards ceremonies, which have become a form of extended paternalism that traps people inside the mental health system for life.

"We're treated like mascots," says Brenda Jones, an early graduate of DMH-sponsored training programs and college-based counseling certificates who can't get the sort of "supported employment" assistance available in Alameda County in California and about twenty other states. "They're pimping us out for gift cards," she says of the endless cycle of short-term volunteer jobs for "consumers." The unemployment rate of people receiving services of various intensity at LA County clinics is close to 90 percent.

As county officials concede, with a few exceptions, they don't use the well-proven "supported employment" approach. "Los Angeles County is terrible," says Dr. Robert Drake. "If you're not helping people find independent, competitive jobs, you're just blowing smoke about recovery." As Keris Myrick, the director of consumer affairs for SAMHSA's Center for Mental Health Services who manages her own schizoaffective disorder with medication, therapy and the life purpose offered by work, told me when I visited LA, "People can't come into the system for treatment because people can't get out, so there's a logjam," seen in long waiting times, overcrowded clinics and harried providers. "There's a fear of letting them go because something bad will happen to them." As a result, while those with life-threatening crises can usually get an emergency response, there are waiting lists for basic psychiatric care as long as ninety days at some clinics.

The worldview of the consumer movement that's supposed to improve treatment, promote alternatives to traditional psychiatry and remove stigma is not widely known outside of the world of mental health care. That has changed somewhat since it has been publicly smeared by critics such as Dr. E. Fuller Torrey as a motley array of crazies funded by SAMHSA taxpayer dollars at "Alternatives" conferences. But it grew out of a desire by "peer advocates" and mental health consumers for a greater say in the care they received. At the same time, there was a growing recognition by academic researchers that peer-to-peer counseling, drop-in centers, and peer-run respite centers as alternatives to visits to the ER were showing increasingly robust evidence that they improved clients' well-being. At The Village, for instance, all the "Full Service Partnerships" include a "peer" with "lived experience," and peer counselors play an increasingly important role in the most effective treatments for serious mental illness, including supported employment.

Yet the value of peers and even the once-accepted goal of "recovery" as part of mainstream psychosocial programs are viewed with disdain by the incoming assistant HHS secretary overseeing SAMHSA, Dr. Elinore McCance-Katz, most recently the chief medical officer of Rhode Island's mental health department and the former top medical officer at SAMHSA until 2015. In controversial 2016 articles in *National Review* and *Psychiatric Times*, she justly took the agency to task for downplaying evidence-based psychiatric services for the most severely mentally ill people in its recent grants to the states. But she also denounced all initiatives for developing a peer workforce as "trivializing" the devastation of untreated mental illness: "Peer support can be an important resource for some, but it is not the answer to the treatment needs of the seriously mentally ill," she declared. In the articles that were thinly disguised job applications to Donald Trump, whose election she described as "an exciting turn of events for people afflicted with mental illness," she ignored altogether the embrace by peers of the leading programs aiding severely mentally ill people developed by the nation's pioneering mental health researchers, including Dr. Robert Drake.

Peer counseling grew out of the mental health consumer movement that by the 1990s had begun to formally organize, echoing the South African disability movement's motto: "Nothing About Us, Without Us." Now, in Los Angeles County and most major mental health departments in the country, at federal agencies such as SAMHSA, and in advocacy groups such as NAMI and Mental Health America, there are peers and consumers in leadership and advisory roles. But that hasn't translated, at least in LA County, to clients' long-term recovery and independence.

• • •

FOR ALL OF THE ABUSES AND CORRUPTION IN THE NATION'S MENTAL health system, there are clear-cut solutions and reforms that could be implemented. They range from stopping the payments for off-label antipsychotic prescribing to incorporating proven treatment programs to cracking down on unregulated "troubled teen" facilities. But those answers have been known for years, even decades, and nothing's been done about it.

There could be a way out of this permanent state of inaction if the lesser-known groups, activists and experts who care deeply about these issues take it on themselves to recruit potential allies among the most influential national advocacy groups, while packaging shocking scandals they know about to win the attention of media outlets. Currently, there is simply no well-organized, powerful national lobbying or legal advocacy group in the country working to halt the dangerous, unproven practices that are so profitable, particularly the overdrugging of children, veterans and the elderly. Top AARP executives, for instance, won't do so unless other experts and advocates figure out a way to shame them or recruit them into taking real action.

On almost every issue raised in this book, there are passionate activists, survivors and experts. Relatively few, however, have the political, legal or media clout to have much impact.

The challenges of fixing the VA and reducing veterans' suicides are among the most intractable problems in mental health care. That's due in no small part to the sharp ideological divides over reform; the sheer size of the VA system, with over 1,200 health-care facilities and 1.6 million veterans receiving specialized mental health treatments annually; and, perhaps most of all, the uniquely poisonous and, at some major VA centers, quasi-criminal leadership willing to cover up fraud and negligent patient care while retaliating against whistleblowers. A good starting point for change is the thoughtful VA Commission on Care report that called for broader patient choice through the private sector and more visionary leadership to promote better quality care and faster access. But it doesn't go far enough, because it assumes on faith that all specialized mental health programs at VA facilities are always better than what's in the private sector, and doesn't provide a mechanism for systematic evaluations from outside evaluators of treatment quality that simply can't be manipulated by VA staff.

Fortunately, the chair of that commission, Nancy Schlichting, the CEO of the successful Henry Ford Health System of Detroit, has unique insights to offer the VA. Under her watch and with her then-chief of behavioral health care, Dr. C. Edward Coffey, they brought suicides down to zero for a patient population of at least 200,000 in the HMO for nearly three years in a row. Even today, their suicide rate of 20 per 100,000 mental health patients is 92 percent less than the national average. Their "Perfect Depression Care" initiative galvanized clinicians and incorporated well-known but rarely used prevention strategies, such as brief screening for depression by primary care providers that led to mental health referrals, and working with patients' families to make sure there weren't weapons at home. But they also encouraged a responsive staff approach of studying suicide tragedies to learn what went wrong, as opposed to downplaying or covering up failures—the hallmark of the VA system.

In the context of the wide-ranging VA scandals, a major shake-up of top administrators at many VA facilities is needed. To make clear that accountability will be imposed on all managers, more funding for agencies outside the VA to investigate wrongdoing is needed since its internal investigative agencies generally can't be trusted. This includes dramatically increasing the staff of the independent federal Office of Special Counsel to investigate whistleblower complaints. Those complaints then can be used by Justice Department prosecutors experienced in health fraud and organized crime to build criminal cases on fraud, perjury and obstruction of justice charges against the most irresponsible administrators if firing proves too time-consuming. Marching several high-profile, bonus-collecting VA executives and their henchmen out of various regional VA hospitals in handcuffs could have a salutary effect. Whistleblowers' hopes for such a crackdown, though, are unlikely to be realized with Shulkin as head of the VA.

Even so, to speed these goals along, I have a few personnel suggestions to prod the new Secretary of the VA to fix the agency and change its culture. Hire Dr. C. Edward Coffey, currently the CEO and President of the prestigious Menninger Clinic, as under secretary of health with a special portfolio for suicide prevention; and appoint Joseph Beemsterboer, the chief of DOJ's Health Care Fraud unit, either as a special prosecutor with a broad mandate to prosecute or force out rogue administrators, or as the Inspector General. These selections involve the traditional good cop/bad cop approach brought to transforming the VA.

For both the VA and the nation's mental health system, one of the thorniest problems is the division between drug treatment and mental health care, which puts both recovery and sanity at risk every day. About 50 percent of the most severely mentally ill people also have a substance abuse problem, while little over half of drug addicts have at least one serious mental illness. The solution is offering effective, personalized, integrated treatment by staff cross-trained in mental health and drug addiction, along with such strategies as "motivational interviewing" to spur change.

The results are striking. Drake led a seven-year follow-up study of inner-city Connecticut residents with schizophrenia and substance abuse who were offered those services—and found that 70 percent later didn't have psychiatric symptoms and over 60 percent were no longer substance abusers. Unfortunately, relatively few state regulators are now paying attention to whether these services are being delivered properly. That could change if an independent assessment system—co-developed by a colleague of Drake at Dartmouth, now at Stanford Medical School, Dr. Mark McGovern, as described in detail in the book *Inside Rehab*—was widely applied across VA and Medicaid programs, as it has been used in the past with select private and government-funded community treatment programs. For several years ending about 2012, there was hope that this could actually happen, because SAMHSA gave roughly fifteen states millions in grants to expand their drug addiction and mental health clinics' capacity to offer quality co-occurring disorder services, largely through far better independent evaluation of programs followed by staff training. This, in turn, inspired more than thirty states overall to adopt in varying degrees these evaluation methods. Then SAMHSA pulled the plug on its incentives.

McGovern's assessment tools have been essential: Going by the names Dual Diagnosis Capability in Addiction Treatment (DDCAT) and Dual Diagnosis Capability in Mental Health Treatment (DD-CMHT), they're used, respectively, for drug treatment and mental health centers. They measure everything from leadership to evidence-based treatments, and then are used to spur improvements.

It takes only a one-day site visit to fully assess and write up any clinic. The reality, though, is that as few as one in ten mental health clinics—and 20 percent of addiction clinics—actually have the capacity to adequately offer these services despite their marketing claims, as he reported in 2014.

Except for a relative handful of states, such as Washington, spending their own funds on it, McGovern's smart method to promote quality dual-diagnosis care isn't widely used anymore. "We had an opportunity to offer good care and save lives," he says. "The human toll is immeasurable," especially with opiate overdoses skyrocketing.

But it seems likely that a lawsuit or new legislation are the only ways to force the VA to accept such independent evaluations in a way they couldn't game—as they've done with all other rating systems.

Virtually every major problem in the mental health system has a solution waiting to be implemented, but virtually no one in power wants to carry it out. At the national level, when it comes to off-label prescribing, some of the smartest thinking comes from groups such as the Lown Institute and its "Right Care" initiative that's developing a community organizing approach to fighting overtreatment of all kinds, a model that's already worked in the UK to bring down antipsychotic overmedication for the elderly. Lown shares a common goal in challenging overmedication with Georgetown University's Pharmed-Out conferences and the "Selling Sickness" campaign, co-developed by Kim Witczak after her husband "Woody" killed himself at age thirty-seven, shortly after starting Zoloft. If they could enlist the Nader-founded Public Citizen Health Research Group to take on this issue with lawsuits, media assaults and grassroots activism, then perhaps the prospects for change in these deadly practices could improve. The Lown Institute's campaign scheduled for the fall of 2017, a "Right Care Top Ten" that highlights five "Do's" and "Don'ts" for different health arenas, including behavioral health care, is a promising start that could be amplified by an alliance with Public Citizen.

For almost every reform that's needed, there is an alliance that could be built to push it forward, anchored by a powerful advocacy group or well-connected community leaders. Judge Steven Leifman in Miami-Dade County constructed over the years a statewide coalition, including leading law enforcement officials that brought about the county's innovative alternatives to jailing the mentally ill. Judge Ginger Lerner-Wren in Broward County, Florida, in 1997 pioneered the nation's first mental health court, which routes mentally ill non-violent misdemeanor offenders into voluntary treatment overseen by the judge instead of into jail. She was backed by mental health advocates and court leaders prodded into action by a grand jury's rebuke of the county jail for warehousing thousands of mentally ill inmates for minor crimes. Over three hundred mental health courts are in operation nationwide now, and when they work well, as a 2015 review of major studies in *Pacific Standard* magazine found, they reduce re-arrests and days in jail by nearly half.

In a similar fashion, the opportunity to promote better, non-drugging, community-based alternatives to juvenile detention for children with emotional problems could become a higher priority issue when already influential reform groups add this goal to their agenda. New attention to the junior division of Incarceration Nation could be won, for example, if the Children's Defense Fund (CDF) and its state chapters took stronger action on this front. (Its influential president, Marian Wright Edelman, has already spoken out against the over-medication of kids.) For instance, CDF could actively promote such well-documented alternative programs as multi-systemic therapy, which slashes re-arrest rates of troubled juveniles by as much as 90 percent, as I found in the SHIELDS program for low-income youth in LA. Their outreach workers did it through parent and child in-home counseling that strengthens the parent's involvement in the child's school, friendships and community. In addition, if CDF decided to square off against CMS on its pro kiddie-drugging policies, children's health and even their lives could be preserved.

Unfortunately, we can't expect the leading national mental health advocacy groups to be agents of change in stopping dangerous practices. The NAMI and Mental Health America organizations receive 19 percent and roughly a third of their funding, respectively, from drug companies. NAMI, for instance, was an early champion of J&J's TMAP program and has fought any efforts to restrict prescribing of antipsychotics. Neither group has taken a strong public stance against the overmedication of children, and leaders of both insist that drug industry funding hasn't compromised their policy positions. Yet when I suggested to one organization's local activist that the national group take a stand against dangerous off-label prescribing that could change their image as being under the thumb of the drug industry, she replied, "We *are* under the thumb of the drug industry."

Laundry lists of proposed reforms, of course, don't bring about change. The governing philosophy of those seeking to change our dangerous and ineffective mental health system could be lifted straight from the Hippocratic Oath: *First, Do No Harm*. And it should be amended to read: *Second, Do What Works*. Yet, sadly, the prospects for the wider use of innovative and effective programs are even bleaker now in the Trump era if indeed insurance coverage shrinks and Medicaid budgets are slashed.

In looking over the landscape of reform, it almost always has come about because someone in power has been forced by a lawsuit, court order, media coverage or public protests to change. In medical care, paying people extra to do the right thing and refusing to pay for bad treatments can also have an impact. Changing the way we treat people with a serious mental illness should be considered a social justice issue that goes beyond just those affected by its devastating impact. And when change does occur, its effect can be profound.

Robert Drake, for example, remembers one of the first mentally ill people he recruited to participate in a trial of supported employment. "He was a guy in a day treatment program and I was his doctor," he says. "He just sat around, saying nothing, for years." With his long-lasting schizophrenia, the patient was so moribund and quiet that Drake sent him for neuropsychological testing, which didn't show any underlying physical disease. Then a colleague working in the supported employment program somehow recruited him and helped him find work. "I thought he was the last guy in the world who could get a job," he says.

"He settled in, took off, and he's gotten better and better over the years," Drake says. "I see him now once in a while around town. He has his own apartment, his own car, a pass to the Skyway. He has friends."

"He doesn't look like the same guy at all."

ENDNOTES

Quotes and facts derived from interviews by the author generally won't be included in the endnotes section. Some documents and websites cited below can be read in full at this book's companion website, www.mentalhealthinc.net, or at the author's Scribd account: https://www.scribd.com/user/9995978/Art-Levine-Mental-Health-Inc.

Full URLs for all endnotes in the book can be found here: https://www .scribd.com/document/350654872/Mental-Health-Inc-Web-Endnotes.

In some cases, well-known events or statistics that have been widely publicized or are easily found via Google may be omitted. Full web addresses for news articles available online from the original publications are generally not included because of the changing nature of web URLs; in cases of online-only documents, lengthy URLs will typically be replaced by the website's homepage.

Introduction

9 *anger*: "Steve Tompkins" [name changed for privacy], interview with author, April 2015.

10 *"not going to do that"*: Redacted South Charleston PD police report on April 16, 2014, disturbance, sent by email from W. Michael Moore, counsel for City of South Charleston, on June 12, 2015.

11 *vets treated by the Department*: Jamie Reno, "Nearly 30% of Vets Treated by VA Have PTSD," *The Daily Beast*, October 21, 2012; Department of Veterans Affairs (VA), National Center for PTSD, *How Common Is PTSD?* as of October 3, 2015, http://www.ptsd.va.gov.

11 *vets could get access*: American Public Health Association, "Removing Barriers to Mental Health Services for Veterans," November 18, 2014, https://www.apha.org.

11 *increased more than 40 percent*: VA, Budget in Brief, 2017, February 18, 2016, http://www.va.gov; Lukas Pleva, "Funding Bill Signed Into Law," *Politifact*, April 5, 2010.

11 *"often unavailable"*: National Alliance on Mental Health (NAMI), "State Mental Health Cuts: A National Crisis," March 2011, https://www.nami.org.

11 *stunning 55 percent*: Pamela Hyde, Administrator, "Report to Congress on the Nation's Substance Abuse and Mental Health Workforce Issues," Substance Abuse and Mental Health Services Administration (SAMHSA), January 24, 2013, 10, http://store.samhsa.gov.

11 *twenty-three million Americans*: Congressional Budget Office (CBO), "American Health Care Act (AHCA), Cost Estimate," May 24, 2017, https://www.cbo.gov.

11 *damage to Obamacare's protections*: Casey Quinlan, "Trump Is Already Taking Actions to Sabotage Obamacare," *ThinkProgress*, March 9, 2017, https://thinkprogress.org.

12 *narrowly passed the House*: Sarah Kliff, "The American Health Care Act: The Obamacare Repeal Bill the House Just Passed, Explained," *Vox*, May 4, 2017, https://www.vox.com/policy.

12 *more than 130 million people*: Emily Gee, "Number of Americans With Pre-Existing Conditions by Congressional District," Center for American Progress (CAP), April 5, 2017, https://www.americanprogress.org.

12 *extra $20,000 a year*: Sam Berger et al., "Latest ACA Repeal Plan Would Explode Premiums for People With Pre-Existing Conditions," CAP, April 20, 2017, https://www.americanprogress.org/issues.

12 *administration's backstage regulatory*: Families USA, "ACA Threat Tracker," http://familiesusa.org; Michael Hiltzik, "Trump Didn't Blow Up Obamacare on Monday, but Left It Hanging by a Thread," *Los Angeles Times*, May 22, 2017, http://www.latimes.com/business/hiltzik.

13 *leave all the ACA marketplaces*: Amy Goldstein, "Aetna Exiting All ACA Insurance Marketplaces in 2018," *Washington Post*, May 10, 2017, https://www.washingtonpost.com/national/health.

13 *about fourteen million people*: Jon Greenberg, "Medicaid Expansion Drove Health Insurance Coverage Under Health Law, Rand Paul Says," *Politifact*, January 15, 2017, http://www.politifact.com/truth-o-meter.

13 *previously uninsured*: Judith Dey et al., "Benefits of Medicaid Expansion for Behavioral Health," ASPE Issue Brief, Office of the Assistant Secretary for Planning and Evaluation (ASPE), Department of Health and Human Services (DHHS), March 28, 2016, https://aspe.hhs.gov; Richard Frank et al., "Keep Obamacare to Keep Progress on Treating Opioid Disorders and Mental Illnesses," *The Hill*, January 11, 2017, http://thehill.com/blogs/.

13 *crafted by Sen. Marco Rubio*: Robert Pear, "Marco Rubio Quietly Undermines Affordable Care Act," *New York Times*, December 9, 2015; Seth Chandler, "Judge's Ruling on 'Risk Corridors' Not Likely to Revitalize ACA," *Forbes*, February 13, 2017.

13 *drastically reduced their involvement*: Reed Abelson, "Humana Plans to Pull Out of Obamacare's Insurance Exchanges," *New York Times*, February 14, 2017.

13 *"if the market is destroyed"*: Timothy Jost, "What's Next for Health Policy," Alliance for Health Reform (AHR), April 4, 2017, http://www.all-health.org.

13 *financially viable*: CBO, "American Health Care Act."

14 *$839 billion from Medicaid*: Benjy Sarlin, "Deep Medicaid Cuts Drive Backlash to House Health Care Bill," NBC News, May 5, 2017, http://www.nbcnews.com/politics.

14 *gutted protections for consumers*: Michael Hiltzik, "All the Horrific Details of the GOP's New Obamacare Repeal: A Handy Guide," *Los Angeles Times*, May 4, 2017, http://www.latimes.com/business/hiltzik.

14 *effort to blackmail*: Gene B. Sperling et al., "Six Ways to Tell If Trump Is Sabotaging Obamacare," *The Atlantic*, March 29, 2017, https://www

.theatlantic.com/politics; Robert Pear, "Trump Threatens Health Subsidies to Force Democrats to Bargain," *New York Times*, April 13, 2017, https://www.nytimes.com.

14 *avoid a government shutdown*: Burgess Everett et al., "White House to Continue Obamacare Payments, Removing Shutdown Threat," *Politico*, April 26, 2017, http://www.politico.com/story.

14 *quadrupled to 960 in 2017*: Sarah Kliff et al., "Nearly 1,000 Healthcare.gov Counties Will Have Just One Insurer Next Year," *Vox*, October 26, 2016, https://www.vox.com/science-and-health.

15 *frontal assaults on the program*: M. J. Lee et al., "Trump Budget: $800 Billion in Medicaid Cuts," CNN, May 22, 2017, http://www.cnn.com.

15 *more than Medicare*: Kate Zernike et al., "In Health Bill's Defeat, Medicaid Comes of Age," *New York Times*, March 27, 2017, https://www.nytimes.com.

15 *leading funder*: Judge David L. Bazelon Center for Mental Health Law, "Medicaid: Lifeline for Children and Adults With Serious Mental Illnesses," http://www.bazelon.org.

15 *administration's "sabotage" efforts*: Families USA, "Affordable Care Act Attack Tracker," April 2017, http://familiesusa.org/; Tony Pugh, "Health Advocates Blast New Trump Proposals to Stabilize Obamacare Marketplace," McClatchy, February 15, 2017, http://www.mcclatchydc.com; AHR, "Materials List: Medicaid Moving Forward," April 3, 2017, http://www.allhealth.org.

15 *federal waivers*: Rachel Gershon, "Waivers Represent a Quieter Way for Republicans to Change Health Care," *STAT*, March 29, 2017, https://www.statnews.com.

15 *lock out Medicaid recipients*: Kaiser Family Foundation, "All About Section 1115 Medicaid Waivers," http://kff.org/tag/waivers; Lisa Gillespie, "State Official Expects Kentucky Medicaid Waiver to Be Approved by June," WFPL (Louisville), March 23, 2017, http://wfpl.org/state-official.

15 *test them for illegal drugs*: Scott Bauer, "Walker Medicaid Director Defends Drug Testing for Medicaid Recipients," Associated Press, April 6, 2017, http://dailyreporter.com; Grant Smith, "Jeff Sessions Will Double Down on Failed Drug War," *The Hill*, February 2, 2017, http://thehill.com.

16 *thirteen million*: Issie Lapowsky, "Obamacare's Demise Is a Looming Disaster for Mental Health," *Wired*, January 15, 2017; Lindsay Holmes, "Trumpcare Will Be Catastrophic for People With Mental Health Issues," *HuffPost,* May 4, 2017, http://www.huffingtonpost.com.

16 *"Healthy Indiana"*: Jake Harper, "Indiana's Model for Medicaid Could Spread—But It's Not Working for Everyone," WFYI (Indianapolis), January 10, 2017, http://www.wfyi.org.

16 *required monthly payment*: Maureen Groppe, "Indiana's Alternative Medicaid Program Shows Tradeoffs of Charging Recipients for Care," *USA Today*, May 8, 2017, https://www.usatoday.com/story.

16 *"block grants"*: Maura Calsyn et al., "The Republicans' Plan for Medi-

caid: A Wolf in Sheep's Clothing," CAP, January 12, 2017, https://www.americanprogress.org.

17 *cut over 350,000*: "2005 TennCare Cuts," Tennessee Justice Center, https://www.tnjustice.org/2005-cuts/; Kristin M. Hall, "Obit Calls Out TennCare Cuts," *Knoxville News Sentinel*, April 12, 2011, online at https://www.scribd.com.

17 *theoretically eligible*: Ione Farrar, *TennCare Reform, One Year Later*, Community Research Council, June 2007, 9,16–17, online at Sribd.com, "Tenncare-Cuts," https://www.scribd.com/

18 *even liberal governors*: Chad Terhune et al., "Why Blue States Might Ditch Beloved Obamacare Protections," *Kaiser Health News*, May 8, 2017, http://khn.org/news.

18 *exorbitant out-of-pocket costs*: NAMI, "Out-of-Network, Out-of-Pocket, Out-of-Options: The Unfulfilled Promise of Parity," November 2016, http://www.nami.org.

18 *potential deathblow*: German Lopez, "The House's Obamacare Repeal Bill Would Strand Drug Addicts Without Access to Care," *Vox*, March 13, 2017, http://www.vox.com; Richard Frank, "Keep Obamacare," *The Hill*, January 11, 2017; Kaiser Family Foundation, "Medicaid's Role in Addressing the Opioid Epidemic," March 17, 2017, http://kff.org/infographic/.

18 *worsened by the impact*: Deirdre Shesgreen, "Trump Administration Missing Mark On Opioids, Advocates Say," *USA Today*, May 15, 2017, https://www.usatoday.com/story; Julia Lurie, "Trump's Health Secretary Says Addiction Meds Are 'Substituting One Opioid For Another,'" *Mother Jones*, May 10, 2017, http://www.motherjones.com/politics/2017/05/tom-price.

19 *second-most common*: Centers for Disease Control and Prevention (CDC), "Suicide: Facts at a Glance," 2015, http://www.cdc.gov/.

19 *33,000 firearm deaths a year*: CDC, National Center for Health Statistics, All Injuries/Mortality/All Firearm Deaths, June 30, 2016, https://www.cdc.gov/nchs/fastats/.

19 *over 60 percent*: Margot Sanger-Katz, "Gun Deaths Are Mostly Suicides," *New York Times*, October 8, 2015, https://www.nytimes.com.

19 *over $4 billion*: Deanna Pan, "MAP: Which States Have Cut Treatment for the Mentally Ill the Most?" *Mother Jones*, April 29, 2013, http://www.motherjones.com.

19 *budgets still remain below 2009 levels*: NAMI, "State Mental Health Legislation 2015: Trends, Themes and Effective Practices," December 2015, http://www.nami.org.

19 *40 percent*: Association for Psychological Science, "Stigma as a Barrier to Mental Health Care," September 4, 2014, https://www.psychologicalscience.org.

19 *ten million*: NAMI, "Mental Health by the Numbers: Prevalence of Mental Illness," 2015, http://www.nami.org.

20 *senseless mass shooting*: Mark Follman et al., "US Mass Shootings, 1982–2016: Data From Mother Jones' Investigation," *Mother Jones*, September 24, 2016, http://www.motherjones.com.

20 *shot or killed in each incident*: Gun Violence Archive, "Mass Shootings—2017," http://www.gunviolencearchive.org.

20 *60 percent*: Jonathan M. Metzl and Kenneth T. MacLeish, "Mental Illness, Mass Shootings, and the Politics of American Firearms," *American Journal of Public Health* 105, no. 2 (February 2015): 240–249, http://ajph.aphapublications.org.

20 *"psychopathic shooters"*: Peter Langman, *School Shooters: Understanding High School, College, and Adult Perpetrators* (Lanham, MD: Rowman & Littlefield, 2015), 1–6.

21 *"D-" rating*: NAMI, "Grading the States: A Report on America's Health Care System for Serious Mental Illness—2006," March 1, 2006, https://www.nami.org.

21 *another potential loophole*: "Congress Moves to Roll Back a Sensible Obama Gun Policy" editorial, *New York Times*, February 7, 2017, https://www.nytimes.com.

21 *eleven times more likely*: Linda A. Teplin, PhD. et al., "Crime Victimization in Adults With Severe Mental Illness," *Archives of General Psychiatry* 62 (August 2005): 911–21, http://jamanetwork.com/journals/jamapsychiatry.

21 *likely to engage in violence*: Seena Fazel et al., "Schizophrenia and Violence: Systematic Review and Meta-Analysis," *PLOS Medicine* 6, no. 8 (August 11, 2009), http://journals.plos.org/plosmedicine/.

21 *major risk factors*: Michael Rezendes et al., "The Desperate and the Dead: Families in Fear," Spotlight, *Boston Globe*, June 23, 2016, https://apps.bostonglobe.com/spotlight.

22 *research on violence*: Seena Fazel et al., "Schizophrenia and Violence"; J. C. Matejkowski et al., "Characteristics of Persons With Severe Mental Illness Who Have Been Incarcerated for Murder," *Journal of the American Academy of Psychiatry and the Law* 36, no. 1 (March 2008): 74–86, http://jaapl.org.

22 *protest of nearly two hundred*: Brian MacQuarrie, "Rally Held to Protest Spotlight Series," *Boston Globe*, August 2, 2016, https://www.bostonglobe.com.

22 *"They demonized us"*: Ruthie Poole, interview and email correspondence with the author, August 2016.

23 *reform bill*: Tim Murphy, U.S. House of Representatives, "Helping Families in Mental Health Crisis Act of 2016," July 2016, https://murphy.house.gov.

23 *rights-oriented mental health advocates*: Susan Rogers et al., "Response to Murphy's Bill: Mental Health Advocates Blast Rep. Tim Murphy's Bill…," Bazelon Center, December 12, 2013, http://www.bazelon.org.

24 *risky antipsychotic*: Julie Robinson, "Veterans' Families Question Cause of Deaths: Post-Traumatic Stress Syndrome Treatment Cited," *Charleston Gazette* (West Virginia), March 1, 2009, online at http://www

.commondreams.org; Department of Justice (DOJ), "Pharmaceutical Giant AstraZeneca to Pay $520 Million for Off-Label Drug Marketing," April 27, 2010, https://www.justice.gov; Bailey Perrin Bailey et al., "Plaintiffs' Omnibus Legal Memorandum Responding in Opposition to AstraZeneca's Summary Judgment Motions...," Seroquel Litigation Documents, November 24, 2008, http://industrydocuments.library .ucsf.edu.

24 *$5 billion a year*: Michelle McNickle, "Drugmakers Face Loss of Exclusivity on Several Blockbuster Brands," *Medical Practice Insider*, March 29, 2012, http://www.medicalpracticeinsider.com.

24 *side effects*: Matthew Perrone, "Deaths Raise Questions on Drugs Given to Sleepless Vets," AP/NBC News, http://www.nbcnews.com; "Highlights of Prescribing Information," *Seroquel, AstraZeneca Medication Guide* (approved by the Food and Drug Administration [FDA]), June 2011, http://www.accessdata.fda.gov.

24 *four hundred combat veterans and other military*: Fred A. Baughman, "Soldiers of the Iraq/Afghanistan Era Dead of What Seem to Be Probable Sudden Cardiac Deaths...," *European Heart Journal*, December 29, 2011, http://proximajmone.altervista.org; also see full document online at https://www.scribd.com/document.

24 *"drug toxicity"*: James Dao et al., "For Some Troops, Powerful Drug Cocktails Have Deadly Results," *New York Times*, February 13, 2011, http://www.nytimes.com; Bob Brewin, "Military's Drug Policy Threatens Troops' Health, Doctors Say," *Nextgov*, January 18, 2011, http://www.nextgov.com.

24 *aggressive marketing*: Martha Rosenberg, "Are Veterans Being Given Deadly Cocktails to Treat PTSD," *AlterNet*, March 5, 2010, http://www.alternet.org.

24 *pharmaceutical-subsidized patient advocacy groups*: David Dayen, "New Report Exposes 'Patient Advocacy' Groups as a Big Pharma Scam," *The Intercept*, December 1, 2016, https://theintercept.com.

25 *(PIER)*: W. R. McFarlane, "Portland Identification and Early Referral: A Community-Based System for Identifying and Treating Youths at High Risk of Psychosis," *Psychiatric Services* 61, no. 5 (May 2010): 512–515, https://www.ncbi.nlm.nih.gov/.

25 *"shambles"*: Michael F. Hogan et al., "Achieving the Promise: Transforming Mental Health Care in America," The President's New Freedom Commission on Mental Health, DHHS publication no. SMA-03-3832, July 2003, http://govinfo.library.unt.edu.

26 *"neurodevelopmental"*: S. Hossein Fatemi and Timothy D. Folsom, "The Neurodevelopmental Hypothesis of Schizophrenia, Revisited," *Schizophrenia Bulletin* 35, no. 3 (2009): 528–548, schizophreniabulletin .oxfordjournals.org.

26 *bedlam era*: Robert Whitaker, *Mad in America: Bad Science, Bad Medicine, and the Enduring Mistreatment of the Mentally Ill* (New York: Basic Books, 2002), 1–38.

26 *"snakepit" hospital era*: Richard D. Lyons, "How Release of Mental Patients Began," *New York Times*, October 30, 1984, http://www.nytimes.com.

27 *less than 40,000 such beds*: Treatment Advocacy Center, "Going, Going, Gone: Trends and Consequences of Eliminating State Psychiatric Beds, 2016," http://www.treatmentadvocacycenter.org.

27 *make up a third*: Treatment Advocacy Center, "Serious Mental Illness and Homelessness," September 2016, http://www.treatmentadvocacycenter.org.

27 *nearly 700,000*: David Grabowski, "Mental Illness in Nursing Homes: Variations Across States," *Health Affairs*, 28, no. 3 (May 2009): 689–700, https://www.ncbi.nlm.nih.gov; Angela M. Greene et al., *Understanding Unlicensed Care Homes: Final Report*, DHHS, ASPE, September 1, 2015, https://aspe.hhs.gov.

27 *Nearly once a month*: Rob Barry et al., "Neglected to Death, Part 1: Once Pride of Florida, Now Scenes of Neglect," *Miami Herald*, April 30, 2011, http://www.miamiherald.com.

27 *potentially fatal side effects*: Robert Whitaker, "Lure of Riches Fuels Testing," *Boston Globe*, November 17, 1998, online at http://psychrights.org/Stories/SusanEndersbe.htm.

27 *exaggerated and false claims*: Steven Brill, "America's Most Admired Lawbreaker," *HuffPost*, Highline, September 2015, http://highline.huffingtonpost.com; Sammy Almashat et al., "Twenty-Five Years of Pharmaceutical Industry Criminal and Civil Penalties: 1991 Through 2015," *Public Citizen*, March 31, 2016, http://www.citizen.org; Steven Sheller et al., *Pharmageddon—A Nation Betrayed: A National Trial Lawyer Reveals an Industry Spinning Out of Control* (Norfolk, VA: Cape Cedar Media, 2016).

27 *devastating independent*: Jeffrey A. Lieberman et al., "Effectiveness of Antipsychotic Drugs in Patients With Chronic Schizophrenia," *New England Journal of Medicine*, 353 (September 22, 2005): 1209–1223, http://www.nejm.org.

28 *essentially rigged*: Whitaker, *Mad in America*, 253–286; Shankar Vendantam, "Comparison of Schizophrenia Drugs Often Favors Firm Funding Study," *Washington Post*, April 12, 2006, http://www.washingtonpost.com.

28 *two to five times*: Peter C. Gotzsche, *Deadly Psychiatry and Organised Denial* (Copenhagen: People's Press, 2015), Kindle ed., chapter 11.

28 *higher risk of suicide*: Jonathan Mahler, "The Antidepressant Dilemma," *New York Times Magazine*, November 21, 2004, http://www.nytimes.com; Benedict Carey, "Antidepressant Paxil Is Unsafe for Teenagers, New Analysis Says," *New York Times*, September 16, 2015, https://www.nytimes.com.

28 *well-hidden*: Simone Pisano et al., "Update on the Safety of Second Generation Antipsychotics in Youths: A Call for Collaboration Among Pediatricians and Child Psychiatrists," *Italian Journal of Pediatrics* 42 (May 21, 2016): 5, https://www.ncbi.nlm.nih.gov; Duff Wilson, "Side Effects May Include Lawsuits," *New York Times*, October 2, 2010, http://www.nytimes.com.

28   *the $711 billion in global net profits*: Almashat et al., "Twenty-Five Years."

29   *dramatic new evidence*: Anissa Abi-Dargham et al., "Dopamine Hypothesis of Schizophrenia," *Biological Psychiatry* 8, no. 1 (January 1, 2017), http://www.biologicalpsychiatryjournal.com; "The Emergence of a New Dopamine Hypothesis of Schizophrenia," press release, Elsevier, January 2, 2017, http://www.biologicalpsychiatryjournal.com/pb/assets.

29   *lack the tools*: Thomas Insel, "Rethinking Schizophrenia," *Nature* 468 (November 2010): 187–193, http://www.nature.com.

29   *debunked this theory*: Jeffrey Lacasse and Jonathan Leo, "Challenging the Narrative of Chemical Imbalance: A Look at the Evidence," in B. Probst, editor, *Critical Thinking in Clinical Assessment and Diagnosis* (New York: Springer, 2015), 275–282, online at http://diginole.lib.fsu.edu/islandora.

30   *almost anyone with problems*: Maia Szalavitz, "Antipsychotic Prescriptions in Children Have Skyrocketed: Study," *Time*, August 9, 2012, http://healthland.time.com.

30   *after nearly ninety reported on-site teen deaths in the last fifteen years*: Jesse Hyde, "Life and Death in a Troubled Teen Boot Camp," *Rolling Stone*, November 12, 2015, http://www.rollingstone.com; Victims, Wiki Fornits, updated through October 2016, https://wiki.fornits.com.

30   *$2 billion in settlements*: Katie Thomas, "J.&J. to Pay $2.2 Billion in Risperdal Settlement," *New York Times*, November 4, 2013, http://www.nytimes.com.

31   *a $158 million settlement*: Janet Elliott, "Johnson and Johnson Settles Texas Medicaid Fraud Lawsuit for $158 Million," *Dallas Morning News*, January 2012, http://www.dallasnews.com.

31   *too disabled to work*: NAMI, "Road to Recovery: Employment and Mental Illness," July 2014, https://www.nami.org.

31   *receiving treatment*: Testimony of Dr. Joseph Parks, *Examining SAMHSA's Role in Delivering Services to the Severely Mentally Ill, Hearing Before the Subcommittee on Oversight and Investigations of the Committee on Energy and Commerce*, 113th Cong. (May 22, 2013), 91–93, https://www.gpo.gov.

31   *sixteen million adults and children*: NAMI, "Prevalence of Mental Illness."

32   *more than 40,000*: CDC, National Center for Health Statistics, Suicide and Self-Inflicted Injury/Mortality, https://www.cdc.gov/nchs/fastats/suicide.htm.

32   *soared to its highest level in thirty years*: Sabrina Tavernise, "U.S. Suicide Rate Surges to a 30-Year High," *New York Times*, April 22, 2016, https://www.nytimes.com.

32   *largest psychiatric facility*: Renee Montagne, "Inside the Nation's Largest Mental Institution," NPR, August 13, 2008, http://www.npr.org.

32   *Over 20 percent of its 17,000 inmates*: Los Angeles County's Sheriff's Department, "Custody Division Year End Review, 2015," updated June 16, 2016, http://www.la-sheriff.org.

32 *death of an inmate, Unique Moore*: Art Levine, "Why Did L.A. County Inmate Unique Moore Die?" *HuffPost,* February 29, 2016, http://www .huffingtonpost.com/art-levine.

33 *jumping off of a Dallas bridge*: Miles Moffeit, "Danger in the Psych Ward," *Dallas Morning News*, March 18, 2016, http://interactives.dallasnews.com.

33 *compromised by drug money*: Ken Silverstein, "Prozac.org," *Mother Jones,* November/December 1999, http://www.motherjones.com; email statements from NAMI and Mental Health America, August 2016, online at https://www.scribd.com.

Chapter 1: Drugging Our Kids

35 *maltreatment of children*: Jeanne Lenzer, "Whistleblower Charges Medical Oversight Bureau With Corruption," *BMJ* 329 (2004): 69, https://www.ncbi.nlm.nih.gov; Mark Scolforo, "Drug Makers Accused of Aiding in Deaths," Associated Press, July 6, 2004, http://usatoday30 .usatoday.com/.

35 *overdrugging death*: Benedict Carey, "Debate Over Children and Psychiatric Drugs," *New York Times*, February 15, 2007, http://www .nytimes.com.

36 *intensive lobbying*: Brill, "America's Most Admired Lawbreaker."

36 *kiddie diagnoses*: Art Levine, "Feds Pay for Drug Fraud: 92 Percent of Foster Care, Poor Kids Prescribed Antipsychotics Get Them for Unaccepted Uses," *HuffPost,* April 30, 2015, http://www.huffingtonpost.com.

36 *doubled among children*: Lisa Rapaport, "Antipsychotic Use Rising Among Teens and Young Adults," Reuters, July 10, 2015, http://www .reuters.com.

36 *already paid billions*: Lena Groeger, "Big Pharma's Big Fines," *ProPublica*, February 24, 2014, http://projects.propublica.org/graphics/bigpharma.

36 *without the approval*: DHHS, OIG, "Second-Generation Antipsychotic Drug Use Among Medicaid-Enrolled Children: Quality-of-Care Concerns," March 2015, https://oig.hhs.gov.

36 *all ages without question*: Eric P. Slade, Ph.D. and Linda Simoni-Wastila, "Forecasting Medicaid Expenditures for Antipsychotic Medications," *Psychiatric Services* 66, no. 7 (July 1, 2015): 713–718, http://ps.psychiatryonline.org.

37 *most dangerous*: Roni Jacobsen, "Should Children Take Antipsychotic Drugs?" *Scientific American,* March 1, 2014, https://www.scientificamerican.com.

37 *one in five*: Ryan D'Agostino, "The Drugging of the American Boy," *Esquire*, April 2014, http://www.esquire.com.

37 *off-label uses*: Mark Olfson et al., "Treatment of Young People With Antipsychotic Medications in the United States," *JAMA Psychiatry* 72, no. 9 (September 2015): 867–874, http://jamanetwork.com.

37 *corrupting influence*: Duff Wilson, "Side Effects May Include Lawsuits," *New York Times*, October 2, 2010, http://www.nytimes.com.

37 *free speech lawsuit*: "Penn Psychiatrist Files Whistleblower Lawsuit—Investigation Confirms Medicare Chief Lied," *Philadelphia Daily News*, July 7, 2004, online at http://ahrp.org.

37 *mounting concerns*: Rob Waters, "Medicating Amanda," *Mother Jones*, May/June 2005, http://www.motherjones.com/politics/2005/05/medicating-amanda; Lenzer, "Whistleblower Charges."

38 *Kruszewski's report*: *Kruszewski v. Gorton*, Second Amended Complaint, U.S. District Court for the Middle District of Pennsylvania, December 2005, https://www.scribd.com.

38 *endangered clients*: Evelyn Pringle, "Makers of Zyprexa Risperdal and Seroquel Under Fire," Lawyers and Settlements, March 9, 2007, https://www.lawyersandsettlements.com.

38 *settled a lawsuit in 2007*: "Psychiatrist Is Awarded Settlement After Fraud Allegations," *BMJ* 335, no. 7614 (August 11, 2007): 267, https://www.ncbi.nlm.nih.gov.

38 *legal actions*: Debra Erdley, "Psychiatric Hospital in Washington County Pays $150,000 to Settle Suit Alleging Abuse, Fraud," *Pittsburgh Tribune-Review*, May 20, 2009, http://triblive.com.

38 *new antipsychotic product*: Kenney Egan et al., "Pfizer Pays a Record Amount to Settle Federal and State Fraud Investigations Into Illegal Off-Label Marketing Practices," PR NewsWire, September 2, 2009, http://www.prnewswire.com.

39 *secretly file*: *Kruszewski et al. v. Pfizer, Inc.*, First Amended Complaint, U.S. District Court for the Eastern District of Pennsylvania, case no. 07-CV, 4106, 2007, online at https://www.scribd.com.

39 *huge federal settlements*: Jim Edwards, "Behind Two Big Drug Company Settlements: Professional Whistleblowers," CBS Moneywatch, April 28, 2010, http://www.cbsnews.com.

39 *uncovered a campaign*: John W. Whitehead, "A Lone Wolf Takes on the Drug Leviathan: An Interview With Allen Jones," Rutherford Institute, October 13, 2005, https://www.rutherford.org.

40 *was forced to resign*: Ben Wallace-Wells, "Bitter Pill," *Rolling Stone*, February 5, 2009, online at http://www.narpa.org/bitter pill.htm.

40 *whistleblower lawsuit*: Janet Elliott, "Johnson & Johnson Settles Texas Medicaid Fraud Lawsuit for $158 Million," *Dallas Morning News*, January 2012, http://www.dallasnews.com.

41 *researchers-for-hire*: Penny Sarchet, "Harvard Scientists Disciplined for Not Declaring Ties to Drug Companies," *Nature,* news blog, July 4, 2011, http://blogs.nature.com/news.

41 *cleared by a grand jury*: John P. Kelly, "Cleared by Grand Jury, Riley Psychiatrist Wants to Practice Medicine Again," *Patriot Ledger* (Quincy, MA), July 2, 2009, http://www.patriotledger.com/; Testimony by Dr. Kifuji in *Commonwealth of Massachusetts vs. Carolyn Riley*, Plymouth Superior Court, docket no. 07-00147, Brockton, MA, January 25–26, 2010, online at Art Levine *Mental Health, Inc.*, https://www.scribd.com and https://www.scribd.com-trial-day-2.

41 *settled a related civil malpractice lawsuit*: Patricia Wen, "Tufts Settles Suit Against Doctor in Girls Death for $2.5m," *Boston Globe*, January 25, 2011, http://archive.boston.com.

41 *has been denounced*: "Expert or Shill," editorial, *New York Times*, November 29, 2008, http://www.nytimes.com.

42 *forty-fold increase*: National Institute of Mental Health (NIMH), "Rates of Bipolar Diagnosis in Youth Rapidly Climbing, Treatment Patterns Similar to Adults," September 3, 2007, https://www.nimh.nih.gov.

42 *no capacity to monitor*: Children's Rights, "Massachusetts Fails to Ensure the Safe Administration of Psychotropic Medications to Children in Foster Care," October 3, 2012, http://www.childrensrights.org; DHHS Children's Bureau, Child Welfare Information Gateway, "Reform Based on Litigation," https://www.childwelfare.gov.

42 *have leveled off*: Stephen Crystal et al., "Rapid Growth of Antipsychotic Prescriptions for Children Who Are Publicly Insured Has Ceased, but Concerns Remain," *Health Affairs* 35, no. 6 (June 2016): 974–82, http://content.healthaffairs.org.

42 *tough new state legislation*: Elaine Korry, "California Moves to Stop Misuse of Psychiatric Meds in Foster Care," NPR, September 2, 2015, http://www.npr.org.

42 *spurred by*: Karen da Sá, "Drugging Our Kids," *Mercury News*, August 24, 2014, http://extras.mercurynews.com/druggedkids.

42 *won new approval*: Fran Lowry, "FDA Expert Panel Approves Use of Atypical Antipsychotic Drugs in Kids," *Medscape*, June 11, 2009, http://www.medscape.com.

43 *prescribed the off-label medications*: Carol Marbin Miller, "Broward Psychiatrist Gets Harsh Letter from FDA," *Miami Herald*, March 15, 2010, online at http://articles.sun-sentinel.com.

43 *guinea pigs for Pfizer*: Marbin Miller, "Broward Psychiatrist."

43 *according to a 2009 lawsuit*: Carol Marbin Miller, "Mother's Lawsuit Against Doctor, Hospital Links Mental-Health Drugs to Child's 2003 Death," *Miami Herald*, June 5, 2009, online at https://gabrielmyers.wordpress.com.

43 *for the deaths or overdoses*: Michael LaForgia, "Troubled Doctors Hired to Treat Kids in State Custody," *Palm Beach Post*, June 19, 2011, online at https://www.pressreader.com; Carol Marbin Miller and Diana Moskowitz, "Boy's County Psychiatrist Has Other Issues," *Miami Herald*, April 23, 2011, online at http://www.thelizlibrary.org.

43 *enormous amounts*: Joel Engelhardt, "State Vows Better Monitoring of Antipsychotics in Juvenile Jails," *Palm Beach Post*, February 27, 2013, http://www.mypalmbeachpost.com.

43 *were lavished with*: Fred Grimm, "In Florida, Zombie Pills for Kids Are an Old Scandal," *Miami Herald*, September 25, 2015, http://www.miamiherald.com.

43 *prescribing remains roughly the same*: Information request reply from Amanda Fortuna, Florida Department of Juvenile Justice (DJJ), email, De-

cember 12, 2015; Florida DJJ, "Use of Psychotropic Medication in DJJ Residential Commitment Programs, Final Draft," October 2015, https://www.scribd.com/document.

44 *for stimulants and antipsychotics*: Office of Child Welfare Data Reporting Unit, Florida Department of Children and Families (DCF), "Psychotropic Medications Report for Children in Out-of-Home Care...," September 1, 2016, http://www.dcf.state.fl.us.

44 *expanded official approval*: Evelyn Pringle, "FDA Throws Lifeline to Antipsychotic Pushers," *CounterPunch*, June 12, 2009, http://www.counter-punch.org.

44 *illegal marketing*: Almashat et al., "Twenty-Five Years."

44 *criminal and civil allegations*: "Eli Lilly Fined Nearly $1.5B in Drug Marketing Case," CNN Money, January 15, 2009, http://money.cnn.com /2009/01/15/news/companies/eli_lilly/.

44 *fraudulent marketing*: Gardiner Harris, "Pfizer Pays $2.3 Billion to Settle Marketing Case," *New York Times*, September 2, 2009, http://www .nytimes.com.

44 *fraudulently selling*: DOJ, "AstraZeneca to Pay $520 Million."

44 *young as ten*: Martha Rosenberg, "Seroquel, Zyprexa and Geodon for Kids? You Bet Says FDA Panel,"*Dissident Voice*, June 13, 2009, http:/ /dissidentvoice.org.

45 *prescribed Seroquel*: Statement of Liza Ortiz, FDA, Center for Drug Evaluation and Research (CDER), Psychopharmacologic Drugs, Advisory Committee Meeting, transcript, June 9, 2009, 387–389, https://www.fda .gov/downloads.

45 *staff report*: Rob Waters, "FDA Was Urged to Limit Kids' Antidepressants," *San Francisco Chronicle*, April 16, 2004, http://www.sfgate.com; Thomas Laughren, LinkedIn, https://www.linkedin.com.

46 *agreement with DOJ*: DOJ, "Justice Department Announces Largest Health Care Fraud Settlement in Its History," news release on Pfizer, September 2, 2009, https://www.justice.gov.

46 *whistleblower fraud lawsuit*: *Booker et al. vs. Pfizer, Inc.*, U.S. District Court, District of Massachusetts, no.1:10-CV-11166-DPW, Fifth Amended Complaint and Demand for Jury Trial, October 2012, online at https://www.scribd.com.

46 *rejected the lawsuit*: Brian Amaral, "Pfizer Beats FCA Suit Over Geodon Marketing," *Law 360*, May 24, 2016, https://www.law360.com; *Booker v. Pfizer*, U.S. Court of Appeals for the First Circuit, No. 16-1805, Appeal from the U.S. District Court for the District of Massachusetts, January 30, 2017, http://media.ca1.uscourts.gov.

47 *worst prescription-monitoring*: Mark Abdelmalek et al., "New Study Shows U.S. Government Fails to Oversee Treatment of Foster Children With Mind-Altering Drugs," ABC News, November 30, 2011, http:/ /abcnews.go.com.

47 *drugging "parameters"*: Department of Family and Protective Services and

The University of Texas at Austin College of Pharmacy, "Psychotropic Medication Utilization Parameters for Foster Children Texas," December 2010, https://www.dfps.state.tx.us.

48   *awash in J&J money*: Janet Elliott and Mark Curriden, "Texas AG Suit Over the Drug Risperdal Goes to Trial Monday," *Dallas Morning News,* January 8, 2012, https://www.dallasnews.com; *Allen Jones et al. v. Jannsen Pharmaceutica et al.,* "False Claims Act Complaint and Demand for Jury Trial," U.S. District Court for the Eastern District of Pennsylvania, March 25, 2004, online at http://highline.huffingtonpost.com/miracleindustry.

48   *troubled eleven-year-old girl*: Michael Barajas, "Big Pharma's Troubling History of Pushing Drugs on Foster Kids," *San Antonio Current,* April 9, 2013, http://www.sacurrent.com; DOJ, Pfizer Plea Agreement, August 31, 2009, https://www.justice.gov.

49   *paid by J&J*: Craig Malislow, "Down the Hatch," *Houston Press,* December 14, 2011, http://www.houstonpress.

49   *ghostwritten*: Allen Jones et al., "False Claims Act Complaint," March 2004; Dr. Roy Poses, "The Texas TMAP Trial as Illustration of a Systematic Stealth Marketing Campaign," *Health Care Renewal,* February 10, 2012, http://hcrenewal.blogspot.com; David Rothman, Expert Witness Report, October 15, 2010, *Jones v. Jannsen,* online at http://psychrights.org.

49   *pro-Risperdal schizophrenia guidelines*: Paula J. Kaplan, "Diagnosisgate: Conflict of Interest at the Top of the Psychiatric Apparatus," *Aporia: The Nursing Journal* 7, no. 1 (January 2015), 30–41, http://www.oa.uottawa.ca; Expert Witness Report, David Rothman, 14–21; Allen Frances, "'Diagnosisgate' Deconstructed and Debunked," *HuffPost,* March 6, 2015, http://www.huffingtonpost.com.

49   *teenage boys*: Ed Silverman, "J&J Sees Male Breasts and Quickly Settles Risperdal Suit," *Forbes,* September 11, 2012, http://www.forbes.com; David Crow, "J&J's legal costs surge in wave of product lawsuits," *Financial Times,* March 7, 2017, https://www.ft.com; Highlights of Prescribing Information, Risperdal, February 2017, page 6 cites gynecomastia, https://www.janssenmd.com.

Chapter 2: Drugging Our Seniors to Death

53   *arrest in 2009*: California Attorney General's Press Office, "Brown Announces Arrests of Nursing Home Employees Who Drugged Patients for Staff's Convenience," February 18, 2009, https://oag.ca.gov/news/press-releases.

53   *after being convicted*: Jason Kotowski, "Former Nursing Director Sentenced to 3 Years for Inappropriately Medicating Patients," *Bakersfield Californian,* January 9, 2013, http://www.bakersfield.com.

53   *abetted in her crimes*: Kotowski, "Former Nursing Director"; *People of the State of California v. Gwen Hughes et al.,* Declaration in Support of Arrest Warrant and Felony, Sup. Ct. of Calif., County of Kern, AG docket

no. FR2007100234, 2009, online at https://www.scribd.com/document/343149802.

53   *finally unmasked*: DOJ, "Johnson & Johnson to Pay More Than $2.2 Billion to Resolve Criminal and Civil Investigations," news release, November 4, 2013, https://www.justice.gov.

53   *nearly 300,000*: Ina Jaffe and Robert Benincasa, "Old and Overmedicated: The Real Drug Problem in Nursing Homes," NPR, December 8, 2014, http://www.npr.org.

54   *90 percent of the drugs*: Center for Medical Advocacy, "Misuse of Antipsychotic Drugs in Nursing Homes: Are We Making Any Progress?" 2013, http://www.medicareadvocacy.org.

54   *"15,000 elderly people"*: Testimony of Dr. David Graham, *The Adequacy of FDA to Assure the Safety of the Nation's Drug Supply*, House Subcommittee on Oversight and Investigations of the Committee on Energy and Commerce, February 13, 2007, https://www.gpo.gov.

54   *without the consent*: Office of the California Attorney General, "Brown Announces Arrest of Nursing Home Employees Who Drugged Patients for Staff's Convenience," February 18, 2009, https://oag.ca.gov/news.

55   *debilitating shots of Haldol*: Marjie Lundstrom and Phillip Reese, "Unmasked: Who Owns California's Nursing Homes?" *Sacramento Bee*, November 9, 2014, http://www.sacbee.com.

56   *and the coroner's report*: Thom Jansen, "Chemical Restraints: Anti-Psychotic Meds Given to Elderly Despite Warnings," ABC 10 (Sacramento), June 17, 2015, http://www.abc10.com and Placer County Coroner Report, November 20, 2013, http://www.scribd.com/doc/268978872.

57   *against the department*: "FATE Concludes Public Interest Lawsuit Against the California Department of Public Health," *FATE: Newsletter of the Foundation Aiding the Elderly* 16, no. 1 (Winter 2016): 2, http://www.4fate.org.

57   *supposedly educates*: Centers for Medicare and Medicaid (CMS), National Partnership to Improve Dementia Care in Nursing Homes, https://www.cms.gov.

57   *CMS assumes*: Ina Jaffe and Robert Benincasa, "Alternatives to Antipsychotics: Nursing Homes Rarely Penalized for Oversedating Patients," NPR, September 12, 2014, http://www.npr.org.

58   *three times for modest amounts*: California Department of Public Health, Facility Information, Roseville Point Health & Wellness Center, http://hfcis.cdph.ca.gov; full references for this book's California nursing home controversies online at https://www.scribd.com/document/343213309/References-CA-Nursing-Homes-Oversight.

58   *five-star rating*: Roseville Point Health & Wellness Center, Nursing Home Profile, www.medicare.gov/nursinghomecompare.

58   *filed a complaint*: FATE letter of complaint re: Roseville Point and Genine Zisso, June 7, 2013, online at https://www.scribd.com and https://www.scribd.com/document.

58   *gamed the Medicare system*: Katie Thomas, "Medicare Star Ratings Allow Nursing Homes to Game the System," *New York Times*, August 24, 2014, https://www.nytimes.com.

58   *openly admitted*: David Martin and Sheila MacVicar, "Drugging Dementia: Are Antipsychotics Killing Nursing Home Patients?" Al Jazeera, March 11, 2015, http://america.aljazeera.com.

58   *better . . . national average*: CMS facility antipsychotic use spreadsheet, 2nd Quarter, 2015, enclosed in email from Tony Chicotel, staff attorney, California Advocates for Nursing Home Reform (CANHR), December 16, 2015.

59   *"low-balling"*: Marjie Lundstrom, "'All They Got Was a Slap on the Hand': Is California Low-Balling Penalties in Nursing Home Death Investigations?" *Sacramento Bee*, January 9, 2017, http://www.sacbee.com.

59   *Class B citation*: Email from Carole Herman, President of FATE, May 9, 2017; California Department of Public Health, Citation of Roseville nursing home, April 25, 2017, 1, https://www.scribd.com/document.

60   *decertified three*: Marjie Lundstrom and Phillip Reese, "California's Largest Nursing Home Owner Under Fire From Government Regulators," *Sacramento Bee,* June 13, 2015, http://www.sacbee.com/news.

61   *setting herself on fire*: Lundstrom and Reese, "Shifting Population in California Nursing Homes Creates 'Dangerous Mix,'" *Sacramento Bee*, April 2, 2016, http://www.sacbee.com.

61   *has defended the quality of care*: "Shlomo Rechnitz vs. California: Key Documents," *Sacramento Bee*, June 13, 2015. http://www.sacbee.com /news/investigations.

61   *facility was raided*: Marjie Lundstrom, "FBI Raids Riverside Nursing Home," *Sacramento Bee,* October 24, 2015, http://www.sacbee.com.

61   *charged with crimes*: Department of Justice, State of California, "Attorney General Kamala D. Harris Files Involuntary Manslaughter Charges Against Skilled Nursing Facility Verdugo Valley, LLC," news release, August 28, 2015, https://oag.ca.gov/news.

62   *"harmful drugging"*: "Recognizing Elder Abuse Awareness Day: Working Together to Curb Misuse of Powerful Antipsychotic Drugs in Nursing Homes," Center for Medicare Advocacy, http://www.medicareadvocacy.org.

62   *joined forces*: "Former Medicare Head Joins TwinMed, LLC as CEO," Business Wire, press release, January 8, 2014, http://www.businesswire.com.

62   *agreed to pay $3.5 million*: Jason Meisner, "Doctor Given Prison for Taking Kickbacks to Prescribe Risky Drug," *Chicago Tribune*, March 11, 2016, http://www.chicagotribune.com.

63   *spread the good news*: Christina Jewett and Sam Roe, "Drugmaker Paid Psychiatrist Nearly $500,000 to Promote Antipsychotic, Despite Doubts About Research," *ProPublica*, November 11, 2009, https://www.propublica.org.

63   *paying kickbacks to Omnicare*: Natasha Singer, "Johnson & Johnson Accused of Drug Kickbacks," *New York Times*, January 15, 2010, http://www .nytimes.com.

64 *leaked internal documents*: Alex Berenson, "Eli Lilly Said to Play Down Risk of Top Pill," *New York Times*, December 17, 2006, http://www.ny-times.com.

64 *urged nursing homes*: Tom Murphy and Marley Seaman, "Lilly Settles Zyprexa Suit for $1.42 Billion," *Seattle Times*, January 15, 2009, http://old.seattletimes.com/html.

64 *2014 lawsuit*: Jeremy Heallen, "AstraZeneca Facing Suit in Texas Over Seroquel Marketing," *Law360*, October 10, 2014, https://www.law360.com.

64 *host of sleazy tricks*: Katherine Hobson, "Whistleblower Twice Over: First Lilly Now AstraZeneca," *Wall Street Journal*, April 28, 2010, http://blogs.wsj.com; DOJ, "AstraZeneca Seroquel Settlement Agreement," April 27, 2010, online at http://psychrights.org.

65 *decrying overmedication*: Daniel R. Levinson, "Overmedication of Nursing Home Patients Troubling," DHHS, OIG, May 9, 2011, https://oig.hhs.gov.

65 *over-drugging the elderly*: DOJ, Northern District of California, "Watsonville Nursing Home Owners, Operators and Manager Agree to Pay $3.8 Million to Settle Allegations of False Claims," news release, May 21, 2015, https://www.justice.gov.

66 *new anti-fraud lawsuits*: Booker v. Pfizer, Appeal, January 30, 2017; Heallen, "AstraZeneca Facing Suit in Texas."

66 *Vermillion Cliffs*: Pam Belluck, "Giving Alzheimer's Patients Their Way, Even Chocolate," *New York Times*, December 31, 2011, http://www.nytimes.com.

67 *royalty payments*: Angie Drobnic Holan, "AARP Profits from Insurance Sales; GOP Calls It a Health Reform Conflict," *Politifact*, September 29, 2009, http://www.politifact.com/.

68 *granted a groundbreaking order*: AARP, "Ventura Facility Residents Successful in Challenging, Illegal Drugging," press release, February 4, 2014 http://www.aarp.org.

Chapter 3: The Secret History of the VA's Tragedies in Tomah and Phoenix

69 *more than thirty patients had died*: Aaron Glantz, "See Results of Government Investigations Into VA in Tomah, Wisconsin," *Reveal* from The Center for Investigative Reporting, March 23, 2015, https://www.revealnews.org.

69 *published influential studies*: Katherine E. Watkins et al., "The Quality of Medication Treatment for Mental Disorders in the Department of Veterans Affairs and in Private-Sector Plans," *Psychiatric Services* 67, no. 4 (April 1, 2016): 391–396, http://ps.psychiatryonline.org.

70 *assessment of the VA's overall quality*: Peter Hussey et al., *Resources and Capabilities of the Department of Veterans Affairs to Provide Timely and Accessible Care to Veterans* (Santa Monica, CA: RAND Corporation), 2015, http://www.rand.org.

70   *deadly wait times*: Curt Devine et al., "Report: Deadly Delays in Care Continue at Phoenix VA," CNN, October 4, 2016, http://www.cnn.com.

70   *pro-privatization agenda*: Alicia Mundy, "The VA Isn't Broken, Yet," *Washington Monthly*, March/April/May 2016, http://washingtonmonthly.com /magazine.

70   *Commission on Care*: Dennis Wagner, "VA Scandal: 'Drastic' Proposal Stirs Fears of Privatizing Veterans' Care," *Arizona Republic*, April 1, 2016, http://www.azcentral.com.

71   *actual reform ideas*: Donald J. Trump, "ICYMI: Trump's Ten Point Plan to Reform the VA" (excerpted from speech given in Virginia Beach, VA), July 11, 2016, https://www.donaldjtrump.com/press-releases.

72   *recklessly overused opiates*: Aaron Glantz, "Opiates Handed Out Like Candy to 'Doped-Up' Veterans at Wisconsin VA," *Reveal* from the Center for Investigative Reporting, January 2, 2015, https://www.revealnews.org.

72   *medication-linked deaths*: Audrey Hudson and Andrea Billups, "Dead Veteran's Kin Demand Inquiry," *Washington Times*, November 13, 2008, http://www.washingtontimes.com.

72   *public about abuses*: Ryan Honl, "Here Are the Facts About the Tomah VA Scandal," *Cap Times* (Madison, WI), May 19, 2016, http://host .madison.com.

73   *March 2014 report*: John Daigh, Jr., "Alleged Inappropriate Subscribing of Controlled Substances and Alleged Abuse of Authority...," VA OIG, MC# 2011-04212-HI-0267, March 12, 2014, https://www.document-cloud.org.

73   *found in his hospital bed*: Patricia Kime, "VA Hospital at Fault in Marine Veteran's Death," *Military Times*, August 19, 2016, http://www.military-times.com.

73   *House-Senate field hearing*: Statement of Dr. Carolyn Clancy, House Committee on Veterans Affairs, March 30, 2015, online at http://docs.house .gov/meetings.

73   *diagnosed 60 percent*: Sarah Childress, "Veterans Face Greater Risks Amid Opioid Crisis," PBS *Frontline*, March 28, 2016, http://www.pbs .org/wgbh/frontline.

73   *"mixed drug toxicity"*: VA OIG, *Unexpected Death of a Patient During Treatment with Multiple Medications, Tomah VA Medical Center, Tomah, Wisconsin*, report no. 15-02131-471, August 6, 2015, https://www.va.gov.

75   *congressional panel*: House–Senate Tomah field hearings, transcript, March 30, 2015, https://www.gpo.gov/.

75   *burgeoning illegal drug trade*: Aaron Glantz, "The Death of Baby Ada Mae and the Tragic Effects of Addicted Veterans," *Reveal* from The Center for Investigative Reporting, March 15, 2015, https://www .revealnews.org.

75   *conducting a criminal investigation*: Sari Lesk, "Criminal Investigation Continues at Tomah," *Stevens Point Journal*, May 7, 2015, http://www .stevenspointjournal.com.

75 *finally fired*: Patricia Kime, "VA: Tomah Chief of Staff Fired Without Settlement," *Military Times*, November 2, 2015, http://www.militarytimes .com.

75 *restored in April 2016*: David Wahlberg, "Former Tomah VA Doctor's Medical License Restored," *Wisconsin State Journal*, April 12, 2016, http://host.madison.com.

75 *permanently surrender*: Bill Glauber and Daniel Bice, "Fired Tomah VA Chief to Surrender Medical License," *Milwaukee Journal-Sentinel*, January 18, 2017, http://www.jsonline.com.

77 *reached an agreement*: Wisconsin Medical Examining Board, Division of Legal Services and Compliance, "Final Decision and Order for Remedial Education in the Matter of the License of Rhonda D. Davis, MD," case no. 15 MED 002, November 8, 2016, https://online.drl.wi.gov.

78 *curb and monitor opiate overprescribing*: *Jason Simcakoski Memorial Opioid Safety Act*, S.1641, 114th Cong. (2015–2016), https://www.congress.gov.

78 *Opioid Therapy Risk Report*: Reynaldo Leal, "VA Accelerates Deployment of Nationwide Opioid Therapy Tool," VA news release, March 9, 2015, http://www.blogs.va.gov.

79 *fail to work*: Kyle Buckley, "VA Electronic Health Records: What Federally Mandated Health Integration Really Looks Like," National Center for Policy Analysis, May 8, 2013, http://www.ncpa.org.

79 *agreed to a legal settlement*: Testimony of Kimberly Stowe Green, House Subcommittee on Health, House Veterans Affairs Committee, October 10, 2013, http://docs.house.gov/meetings; interviews and email correspondence with Green's attorney, Brant Mittler, October–November, 2015.

79 *little-noticed assessments*: "VA Code in Flight: Pharmacy Reengineering Data Update (PRE DATUP) 2.0," Open Source Health Record Alliance, 2014, https://www.osehra.org/blog; Assessment H (Health Information Technology), MITRE Corporation, September 1, 2015, https://www.va .gov/opa.

80 *forced out of his post*: Jacqueline Klimas, "VA Inspector General Steps Down Amid Controversy, Claims of Whitewashing," *Washington Times*, June 30, 2015, http://www.washingtontimes.com.

80 *The Senate governmental affairs committee*: Majority Staff Report of the Committee on Homeland Security and Governmental Affairs, U.S. Senate, *The Systemic Failure and Preventable Tragedies at the Tomah VA Medical Center*, May 31, 2016, http://www.hsgac.senate.gov.

81 *pattern of revenge*: Dan Elliott, "Veterans Affairs Whistleblower Resigns, Citing Retaliation," Military.com, November 17, 2016, http://www .military.com.

81 *corrosive culture"*: Carolyn Lerner, "Continued Deficiencies at the Department of Veterans Affairs' Facilities," Letter to the President from the Office of Special Counsel, June 23, 2014, https://osc.gov.

81 *50 percent increase*: Pauline Jelinek, "Number of Troops with PTSD up

50 Percent," Associated Press, May 28, 2008, http://www.sandiegounion-tribune.com.

81 *only half of veterans*: "Only Half the Vets With PTSD Are Getting Treatment: Report," CBS News, June 20, 2014, http://www.cbsnews.com.

81 *evidence-based treatment*: VA OIG, "Veterans Health Administration (VHA): Review of Veterans' Access to Mental Health Care," April 23, 2012, https://www.va.gov/oig/pubs/VAOIG-12-00900-168.pdf.

82 *nation's leading hospitals*: Adam Oliver, "The Veterans Health Administration: An American Success Story?" *Milbank Quarterly* 85, no. 1 (March 2007): 5–35. https://www.ncbi.nlm.nih.gov/pmc/articles/PMC2690309/.

82 *forty veterans had died*: "Timeline: The Road to VA Wait-Time Scandal," *Arizona Republic*, May 9, 2014, http://www.azcentral.com.

82 *new VA scandals*: VA, "Access Audit: System-Wide Review of Access, Results of Access Audit," May 12, 2014–June 3, 2014, https://www.va.gov/health/docs.

82 *reward administrators*: Chelsea J. Carter, "Were Bonuses Tied to VA Wait Times: Here's What We Know," CNN, May 30, 2014, http://www.cnn.com/2014/05/30/us/va-bonuses-qa/index.html.

83 *received a trip to Disneyland*: Dennis Wagner, "Fired Phoenix VA Chief Helman Took Secret Gifts," *Arizona Republic*, December 23, 2014, http://www.azcentral.com.

83 *sentenced in May 2016*: Dennis Wagner, "Judge Sentences Former Phoenix VA Director Sharon Helman to Probation," *Arizona Republic*, May 16, 2016, http://www.azcentral.com.

83 *overturned her firing*: Dennis Wagner, "Former Phoenix VA Director's Firing Overturned by Federal Appeals Court," *Arizona Republic*, May 9, 2017, http://www.azcentral.com/story.

83 *authority to fire*: Eric Katz, "Support Grows for Bills to Boost VA Firing, Restrict Its Unions," *Government Executive*, May 17, 2017, http://www.govexec.com.

83 *AFGE president denounced*: Brandon Coleman, "Veterans Affairs Whistleblower to Trump: Clean Up This Agency," *Daily Caller*, December 15, 2016, http://dailycaller.com.

84 *Openly declared*: Travis J. Tritton, "VA Abandons Law Aimed at Firing Employees," *Stars and Stripes*, June 17, 2016, https://www.stripes.com.

84 *reform legislation*: House Committee on Veterans Affairs, *The Veterans Access, Choice and Accountability Act of 2014*, Highlights, https://veterans.house.gov. CK check text https://www.congress.gov/bill/113th-congress/house-bill/3230

84 *same pattern continued*: Bill Theobald, "More Bonuses for VA Employees Despite Ongoing Problems at the Agency," *USA Today*, October 28, 2016, http://www.usatoday.com.

84 *two hundred veterans died*: Stephen Dinan, "200 Veterans Die Waiting for Care as Troubled Phoenix VA Builds New Backlog," *Washington Times*, October 4, 2016, http://www.washingtontimes.com.

85 *quick removal of the director*: Joshua Barajas, "VA Secretary Shulkin Addresses Report That VA Hospital in D.C. Puts Patients at 'Unnecessary Risk'," PBS *NewsHour*, April 13, 2017, http://www.pbs.org/newshour/.

85 *new website*: Donovan Slack, "New VA Chief on Public Scrutiny: Bring It," *USA Today*, April 12, 2017, https://www.usatoday.com.

85 *contrived criminal investigation*: Testimony of Shea Wilkes, *Improving VA Accountability: Examining First-Hand Accounts of Department of Veterans Affairs Whistleblowers*, Senate Committee on Homeland Security and Governmental Affairs, September 22, 2015, https://www.hsgac.senate.gov/hearings/.

86 *mental health legislation*: *Clay Hunt SAV Act*, Pub. L. No.: 114-2 (2015), https://www.congress.gov.

Chapter 4: The Secret History of the VA Scandals, Part II

87 *smears against Laney*: Dennis Wagner, "Phoenix VA Fiscal Officer Wins Whistleblower Reprisal Case," *Arizona Republic*, October 16, 2015, http://www.azcentral.com; Merit System Protection Board (MSPB), Denver Field Office, Initial Decision, October 15, 2015, https://www.scribd.com.

87 *"Did you have threesomes?"*: Appellant's Response to Order on Jurisdiction and Proof Requirements [supplemented with Laney emails to VA on "threesomes," June 2015], MSPB, 7–8, 19–23, July 6, 2015, https://www.scribd.com Laney-Timeline-of-VA-Harassment.

88 *belatedly filed*: Lisa Rein, "VA Manager Indicted on 50 Counts of Falsifying Records of Veterans Waiting for Medical Care," *Washington Post*, July 20, 2015, https://www.washingtonpost.com.

88 *public vows*: Bobbie O' Brien, "Veterans Secretary Wants VA Whistleblowers," WUSF (Tampa Bay), October 3, 2014, http://wusfnew .wusf.usf.edu.

88 *retaliated against*: Dennis Wagner, "Phoenix VA Bosses Mired In Personal Conflicts," *Arizona Republic*, May 23, 2015, http://www.azcentral.com.

90 *dog-and-pony show*: "President Trump Signs VA Accountability Executive Order," *Fox and Friends*, April 28, 2017, http://video.foxnews.com.

91 *suicidal patients were ignored*: Testimony of Jose Mathews, MD, House Committee on Veterans' Affairs, July 8, 2014, https://veterans.house.gov/witness-testimony/jose-mathews-md.

91 *"ensures leadership accountability"*: VA Claims on Increasing Transparency and Accountability, August 23, 2016, https://www.scribd.com.

91 *blood-and-bone splattered*: Mark Greenblatt et al., "Exclusive: Whistleblowers Cite Disorder at VA Hospital," WCPO, (Cincinnati), February 16, 2016, http://www.wcpo.com.

91 *raked in over $300,000*: Benjamin Krause, "Why Do Skeletons Follow Cincinnati VA's Dr. Barbara Temeck," *DisabledVeterans.org*, February 26, 2016, http://www.disabledveterans.org.

92 *prescribing opiates*: Mark Greenblatt et al., "Department of Veterans Af-

fairs Takes Action Against Barbara Temeck, Jack Hetrick at Cincinnati VA," WCPO, February 25, 2016, http://www.wcpo.com.

92 *denies any wrongdoing*: Anne Saker, "Who Runs the VA Here? UC, One Official Charges," May 13, 2016, http://www.cincinnati.com.

92 *congressman complained*: Mark Greenblatt et al., "Records: Dirty and Broken Surgical Tools, Holes in Sterile Wrappers Documented at Cincy VA," WCPO, June 23, 2016, http://www.wcpo.com.

92 *threatened by the VA hospital*: Al Letson, "No Choice: Failing America's Veterans," *Reveal* from The Center for Investigative Reporting, September 17, 2016, https://www.revealnews.org.

92 *high quality, safe services*: Emailed statement from Paula Paige, VA Media Relations, March 10, 2017.

93 *suicide prevention plans*: Patricia Kime, "VA: Veterans Suicide Must Be a Top Priority," *Military Times*, February 4, 2016, http://www.military-times.com; VA, "VA Releases Report on Nation's Largest Analysis of Veteran Suicide," press release, August 3, 2016, https://www.va.gov/opa.

93 *Clay Hunt*: U.S. House, H.R.203, *Clay Hunt SAV Act*, 114th Cong., (2015–2016), https://www.congress.gov.

93 *rubber-stamping*: Andis Robeznieks and Matthew DoBias, "Joint Commission Under Fire: Questions Arise After Walter Reed, West Texas Scandals," *Modern Healthcare*, March 12, 2007 http://www.modernhealthcare.com.

94 *once a month*: Mark Brunswick, "Cut Off Veterans Struggle to Live with VA's New Painkiller Policy," *Minneapolis Star Tribune*, July 12, 2015, http://www.startribune.com.

94 *twice as likely to die*: Aaron Glantz, "VA's Opiate Overload Feeds Veterans' Addictions, Overdose Deaths," *The Center for Investigative Reporting*, September 28, 2013, http://cironline.org.

94 *$200,000 grant from Purdue Pharma*: Dr. Andrew Kolodny, "Making a U-Turn, Clinical Application of Opioid Guidelines," presentation to the American Society of Addiction Medicine, April 6, 2017, 11–14, excerpt online at https://www.scribd.com.

94 *consultant for Purdue*: American-Statesman Investigative Team, "Critics Say Pharmaceutical Firms Spurred the Increase in Prescriptions for Narcotic Painkillers," *Austin American-Statesman*, September 29, 2012, http://www.statesman.com/news/.

94 *25 percent drop*: Emily Wax-Thibodeaux, "New Rules on Narcotic Painkillers Cause Grief for Veterans and VA," *Washington Post*, February 28, 2015, https://www.washingtonpost.com.

95 *increased 55 percent*: Eric Newhouse, "VA Says 68,000 Vets Addicted to Opioid Painkillers," *Psychology Today*, January 23, 2017, https://www.psychologytoday.com.; Childress, "Veterans Face Greater Risks."

95 *No one disciplined [until November2015]*: Bill Glauber and Daniel Bice, "Fired Tomah VA Chief To Surrender Medical License," *Milwaukee Journal Sentinel*, January 18, 2017, http://www.jsonline.com.

95 *twenty a day*: VA, "VA Fact Sheet: Suicide Prevention," July 2016, https://www.va.gov.

95 *one attempt every half hour*: Wes Moore, "Coming Back With Wes Moore," PBS, May 13, 2014, http://www.pbs.org.

95 *44 percent increase*: Janet E. Kemp, "Suicide Rates in VHA Patients Through 2011 With Comparisons With Other Americans and Other Veterans Through 2010," VHA, January 2014, http://www.mentalhealth.va.gov.

96 *one call a day*: Patricia Kime, "VA Crisis Line Director Resigns, Text Messages Go Unanswered," *Military Times*, June 29, 2016, http://www.militarytimes.com.

96 *busy suicide calls*: "VA Defends Work to Fix Troubled Veteran Suicide Hotline," Associated Press, April 4, 2017, https://www.mprnews.org/story.

96 *As many as half*: Terri Tanielen et al., "Invisible Wounds: Mental Health and Cognitive Care Needs of America's Returning Veterans," *RAND*, 2008, http://www.rand.org.

97 *75,000 veterans killed themselves*: VA, "Suicide Prevention Fact Sheet," August 3, 2016, https://www.va.gov.

97 *better than no treatment*: VA, "Suicide Among Veterans and Other Americans 2001–2014," Data Report, August 3, 2016, http://www.mentalhealth.va.gov.

97 *twelve times higher*: Alan Zarembo, "Suicide Rate of Female Military Veterans Is Called 'Staggering,'" *Los Angeles Times*, June 8, 2015, http://www.latimes.com.

98 *disturbing trends*: *American-Statesman* Investigative Team, "Prescription Drug Abuse, Overdoses Haunt Veterans Seeking Relief From Physical, Mental Pain," *Austin American-Statesman*, September 30, 2012, http://www.statesman.com.

98 *four hundred active-duty soldiers*: Baughman, "Soldiers of the Iraq/Afghanistan Era Dead."

98 *accidental prescription drug overdoses*: Amy S. B. Bohnert, "Association Between Opioid Prescribing Patterns and Opioid Overdose-Related Deaths," *JAMA* 205, no. 13 (2011): 1315–1321, http://jamanetwork.com.

98 *follow-up research showed*: Amy Bohnert et al., "Risk of Death From Accidental Overdose Associated With Psychiatric and Substance Use Disorders," *American Journal of Psychiatry* 169, no. 1 (January 2012): 64–70, https://www.ncbi.nlm.nih.gov.

98 *psychiatric drug overdoses*: Rose Rudd et al. "Increases in Drug and Opioid-Involved Overdose Deaths—United States, 2010–2015," *Morbidity and Mortality Weekly Report* 65, no. 50–51 (December 30, 2016): 1445–52, https://www.cdc.gov/mmwr.

98 *272 percent increase*: Glantz, "VA's Opiate Overload."

99 *shot up 4,100 percent*: John Ramsey, "Painkiller Epidemic Especially Pronounced Near Fort Bragg," *Fayetteville Observer*, July 14, 2013, online at http://www.wral.com.

99 *increased nearly 500 percent*: Nicola Davis, "US Heroin Use Has In-

creased Almost Fivefold in a Decade, Study Shows," *Guardian*, March 29, 2917, https://www.theguardian.com.

99   *manufacturers hid those risks*: Peter Loftus, "Pfizer Settles Neurontin Wrongful-Death Suit" *Wall Street Journal*, April 5, 2010, https://www.wsj.com; Katie Thomas and Michael Schmidt, "Glaxo Agrees to Pay $3 Billion in Fraud Settlement," *New York Times*, July 2, 2012, http://www.nytimes.com.

99   *competing "meta-analysis"*: Scott Stossel, "Should We Still Listen to Prozac? Peter D. Kramer Jumps Back Into the Antidepressant Debate," *New York Times*, July 7, 2016, https://www.nytimes.com; F. Hieronymus et al., "Consistent Superiority of Selective Serotonin Reuptake Inhibitors Over Placebo...," *Molecular Psychiatry*, 21 (2016): 523–530, http://www.nature.com.

99   *marshaled in books*: See, for instance, Irving Kirsch, *The Emperor's New Drugs: Exploding the Antidepressant Myth*, (New York: Basic Books, 2011).

100   *70 percent of patients*: Khalid Saad Al-Harbi, "Treatment-Resistant Depression: Therapeutic Trends, Challenges, and Future Directions," *Patient Preference and Adherence* 6 (May 1, 2012): 369–88, https://www.ncbi.nlm.nih.gov; Institute for Quality and Efficiency in Health Care, "Depression: How Effective Are Antidepressants?" Informed Health Online, January 12, 2017, https://www.ncbi.nlm.nih.gov.

100   *eleven times*: Sarah Boseley, "Seroxat Study Under-Reported Harmful Effects on Young People, Say Scientists," *Guardian*, September 16, 2015, https://www.theguardian.com.

100   *suicidal behavior and aggression*: T. Sharma et al. "Suicidality and Aggression During Antidepressant Treatment: Systematic Review and Meta-Analyses Based on Clinical Study Reports," *BMJ* 352 (2016): i65, https://www.ncbi.nlm.nih.gov/pubmed/26819231.

100   *clearly benefit*: Joan Raymond, "'Black Box' Warning on Antidepressants Raised Suicide Attempts," NBC News, April 19, 2013, http://www.nbcnews.com.

100   *justifying their use*: Zhai Yun Tan, "Depression Treatment Often Doesn't Go to Those Most in Need," NPR, August 29, 2016, http://www.npr.org.

100   *thirty-year high*: Sabrina Tavernise, "U.S. Suicide Rate Surges to a 30-Year High," *New York Times*, April 22, 2016, https://www.nytimes.com.

101   *never had major depression*: Yoichiro Takayanagi et al., "Antidepressant Use and Lifetime History of Mental Disorders in a Community Sample," *Journal of Clinical Psychiatry* 76, no. 1 (2015): 40–44, http://www.psychiatrist.com.

101   *one out of every 100 patients*: David Healy et al., "Antidepressants and Violence: Problems at the Interface of Medicine and Law," *PLOS Medici* 3, no. 9 (2006): 1478–1487, http://journals.plos.org.

101   *lawsuits have sharply dropped*: Jeff Swiatek, "'Black Box' Warning on Antidepressants Vastly Reduced Lawsuits Against Eli Lilly, Others," *IndyStar–USA Today*, August 24, 2014, http://www.indystar.com.

101   *clinically depressed*: Katinka Blackford Newman, *The Pill That Steals Lives*, http://www.thepillthatsteals.com/; Katinka Blackford Newman,

"'Depression Pills Made Me Unfit to Be a Mother,'" *Daily Mail*, July 4, 2016, http://www.dailymail.co.uk.

102 omit *"major depression"*: Mark Brunswick, "The VA Incorrectly Reports Suicide Data and Does a Poor Job of Tracking Vets at Risk, GAO Finds," *Minneapolis Star Tribune*, January 5, 2015, http://www.startribune.com/.

102 *veterans shooting themselves*: Kristina Rebelo, "Veteran Kills Himself in Parking Lot of VA Hospital on Long Island," *New York Times*, August 24, 2016, https://www.nytimes.com.

102 *undercounted by the VA*: Kevin Graman, "VA Center Wasn't Aware of Many Veteran Suicides," *Spokane Spokesman-Review*, August 9, 2009, http://www.spokesman.com.

102 *missing in most VA hospitals*: Jeanette Steele, "Veteran Suicides: What Might Have Saved Them?" *San Diego Union-Tribune*, February 4, 2016, http://www.sandiegouniontribune.com.

102 *under the watch of the hospital director*: Cristina Corbin, "Arizona VA Boss Accused of Covering Up Veterans' Deaths Linked to Previous Scandal," *Fox News*, April 24, 2014, http://www.foxnews.com; Dennis Wagner, "Arizona Suicides a Tragic Cost of Broken System," *Arizona Republic*, August 24, 2014, http://www.azcentral.com.

103 *Less than a third*: *Veterans for Common Sense v. Shinseki*, United States Court of Appeals, Ninth Circuit, no. 08-16728, May 10, 2011, http://caselaw.findlaw.com.

103 *1,400 veterans died*: Jamie Reno, "Court Rejects Iraq and Afghanistan Veterans' Demand for Better VA Care," *Daily Beast*, May 9, 2012, http://www.thedailybeast.com.

103 *far back as 2005*: Ron Zapata, "VA Hit With Massive Class Action," *Law 360*, July 23, 2007, https://www.law360.com.

103 *unchecked incompetence*: Carol Williams, "Court Orders Major Overhaul of VA's Mental Health System," *Los Angeles Times*, May 11, 2011, http://articles.latimes.com.

104 *new law in 2008*: Peter Katel, "Caring for Veterans: Does the VA Adequately Serve Wounded Vets?" *CQ Researcher*, April 23, 2010, http://library.cqpress.com.

104 *suicide prevention specialist*: "Evaluation of Suicide Prevention Program Implementation in VHA Facilities, Jan–June, 2009," September 22, 2009, https://www.va.gov.

104 *malingerers*: Tara McKelvey, "God, the Army, and PTSD: Is Religion an Obstacle to Treatment?" *Boston Review*, November/December 2009, http://bostonreview.net.

104 *openly critical*: Erica Goode, "Suicide's Rising Toll: After Combat, Victims of an Inner War," *New York Times*, August 1, 2009, http://www.nytimes.com.

105 *"personality disorder"*: James Dao, "Branding a Soldier with 'Personality Disorder,'" *New York Times*, February 24, 2012, http://www.nytimes.com.

105 *shady diagnostic practices*: "U.S. Military Illegally Discharging Veterans with Personality Disorder, Report Says," *Denver Post*, March 22, 2012, http://www.denverpost.com.

105 *"Other Than Honorable"*: Umar Moulta-Ali and Sidath Viranga Panangala, "Veterans' Benefits: The Impact of Military Discharges on Basic Eligibility," *Congressional Research Service*, R43928, March 6, 2015, https://fas.org.

105 *6 percent*: Veterans Legal Clinic (Harvard Law School), "Underserved: How the VA Wrongfully Excludes Veterans With Bad Paper," Swords to Plowshares and National Veterans Legal Services Program, March 2016, https://www.swords-to-plowshares.org.

106 *twice the rate*: Veterans Legal Clinic, "Underserved."

106 *300,000 jobless veterans*: American Public Health Association, "Removing Barriers to Mental Health Services for Veterans," November 18, 2014, https://www.apha.org.

106 *$4.5 billion in medical care*: Chris Coughlin, "Money Saved at Misdiagnosed Vets' Expense," *Courthouse News Service*, December 30, 2011, http://www.courthousenews.com.

106 *to just under 100,000*: VA, "VA Claims Backlog Now Under 100,000—Lowest in Department History...," *VAntage Point*, August 24, 2015, http://www.blogs.va.gov.

106 *480,000 appeals*: Interview with Gerald Manar, October 2016; Statement of Manar, Veterans of Foreign Wars, House Subcommittee on Disability and Memorial Affairs, *Veterans' Dilemma: Navigating the Appeal System for Veterans Claims,* January 22, 2015, https://veterans.house.gov.

107 *stuck in file drawers*: "Whistleblowers: Veterans Cheated Out of Benefits," CBS News, February 25, 2015, http://www.cbsnews.com.

107 *massive failures*: Benjamin Krause, "OSC Busts Oakland VA Regional Office 14,000 Claim Blunder," *DisabledVeterans.org*, October 14, 2016, http://www.disabledveterans.org.

107 *returned to their high-ranking posts*: Bryant Jordan, "Judge Overturns Demotion of Second VA Official Accused in Job Scam," *Military.com*, February 1, 2016, http://www.military.com.

108 *boondoggle*: Lee Romney, "Veterans Choice Didn't Ease Health Care Woes, Especially in Alaska," *from The Center for Investigative Reporting*, September 15, 2016, https://www.revealnews.org.

108 *rush schedule*: Quill Lawrence, "For Doctors and Patients, 'Veterans Choice' Often Means Long Waits," NPR, June 6, 2016, http://www.npr.org.

110 *legislative*: Steve Walsh, "How Congress and the VA Left Many Veterans Without a 'Choice,'" NPR, May 17, 2016, http://www.npr.org.

110 *"high-performing network"*: David Shulkin, "Beyond the VA Crisis: Becoming a High-Performance Network," *New England Journal of Medicine* 374 (2016): 1003–1005, http://www.nejm.org.

111 *bothered to warn*: No warning regarding quetiapine [the chemical name

for Seroquel] or Seroquel cardiac risk has yet been issued by the VA Center for Medication Safety, as of April 1, 2017, https://www.pbm.va.gov.

Chapter 5: A Marine's Descent Into PTSD Hell

113   *decided to join the Marines*: Most of the personal material in the chapters on Andrew White, Shirley White and Stan White is derived from extensive phone and in-person interviews with Stan and Shirley White, starting in March 2010.

114   *experiences intrusive thoughts*: All medical record quotes come from confidential "Progress Notes" from Huntington VAMC, VISTA Electronic Medical Documentation, March 01, 2007–February 12, 2008, with permission of Stan and Shirley White. Some documents related to Andrew White can be viewed at mentalhealthinc.net or at the author's scribd.com account.

114   *were burned to death*: Ellen Knickmeyer, "Demise of a Hard-Fighting Squad," *Washington Post*, May 12, 2005, http://www.washingtonpost.com.

115   *came so suddenly*: Julie Robinson, "The Cost of War: One Son's Life Was Claimed in Combat; Another by the Trauma That Followed It," *Charleston Gazette-Mail*, March 16, 2008, online at http://veteransforcommonsense.org.

115   *nineteen different*: Douglas Kennedy, "Powerful Psychiatric Drugs Harmful to Veterans?" Fox News, May 27, 2013, Online at http://www.cchr.pt.

116   *promoted Seroquel's off-label use*: Martha Rosenberg, "Are Veterans Being Given Deadly Cocktails to Treat PTSD?" *Alternet*, http://www.alternet.org.

116   *early stages*: Brian C. Lund, "Declining Benzodiazepine Use in Veterans With Posttraumatic Stress Disorder," *Journal of Clinical Psychiatry* 73, no. 3 (March 2012): 292–296, https://www.ncbi.nlm.nih.gov.

116   *more than 770*: Matthew Perrone, "Questions Loom Over Drug Given to Sleepless Vets," Associated Press, August 30, 2010, online at http://www.nbcnews.com.

116   *growth in antipsychotic use*: "Medicating the Military: Use of Psychiatric Drugs Has Spiked; Concerns Surface About Suicide, Other Dangers," *Military Times*, March 29, 2013, http://www.militarytimes.com.

117   *"higher risk of becoming fear-conditioned"*: Email correspondence with Dr. Richard Friedman, May 2017; Friedman, "Why Are We Drugging Our Soldiers," *New York Times*, April 21, 2012, http://www.nytimes.com; Friedman, "Wars on Drugs," *New York Times*, April 6, 2013, http://www.nytimes.com.

117   *five times more likely to have PTSD*: Alan Zarembo, "Pentagon Study Links Prescription Stimulants to Military PTSD Risk," *Los Angeles Times*, November 19, 2015, http://www.latimes.com/science.

117   *second-largest drug expenditure*: Perrone, "Questions Loom Over Drug."

117   *lost its patent protection*: Martha Rosenberg, "Controversial Drug Receives Military Restrictions and FDA Warnings as Its Patent Expires," *Truthout*, June 27, 2012, http://www.truth-out.org.

117 *damning 2011 Journal*: John Krystal et al., "Adjunctive Risperidone Treatment for Antidepressant-Resistant Symptoms of Chronic Military Service–Related PTSD," *JAMA* 306, no. 5 (August 3, 2011): 493–502, http://jamanetwork.com.

117 *payouts of over $1 billion*: Duff Wilson, "AstraZeneca Settles Most Seroquel Suits," *New York Times*, July 28, 2011, https://prescriptions.blogs.nytimes.com.

117 *nearly 800,000*: "VA Data Spread Sheet FY 2011–FY 2015 Atypicals," 3, https://www.scribd.com/document/342907650.

117 *found "dead in bed"*: Baughman, "Soldiers of the Iraq/Afghanistan Era Dead."

118 *needed a waiver*: "DoD Cracks Down on Off-Label Drug Use," *Military Times*, March 29, 2013, http://www.militarytimes.com.

118 *long after his death*: See medical literature search at *PubMed*, for "quetiapine" and "monotherapy," https://www.ncbi.nlm.nih.gov; "Seroquel for Insomnia: A Risky Off-Label Treatment," *Mental Health Daily*, May 23, 2015, online at http://mentalhealthdaily.com.

119 *various sleazy strategies*: DOJ, "AstraZeneca Seroquel Settlement Agreement."

119 *alleged illegal sales techniques*: DOJ, "AstraZeneca to Pay $520 Million."

119 *whistleblower*: Ed Silverman, "Texas AG Lawsuit Claims AstraZeneca Improperly Marketed Seroquel," *Wall Street Journal*, October 10, 2014, http://blogs.wsj.com.

119 *official guidelines*: VA and DoD, "VA/DoD Clinical Practice Guidelines for the Management of Post-Traumatic Stress," 2004, https://www.healthquality.va.gov/.

120 *in-depth scrutiny*: John Nardo, "Seroquel 1: Introduction of an Atypical…," *1Boring Old Man*, 12-Part Series, February 8, 2011, http://1boringoldman.com.

121 *cognitive therapies for PTSD available*: VA OIG, "Healthcare Inspection: Progress in Implementing the Veterans Health Administration's Uniform Mental Health Services Handbook," May 4, 2010, 33–40, https://www.va.gov/oig.

121 *repeatedly confirmed*: See sample search at Sunlight Foundation's Inspectors General portal for "evidence-based," "PTSD" and "poor," https://oversight.garden/reports.

122 *little improvement*: Institute of Medicine, "Effectiveness of PTSD Treatment Provided by Defense Department and VA Unknown…," news release, June 20, 2014, http://www8.nationalacademies.org.

125 *medical licensing board*: Minnesota Board of Medical Practice, "In the Matter of the Medical License of Marlin Gustav Thomas Schauland," September 12, 2009, online at http://psychsearch.net/psychs/mn/9122009.pdf.

125 *Suzie Q*: Patricia Wen, "Psychiatric Drug Sought on Streets," *Boston Globe*, July 13, 2009, http://archive.boston.com.

125 *without needing a DEA permit*: Background interviews with state and federal officials, June 2015; correspondence with Huntington VAMC, DOJ/DEA, West Virginia pharmacy and osteopathic boards, June 2015–

October 2016, online at https://www.scribd.com/document/343754066/HUNTINGTON-VA-Prescribing-Info.

125 *long exceeded*: Benedict Carey, "Drugs Found Ineffective for Veterans' Stress," *New York Times*, August 2, 2011, http://www.nytimes.com.

129 *received roughly $30,000*: See Lawrence B. Kelly or Lawrence Bennett Kelly, Charleston, at *ProPublica* Dollars for Docs, http://projects.propublica.org.

129 *up to 1,600 mg*: Confidential medical records of Andrew White, notes by Dr. Lawrence B. Kelly, November 20, 2007.

131 *took the risky step*: C. Heather Ashton, "Benzodiazepines: How They Work and How to Withdraw," *The Ashton Manual*, online at http://www.benzo.org.uk/manual/; Shirley White, "Andrew Ryan White, January 1, 1985–February 12, 2008," full text of testimony prepared for FDA hearing, April 2009.

135 *Corporal Nicholas Endicott*: Julie Robinson, "Couple Continues Battle After Soldier Son's PTSD Treatment-Related Death," *Charleston Gazette-Mail*, May 28, 2012, http://www.wvgazettemail.com.

136 *amount of methadone alone*: VA OIG, "Healthcare Inspection: Quality of Care of Two Deceased West Virginia Veterans," August 14, 2008, https://www.va.gov; Søren Fanøe, "Risk of Arrhythmia Induced by Psychotropic Medications: A Proposal for Clinical Management," *European Heart Journal* 35, no. 20 (2015): 1306–1315, https://academic.oup.com.

136 *sharply raises the blood plasma*: C. Uehlinger et al., "Increased (R)-Methadone Plasma Concentrations by Quetiapine in Cytochrome P450s and ABCB1 Genotyped Patient," *Journal of Clinical Psychopharmacology* 27, no. 3 (June 2007): 273–278, https://www.ncbi.nlm.nih.gov.

136 *revise the warning label*: Wilson, "Heart Warning Added to Label on Popular Antipsychotic Drug," *New York Times*, July 18, 2011.

136 *multiple prescriptions*: Pauline Jelinek, "Military Eyeing Mysterious Deaths," Associated Press, February 7, 2008, http://www.foxnews.com.

136 *over one hundred studies*: See, for instance, Wayne A. Ray et al., "Atypical Antipsychotic Drugs and the Risk of Sudden Cardiac Death," *New England Journal of Medicine* 360, no. 3 (January 15, 2009): 225–235, https://www.ncbi.nlm.nih.gov; and search "atypical antipsychotic" and "QT" at PubMed: https://www.ncbi.nlm.nih.gov.

Chapter 6: Stan White and the Veterans' Search for Truth and Answers

138 *"That's not supposed to happen"*: Sara Gavin, "Military Men Mysteriously Dying," WOWK (TV 13), March 12, 2008, online at http://www.disabilityrightsca.org.

139 *psychiatric medication crisis*: Robinson, "Cost of War."

140 *"Sudden cardiac death"*: Serge Sicouri and Charles Antzelevitch, "Sudden Cardiac Death Secondary to Antidepressant and Antipsychotic Drugs," *Expert Opinion on Drug Safety* 7, no. 2 (March 2008): 181–194, https://www.ncbi.nlm.nih.gov.

140 *issued a press release*: Dr. Fred Baughman Jr., "A Cluster of Veterans Deaths," PRNewswire, June 20, 2008, http://www.prnewswire.com.

141 *White and Layne deaths*: VA OIG, "Healthcare Inspection: Quality of Care of Two Deceased West Virginia Veterans."

141 *in nearly seventy medical studies*: See search for "QT" [prolongation] and atypical antipsychotic at Pub Med, filtered by date: https://www.ncbi.nlm.nih.gov.

141 *electrocardiograms be given*: Wayne A. Ray et al., "Atypical Antipsychotic Drugs and the Risk of Sudden Cardiac Death," *New England Journal of Medicine* 360, no. 3 (January 15, 2009): 225–235, https://www.ncbi.nlm.nih.gov.

142 *"no association"*: Alexander H. Glassman and J. Thomas Bigger, Jr., "Antipsychotic Drugs: Prolonged QT Interval, Torsades de Pointes, and Sudden Death," *American Journal of Psychiatry* 158 (November 2001): 1774–1782, https://www.ncbi.nlm.nih.gov.

143 *up to 1,200 mg of off-label Seroquel*: Confidential medical records of Andrew White.

143 *maximum recommended dosage*: A. Sparshatt, "Quetiapine: Dose–Response Relationship in Schizophrenia," *CNS Drugs* 22, no. 1 (2008): 49–68, https://www.ncbi.nlm.nih.gov.

143 *sleep aid on the battlefield*: Brewin, "Drug Policy Threatens Troops."

144 *"our heroes we are mistreating"*: Letter by Georgeann Underwood to House and Senate veterans' committees on grandson Derek Johnson, April 2009, online at https://www.scribd.com-Johnson-1 and https://www.scribd.com-2; Julie Robinson, "Vets Taking PTSD Drugs Die in Sleep," *Charleston Gazette*, May 24, 2008, online at http://www.gulfwarvets.com.

Chapter 7: Mr. White Comes to Washington

146 *request from AstraZeneca*: FDA, Center for Drug Evaluation and Research, Psychopharmacologic Drugs Advisory Committee Hearing on April 8, 2009, transcript, 71–72, https://www.fda.gov.

146 *Jorge Armenteros*: Miriam Hill, "Conflicts for FDA Committee Set to Weigh Risks of Seroquel," *Philadelphia Inquirer,* April 4, 2009, online at http://psychrights.org.

147 *thoroughly discredited*: Duff Wilson, "Drug Maker's E-Mail Released in Seroquel Lawsuit," *New York Times,* February 27, 2009, http://www.nytimes.com.

147 *alleged illegal marketing campaign*: DOJ, "AstraZeneca settlement."

147 *"cursed study"*: Shanker Vedantam, "A Silenced Drug Study Creates an Uproar," *Washington Post,* March, 18, 2009, http://www.washingtonpost.com.

148 *cardiac death*: Wayne Ray et al., "Atpical Antipsychotic Drugs," NEJM, January 15, 2009.

148 *reportedly misled*: Waters, "Drug Report Barred by FDA," *San Francisco Chronicle,* February 1, 2004.

148 *Laughren had a new chance*: FDA, Psychopharmacologic Drugs Advisory

Committee, Meeting Transcript, April 8, 2009, https://www.fda.gov.

148 *first-line "monotherapy"*: FDA, AstraZeneca Briefing Document, Drugs Advisory Committee, April 8, 2009, https://www.fda.gov.

149 *nearly 10 percent of adult*: NIMH, "Generalized Anxiety Disorder Among Adults," https://www.nimh.nih.gov.

149 *Seroquel XR was then over $12,000*: Ken O' Day et al., "Long-Term Cost-Effectiveness of Atypical Antipsychotics in the Treatment of Adults With Schizophrenia in the US," *ClinicoEconomics and Outcomes Research* 5 (September 12, 2013): 459–470, https://pdfs.semanticscholar.org.

149 *the drug was safe*: FDA, Drugs Advisory Committee, transcript, April 8, 2009 4–6.

149 *couldn't kill you*: FDA, Drugs Advisory Committee, transcript, 21–27.

150 *seven times*: Advisory Committee, "4.4.6 Mortality From All Causes in Clinical Studies," AstraZeneca briefing document, 90–92.

150 *170 percent higher risk*: FDA, "Information for Healthcare Professionals: Conventional Antipsychotics," June 16, 2008, https://www.fda.gov.

150 *adjunct treatment for depression*: "Seroquel Gets the Abilify Treatment," *The Carlat Psychiatry Blog*, April 14, 2009, http://carlatpsychiatry .blogspot.com.

151 *short trial of Seroquel*: Mark Hamner, "Quetiapine Treatment In Patients With Posttraumatic Stress Disorder: An Open Trial Of Adjunctive Therapy," *Journal of Clinical Psychopharmacology* 23, no. 1 (February 2003), 15–20, https://www.ncbi.nlm.nih.gov.

151 *broadening the use*: Charles Schulz et al., "Broadening the Horizon of Atypical Antipsychotic Applications," *Medscape*, June 15, 2004, http://www.medscape.org.

151 *two additional twelve-week studies*: Mark Hamner, "A Placebo-Controlled Trial of Adjunctive Quetiapine for Refractory PTSD," May 2009, https://clinicaltrials.gov; Hamner, "Quetiapine Treatment for Post-Traumatic Stress Disorder (PTSD)," December 2007, https://clinicaltrials.gov.

151 *half of all clinical trials*: "What Does All Trials Registered and Reported Mean?" Alltrials.net, http://www.alltrials.net/find-out-more/all-trials/.

152 *stopped recommending*: VA, "VA/DoD Clinical Practice Guidelines for Management of Post-Traumatic Stress," 2010, https://www.healthquality .va.gov.

152 *finally co-authored*: Gerardo Villareal, Mark B. Hamner et al., "Efficacy of Quetiapine Monotherapy in Posttraumatic Stress Disorder: A Randomized, Placebo-Controlled Trial," *American Journal of Psychiatry* 173, no. 12 (December 1, 2016): 1205–1212, https://www.researchgate.net.

153 *Pfizer visiting professor in 2011*: Martha Rosenberg, *Born With a Junk Food Deficiency: How Flaks, Quacks and Hacks Pimp the Public Health* (Amherst, NY: Prometheus Books, 2012), 96–97.

153 *damning 2011 study*: Benedict Carey, "Drugs Found Ineffective for Veterans' Stress," *New York Times*, August 2, 2011, http://www.nytimes.com /2011/08/03/health/research/03psych.html.

153 *$846 million for Seroquel*: Bob Brewin, "Mental Illness Is the Leading Cause of Hospitalization for Active-Duty Troops," *Nextgov*, May 17, 2012, http://www.nextgov.com.

154 *800,000 prescriptions for Seroquel*: VA, Office of Public Affairs, "VA Data Spread Sheet, FY 2011–FY 2015, Atypicals," 2015, https://www.scribd.com.

154 *over $1.5 billion*: Bob Brewin, "Mental Illness Is the Leading Cause," *Nextgov*; VA, "VA Data Spread Sheet, Atypicals," 2015.

154 *boasted to a congressional hearing*: Statement of Dr. Carolyn Clancy, Interim Under Secretary for Health, VA, House Subcommittee on Oversight and Investigations, Committee on Veterans' Affairs, , June 10, 2015, https://veterans.house.gov.

154 *any known mental illness*: Allison Bond Kotru, "Many Vets Given Psychiatric Drugs Without Diagnosis," Reuters, October 31, 2013, http://www .reuters.com.

154 *a new FDA-required warning*: Duff Wilson, "Heart Warning Added to Label on Popular Antipsychotic Drug," *New York Times*, July 18, 2011, http:/ /www.nytimes.com.

156 *killing herself three times*: Patricia Kime, "Sailor's Suicide Triggers Lawsuit," *USA Today*, December 7, 2012, http://www.usatoday.com; Deposition of Dr. William McDaniel, *Darla Grese vs. United States of America*, U.S. District Court for the Eastern District of Virginia, Civil Action no. 4:12 cv-49, July 12, 2012, online at https://www.scribd.com.

157 *Sister Surrendered*: Darla M. Grese, *Sister Surrendered*, Amazon Digital Services, April 2014. https://www.amazon.com.

157 *is 23 percent*: Author's correspondence with Huntington VA, June 2015.

158 *A 2012 JAMA*: James Dao, "For Veterans With Post-Traumatic Stress, Pain Killers Carry Risks," *New York Times*, March 7, 2012, https://atwar .blogs.nytimes.com.

158 *VA's weren't sharing data*: *VA Opioid Prescription Policy, Practice, and Procedures*, U.S. Senate Committee on Veterans Affairs, March 26, 2015, https://www.gpo.gov, 20.

159 *120,000 opiate deaths*: C. J. Arlotta, "Has Obama Neglected America's Growing Opioid, Heroin Epidemic?" *Forbes*, August 26, 2015, https://www.forbes.com.

159 *personally honored in 2010*: Huntington VA, "Huntington VA Medical Center Director Recognized by the President," July 2010, http://www .huntington.va.gov/news/director.asp.

Chapter 8: Drug-Free PTSD Recovery
(The information in this chapter is based largely on personal interviews and observations by the author of an Operation Tohidu retreat, February 2015.)

164 *"Operation: Tohidu"*: Carol Costello, "Are Medications an Effective PTSD Treatment?" CNN, July 25, 2015, https://www.youtube.com.

164 *Center for Advanced Warfighter Reintegration*: "History," Warfighter Ad-

vance, http://www.warfighteradvance.org/history.html.

167 *Navy Medicine*: Mary Vieten et al., *Navy Medicine* 95, no. 5 (September–October, 2004): 14–16, https://ia801700.us.archive.org.

168 *rapport is a critical ingredient*: John Norcross et al., "Psychotherapy Relationships That Work II," *Psychotherapy* 48, no. 1 (March 2011): 4–8, https://www.researchgate.net.

Chapter 9: How LA County's Mental Health Officials Neglect Inmates and Ignore Violence

170 *severe mental illness*: Unique Keyona Moore, case no. 2014-07600, Department of Coroner, County of Los Angeles, online at https://www.scribd.com; Levine, "Why Did L.A. County Inmate Unique Moore Die?" *HuffPost*, February 28, 2016.

170 *lawsuit*: *Elaine Bridges and Jimmie Lee Moore v. County of Los Angeles et al.*, Sup. Ct., Co. of Los Angeles, South Central District, case no. TC028303, November 6, 2015, https://www.scribd.com/doc.

170 *nearly 700,000 adults*: Los Angeles County Department of Mental Health (DMH), "Estimated Prevalence of SED & SMI Among Total Population By Age Group and Service Area 2015," online at https://www.scribd.com.

171 *"decedent went into cardiac arrest"*: Unique Keyona Moore report, Department of the Coroner.

172 *the once-powerful Baca*: Celeste Fremon, "The Retrial of Lee Baca: How LA County's Popular Sheriff Got Convicted," *Witness LA*, March 17, 2017, http://witnessla.com.

172 *federally-appointed monitor*: Cindy Chang and Joel Rosen, "After Years of Scandal, L.A. Jails Get Federal Oversight, Sweeping Reforms," *Los Angeles Times*, August 5, 2015, http://www.latimes.com.

172 *class-action ACLU lawsuit*: ACLU of Southern California, "Inmate Abuse Timeline," https://www.aclusocal.org.

172 *commonplace violence*: Human Rights Watch (HRW), "Callous and Cruel: Use of Force Against Inmates with Mental Disabilities in US Jails and Prisons," May 2015, https://www.hrw.org.

173 *60 percent*: Ram Subramanian et al., *Incarceration's Front Door: The Misuse of Jails in America*, VERA Institute of Justice, Center on Sentencing and Corrections, February 2015, http://archive.vera.org.

173 *mentally ill inmate*: Joel Rubin, "A Top L.A. Sheriff's Recruit Was Just Days on the Job When He Says Deputies Beat an Unresisting Inmate," *Los Angeles Times*, May 16, 2016, http://www.latimes.com.

173 *handcuffed nearly naked*: HRW, "Callous and Cruel."

174 *moved to strip*: County of Los Angeles, Chief Executive Office, "Approval of Proposed Jail Health Services Structure," June 9, 2015, http://file.la-county.gov.

174 *ten times*: Dr. E. Fuller Torrey et al., "More Mentally Ill Persons Are in Jails and Prisons Than Hospitals: A Survey of the States," Treatment Advocacy Center, May 2010, http://www.treatmentadvocacycenter.org.

175 *court-ordered consent decree*: Ian Lovett, "Los Angeles Agrees to Overhaul Jails to Care for Mentally Ill and Curb Abuse," *Los Angeles Times*, August 5, 2015, https://www.nytimes.com.

175 *less than a month*: Email from Lt. David Dolson, Los Angeles Sheriff's Department (LASD), Homicide Bureau, November 4, 2015, online at https://www.scribd.com.

176 *80 percent are homeless*: Los Angeles County Sheriff Jim McDonnell, *Testimony Before the 21st Century Policing Task Force*, February 24, 2015, https://cops.usdoj.gov.

177 *citizens commission*: Lourdes Baird et al., *Report of the Citizens' Commission on Jail Violence*, Los Angeles County, September 2012, http://www.lacounty.gov.

177 *convicted*: Alene Tchekmedyian, "L.A. Sheriff's Deputies Sentenced to Prison for Beating a Mentally Ill Inmate and Covering Up the Attack," *Los Angeles Times*, November 28, 2016.

178 *eyewitness accounts*: ACLU National Prison Project and the ACLU of Southern California, "Cruel and Usual Punishment: How a Savage Gang of Deputies Controls L.A. County Jails," September 2011, https://www.aclu.org.

179 *"reign of terror"*: Peter Eliasberg and Margaret Winter, "The Reign of Terror Ends at L.A. County Jails," ACLU of Southern California, December 16, 2014, https://www.aclusocal.org.

179 *40 percent*: Citizen's Commission on Jail Violence, LASD, *Status of Recommendations*, October 21, 2014, http://file.lacounty.gov.

179 *significant problems continue*: LASD, "Force by Category," 2015–2016, online at https://www.scribd.com.

180 *stinging report*: DOJ, "Mental Health Care and Suicide Prevention Practices at Los Angeles County Jails," DJ 168-12C-43, June 4, 2014, https://www.justice.gov.

180 *dumping mentally ill*: Abby Sewell and Cindy Chang, "Ex-Inmates Want L.A. County to Stop Dumping Mentally Ill Inmates on Skid Row," *Los Angeles Times*, September 28, 2015, http://www.latimes.com; Nationally, the lack of proper discharge services can increase suicides: Jennifer Gonnerman, "Kalief Browder Learned How to Commit Suicide on Rikers," *New Yorker*, June 2, 2016, http://www.newyorker.com.

180 *used restraints*: Office of Inspector General, County of Los Angeles, OIG, *Overview and Policy Analysis of Tethering in Los Angeles County Jails*, June 2016, 10, https://oig.lacounty.gov; Maya Lau, "After Four Recent Inmate Deaths, Protesters Call for Changes in L.A. County Jails," *Los Angeles Times*, March 10, 2017, http://www.latimes.com.

181 *roughly 1,900*: LASD, Custody Division Year-End Review 2015, updated June 16, 2016, http://www.la-sheriff.org; Carimah Townes, "The Tragedy of Being a Woman in Jail," Think Progress, https://thinkprogress.org.

181 *degrading experiences*: Alejandro Caceres-Monroy et al., *Breaking the Silence: Civil and Human Rights Violations Resulting from Medical Neglect*

and Abuse of Women of Color in Los Angeles County Jails, Dignity and Power Now, August 4, 2015, http://dignityandpowernow.org.

181 *causing serious injury*: For Ronnquist testimony, see Meeting Transcript of the Meeting of the Los Angeles County Board of Supervisors, May 6, 2014, 140, http://file.lacounty.gov.

181 *leading cause of death*: Victoria Bekiempis, "Suicide Rate in U.S. Jails Jumps," August 4, 2015, http://www.newsweek.com.

182 *$1.6 million settlement*: Cindy Chang, "L.A. County Settles Jail Suicide Case for $1.6 Million," *Los Angeles Times*, September 1, 2015, http://www.latimes.com.

182 *commit crimes again*: John K. Inglehart, "Decriminalizing Mental Illness: The Miami Model," *New England Journal of Medicine*, May 5, 2016, http://www.nejm.org/; Sarah Liebowicz et al., *A Way Forward: Diverting People with Mental Illness from Inhumane and Expensive Jails into Community-Based Treatment That Works*, Report by ACLU of Southern California and the Bazelon Center for Mental Health Law, July 2014, 7, https://www.aclusocal.org.

182 *high-quality services to some*: LA County DMH, *MHSA Annual Update Fiscal Year 2016–2017*, September 20, 2016, http://file.lacounty.gov.

183 *no-confidence vote*: County of Los Angeles Chief Executive Office "Approval of Proposed Jail Health Services Structure," June 9, 2015, http://file.lacounty.gov.

Chapter 10: To Live and Die In LA

185 *more than one a day*: Christopher Ingraham, "We're Now Averaging More Than One Mass Shooting per Day in 2015," *Washington Post*, August 26, 2015, https://www.washingtonpost.com.

186 *stopped dozens*: Art Levine, "Could a LA-Style Threat Assessment Team Have Thwarted the Isla Vista, Seattle or Oregon Shooting Sprees?" *HuffPost*, August 21, 2014, http://www.huffingtonpost.com.

186 *magical powers*: Alison Knopf, "AOT Cost-Effectiveness Study Stirs National Debate," *Behavioral Healthcare Executive*, Aug 22, 2013, http://www.behavioral.net.

187 *repeatedly been hospitalized*: "Implementing AOT Laws," Treatment Advocacy Center, http://www.treatmentadvocacycenter.org.

187 *review of mandated treatment*: S. R. Kisely and L. A. Campbell, "Compulsory Community and Involuntary Outpatient Treatment for People With Severe Mental Disorders," Cochrane Collaboration, December 4, 2014, http://www.cochrane.org.

187 *wouldn't be able to identify*: Email to author from D. J. Jaffe, executive director of Mental Illness Policy Org., December 30, 2015, online at https://www.scribd.com.

187 *can't afford to wait*: Erica Goode, "Focusing on Violence Before It Happens," *New York Times*, March 14, 2013, http://www.nytimes.com.

188 *well over fifty planned school and campus attacks*: DMH, School Threat

Assessment Team (START), Application for 2013 Quality and Productivity Awards, Quality and Productivity Commission (LA County), June 27, 2013, http://qpc.lacounty.gov.

188 *already halted*: Levine, "Could a LA-Style Threat"; DMH, START, Application for 2013 Quality and Productivity Awards.

188 *authority to seize weapons*: Kelly Ward, "The Gun Violence Restraining Order: An Opportunity for Common Ground in the Gun Violence Debate," *Developments in Mental Health Law* 34, no. 3 (October 2015): 1–2.

188 *get their guns back*: Michele Luo, "In Some States, Gun Rights Trump Orders of Protection," *New York Times*, March 17, 2013, http://www.nytimes.com.

189 *copycat threat*: Mark Follman and Becca Andrews, "How Columbine Spawned Dozens of Copycats," *Mother Jones,* October 5, 2015, http://www.motherjones.com.

190 *crime victimization survey*: Linda Teplin et al., "Crime Victimization in Adults With Severe Mental Illness," *Archives of General Psychiatry*, 62, no. 8 (August 2005): 911–912.

190 *three to five times*: Seena Fazel et al., "Schizophrenia and Violence: Systematic Review and Meta-Analysis," *PLOS Medicine*, August 11, 2009, http://journals.plos.org/plosmedicine/article?id=10.1371/journal.pmed.1000120.

190 *debunked claims*: Jeffrey W. Swanson et al., "Mental Illness and Reduction of Gun Violence and Suicide: Bringing Epidemiologic Research to Policy," *Annals of Epidemiology* 25 (2015): 368, https://www.ncbi.nlm.nih.gov/pubmed/24861430.

192 *joint pairings*: LA DMH, Emergency Outreach Bureau, Field Response Operations, http://file.lacounty.gov.

193 *its officers shot thirty-eight people*: Kate Mather and James Queally, "More Than a Third of People Shot by L.A. Police Last Year Were Mentally Ill, LAPD Report Finds," *Los Angeles Times*, March 1, 2016, http://www.latimes.com.

194 *shot a homeless, mentally ill man*: For video of shooting, go to https://www.youtube.com/watch?v=vxyy8mMh2JM.

194 *teams shouldn't get involved*: See #3, demand for LAPD use of SMART teams in Skid Row in Clergy and Laity United for Economic Justice et al., "Open Letter to City of LA Elected Officials, Los Angeles Police Department. . . .," March 12, 2015, online at https://cangress.files .wordpress.com.

194 *quarter of all fatal shootings*: Kimberly Kindy et al., "Fatal Shootings by Police Are Up in the First Six Months of 2016, *Post* Analysis Finds," *Washington Post,* July 7, 2016, https://www.washingtonpost.com/national.

195 *every thirty-six hours*: Wesley Lowery et al., "Distraught People, Deadly Results," *Washington Post,* June 30, 2015, http://www.washingtonpost.com.

195 *confrontations dropped 80 percent*: "Memphis Model: Police Pioneer Use of Crisis Intervention Teams to Deal with Mentally Sick," Democracy

Now, October 22, 2013, https://www.democracynow.org; Art Levine, "The Calm Arm of the Law," *City Link,* March 27–April 2, 2002.

Chapter 11: Torture In Alabama

199 *multibillion-dollar residential treatment industry:* Nina Flanagan, "The Ripeness for the Behavioral Health Market Is Now," *Healthcare Dive,* October 19, 2015, http://www.healthcaredive.com; Sebastian Murdock, "The Troubled Teen Industry Has Been a Disaster for Decades. And It's Still Not Fixed," *HuffPost,* August 23, 2016, http://testkitchen.huffing-tonpost.com/island-view.

200 *whippings, beatings and alleged rapes:* Kathryn Jones, "Horror Stories From Tough-Love Teen Homes," *Mother Jones,* July/August 2011, http://www.motherjones.com; Brandy Zadrozny, "Rapes, Daily Beatings, and No Escape: Christian School Was Hell For These Boys," *Daily Beast,* June 12, 2016, http://www.thedailybeast.com.

200 *brink of death:* Alexandra Zayas, "Military School 'Cadet' Exercised to Brink of Death," *Tampa Bay Times,* October 26, 2012, http://www.tampabay.com, part of series, "In God's Name: Unlicensed Religious Children's Homes," at http://www.tampabay.com/faccca/.

200 *more moderate approach:* Jennifer Rich, "Gateway Academy Takes New Path to Progress," *Washington County News–Holmes County Times Advertiser,* July 21, 2015, http://www.chipleypaper.com/1.497931.

200 *Teen Challenge:* Global Teen Challenge, http://globaltc.org/our-story/.

200 *Florida, Alabama and Missouri:* Alexandra Zayas and Kathleen Flynn, "Unlicensed Youth Homes," *Tampa Bay Times,* February 22, 2013, http://www.tampabay.com/faccca/; Matthew Franck, "Acting on Faith: A Look Inside Reform School in Missouri," *St. Louis Post-Dispatch,* November 17, 2002, online at https://www.culteducation.com; Anna Claire Vollers, "3 Convicted for Child Abuse at Religious Alabama Private School," *Mobile Press-Register,* January 24, 2017, http://www.al.com.

200 *no requirements:* U.S. Department of Education, State Regulation of Private Schools, July 2009, https://www2.ed.gov.

200 *convicted sex offender:* For Teen Challenge in the U.S., go to https://www.teenchallengeusa.com; "Teen Challenge Exposed by Action 9 News," Topix (Orlando), February 5, 2008, online at http://www.topix.com; "Convicted Sex Offender Heads Teen Challenge Augusta," *Topix* (Orlando), February 21, 2008, http://www.topix.com.

200 *"spitting in the face of Jesus":* "Teen Challenge: Coercive Groups Disguised as Rehab," *Daily Kos,* April 27, 2008, http://www.dailykos.com.

201 *chief enforcer of sadistic beatings:* William Knott, manager and co-founder of Restoration Youth Academy (now closed), online at http://www.heal-online.org/rya.htm.

203 *"put in shackles":* See video display of letters accompanying Art Levine, "The Harrowing Story of Life Inside Alabama's Most Sadistic Christian Bootcamp," *Newsweek,* March 2, 2017, http://www.newsweek.com.

203 *vicious corporal punishment*: Kathryn Joyce, "Horror Stories From Tough-Love Teen Homes," *Mother Jones,* July/August 2001, http://www.motherjones.com.

204 *Change.org*: Racheal Anthony, "The State of Missouri, the City of La Russell, Missouri: Stop the Abuse at New Beginnings Ministries Run by Bill and Jennifer McNamara," Petition, Change.org, https://www .change.org.

204 *Lester Roloff*: Pam Colloff, "Remember the Christian Alamo," *Texas Monthly,* December 2001, http://www.texasmonthly.com.

204 *200,000 or more youths*: *Residential Facilities: State and Federal Oversight Gaps May Increase Risk to Youth Well-Being,* GAO-08-696T, April 24, 2008, http://www.gao.gov; Frank Ainsworth, "An Exploration of the Differential Usage of Residential Childcare Across National Boundaries," *International Journal of Social Welfare*, 23, no. 1 (January 2014): 16-24, online at https://www.scribd.com.

204 *Independent Fundamental Baptist*: Susan Donaldson James, "Biblical Reform School Discipline: Tough Love or Abuse?" ABC News, April 12, 2011, http://abcnews.go.com; Angela

204 Smith, memo, "Private School Requirements (Or Lack Thereof)," online at https://www.scribd.com/document.

204 *Restoration Youth Academy*: Anna Claire Vollers, "Former Students Share Harrowing Stories of Life Inside Alabama's Worst Religious Private School," *Mobile Press-Register*, June 30, 2016, http://www.al.com.

207 *institutional suicide*: ACLU, "Alone & Afraid: Children Held in Solitary Confinement and Isolation in Juvenile Detention and Correctional Facilities," August 9, 2013, https://www.aclu.org/report/alone-afraid.

207 *police reports*: A sample, see Holmes County Sheriff's Department, Incident Reports, Teen Challenge, late 1990s–2011, online at http://www.heal-online.org/policereports.pdf.

210 *"residency has no impact"*: Letter via email from Luther Strange, Office of Alabama Attorney General, July 26 2016, online at https://www .scribd.com.

210 *police report*: Prichard, AL Police Department incident report by "Eric" Reyes charging William Knott with assault, August 7, 2012, https://www.scribd.com.

213 *abuse allegations*: Vollers, "Alabama Removes 22 Boys From Religious Boarding School Amid Allegations of Abuse," *Mobile Press-Register*, December 9, 2016, http://www.al.com.

213 *"demon out of you"*: County Sheriff's Office Offense/Incident Report, case no. 2105-066773, September 12, 2015, 4, https://www.scribd .com/document.

216 *regulate all private residential*: Chip Brownlee, "House Votes to Crack Down on Extremist Gay Conversion, Behavioral Bootcamps," *Alabama Political Reporter*, May 5, 2017, http://www.alreporter.com.

217 *few mental health professionals*: Victoria Pelham and Brett Kelman,

"Mental Health Shortages Reach Crisis Levels," *Desert Sun* (Palm Springs), May 21, 2015, http://www.desertsun.com.

217   *Survivors of Institutional Abuse*: For SIA website, go to http://www.sia-now.org.

217   *helping close*: Alexandra Zayas, "Christian Girls' Reform Home Closes After Times Investigation," *Tampa Bay Times*, February 13, 2013, http://www.tampabay.com.

218   *at least nominal oversight*: (California) SB-524, *Private Alternative Boarding Schools and Outdoor Programs*, September 30, 2016, https://leginfo.legislature.ca.gov.

Chapter 12: Profits and Losses from Residential Treatment/Bain Capital

219   *Dana Blum*: Art Levine, "The Dark Side of a Bain Success," *Salon*, July 18, 2012, http://www.theinvestigativefund.org.

220   *water, Sprite and Pepto-Bismol*: "Wrongful Death Case Settled Against Youth Treatment Center," Spence Law Firm, October 10, 2011, http://www.spencelawyers.com; *State of Utah v. Deborah Cole and Jorge Alberto Ramirez*, "Information [filed by DA to support charges for felony abuse or neglect]," in the 3rd District Court, West Jordan Department, Salt Lake County, UT, no. 07019475, October 11, 2007, online at https://www.scribd.com; "Charges Against Youth Counselors in Teen's Death Dismissed," *Deseret News*, September 12, 2008, http://www.deseretnews.com.

220   *online magazine Momlogic*: Gina Kaysen Fernandes, "Saving Troubled Teens: A Greedy Industry?" *Momlogic*, December 10, 2009, online at http://www.heal-online.org.

220   *wrongful death settlement*: "Wrongful Death Case," Spence Law Firm, 2011.

221   *sold for $1.3 billion to Acadia Healthcare*: Caroline Chen, "Acadia Healthcare to Buy CRC Health in $1.18 Billion Deal," *Bloomberg*, October 29, 2014, https://www.bloomberg.com.

221   *Jerry Rhodes*: "CRC Health Group to Be Acquired by Acadia Healthcare," PR Newswire, Oct 29, 2014, http://www.prnewswire.com.

221   *scandal-plagued Universal Health Services*: Gina Chon and Anupreeta Das, "UHS Agrees to Acquire Psychiatric Solutions," *Wall Street Journal*, May 17, 2010, https://www.wsj.com; Miles Moffeit, "Danger in the Psych Ward," *Dallas Morning News*, March 18, 2016, http://interactives.dallasnews.com.

221   *disputed allegations of neglect*: Comments to *ProPublica* from Joey Jacobs, Chairman, President and CEO, Psychiatric Solutions, Inc., November 14, 2008, http://s3.amazonaws.com; *Garden City Employees' Retirement System v. Psychiatric Solutions, Inc.*, U.S. District Court, M.D. Tennessee, Nashville Div., no. 3:09-00882. March 31, 2011, http://securities.stanford.edu; Christina Jewett, "Despite Probe, Problems Continue at Psych Facility," *Chicago Tribune*, February 26, 2009, http://www.chicagotribune.com.

221 *$9 million settlement in 2014*: DOJ, "Tennessee Substance Abuse Treatment Facility Agrees to Resolve False Claims Act Allegations for $9.25 Million," April 16, 2014, https://www.justice.gov.

221 *four patients in less than two years*: Stephanie Innes, "Sierra Tucson Fined Over Deficiencies in Psychiatric Care," *Arizona Daily Star,* July 4, 2016, http://tucson.com.

221 *most recently in August 2015*: Innes, "Second Suicide Reported This Year at Rehab Facility," *Arizona Daily Star,* September 18, 2015, http://tucson.com; Pinal County Sheriff's Office, "Incident Report: Suicidal Subject," September 16, 2015, online at https://www.scribd.com.

222 *unconscious but still breathing*: Innes, "Third Sierra Tucson Patient Death in 13 Months," *Arizona Daily Star*, February 7, 2015, http://tucson.com; Innes, "Lax Care at 'Rehab to Stars' Cost Patient His Life, Lawsuit Says," *Arizona Daily Star*, December 14, 2015, http://tucson.com.

222 *hanged himself in his bathroom closet*: Innes, "Second Suicide."

222 *loosened oversight*: Innes, "Exclusive Tucson Rehab Center Gets License Back," *Arizona Daily Star,* October 31, 2015, http://tucson.com.

222 *corpse was found on the grounds*: Innes, "State Probing Sierra Tucson," *Arizona Daily Star,* October 16, 2011, http://tucson.com.

224 *two weeks to find his body*: Innes, "Rehab Center Sued Over Patient Who Strayed Off, Died," *Arizona Daily Star,* January 17, 2012 http://tucson.com.

224 *mother filed a wrongful death lawsuit*: Innes, "Mother Sues Tucson-Area Rehab Center Over Son's Death," *Arizona Daily Star,* April 15, 2016, http://tucson.com.

225 *promised again*: Innes, "Exclusive Tucson Rehab"; Innes, "Sierra Tucson Fined Over Deficiencies in Psychiatric Care," *Arizona Daily Star,* July 4, 2016, http://tucson.com.

NOTE: See full list of references for articles and documents on Sierra Tucson on pages 222–225, citing more specifics on reported deaths and government citations, here: https://www.scribd.com.

225 *"crown jewel"*: Teya Vitu, "CRC Health Buys Sierra Tucson for $130M," *Tucson Citizen,* May 31, 2005, http://tucsoncitizen.com.

225 *even before Litwak's 2011 death*: Innes, "Third Patient in 13 Months Dies at Sierra Tucson Center," *Arizona Daily Star,* February 7, 2015.

226 *customary practice*: David Corn, "New Romney Video: In 1985, He Said Bain Would 'Harvest' Companies for Profits," *Mother Jones,* September 27, 2012, http://www.motherjones.com.

226 *$220 billion behavioral health field*: DHHS, SAMHSA, "Behavioral Health Spending & Use Accounts 1986–2014," no. SMA-16-4975, http://store.samhsa.gov. Note: Total MH/substance abuse spending amounts to 7.5 percent of total health spending.

226 *dispute the allegations*: Jesse Hyde, "Life and Death in a Troubled Teen Boot Camp," *Rolling Stone,* November 12, 2015, http://www.rollingstone.com; Justin Horwath, "Ranch Owner Sues Over Treatment by State

Officials," *Santa Fe New Mexican,* September 3, 2016, http://www .santafenewmexican.com; D. *Diego Zamora et al. v. James Scott Chandler et al.,* "Complaint for Damages...," County of Santa Fe, First Judicial District, February 2, 2014, https://assets.documentcloud.org.

226   *broader corporate culture at CRC Health Group:* Levine, "Dark Side of a Bain Success."

226   *wrongful death and abuse:* Claire Withycombe, "Mount Bachelor Academy Suits Resolved Privately," *Bend Bulletin,* February 23, 2015, http://www.bendbulletin.com.

226   *former staff and clients:* Levine, "Dark Side of a Bain Success"; Art Levine, "Romney Profits from Bain-Owned Health Company Facing Wrongful Death, Neglect Allegations," *HuffPost,* July 25, 2012, http://www.huffingtonpost.com.

227   *2015 financial statement:* "Acadia Healthcare Reports Third Quarter Financial Results Consistent with Previously Announced Preliminary Financial Results," Business Wire, press release, November 1, 2016, http://www.acadiahealthcare.com.

227   *Mel Sembler:* Molly Redden, "GOP Gov. Rick Scott Raising Big Bucks With Founder of Abusive Teen Boot Camps," *Mother Jones,* April 1, 2014, http://www.motherjones.com.

227   *(WWASPS):* Timothy Williams, "Students Recall Special Schools Run Like Jails," *New York Times,* July 23, 2013, http://www.nytimes.com.

227   *"Romney, Torture and Teens":* Maia Szalavitz, "Romney, Torture and Teens," *Reason,* June 27, 2007, http://reason.com.

227   *more than $450 million:* Chen, "Acadia Healthcare."

227   *30,000 clients daily:* CRC Health, Success Stories (website), http://www .crchealth.com/get-help/success-stories/; Acadia Healthcare, 10-K, Annual Report ending December 31, 2016, available at http://www.acadiahealthcare.com/investors/sec-filings.

228   *massive debt of well over $600 million:* CRC Health Corporation, Form 10-K, Fiscal Year Ended December 31, 2006, https://www. sec.gov.

228   *largest collection:* "Private Equity Descends on Addiction Treatment Centers," *Treatment Magazine,* February 2006, http://www.treatmentmagazine.com.

228   *UHS chain:* SEIU, "Criminal Investigation of UHS Facilities Widens to Include Parent Company," *UHS Behind Closed Doors: The Hidden Harm of Maximizing Profits,* http://uhsbehindcloseddoors.org/investigations; Rosalind Adams, "Locked on The Psych Ward," *BuzzFeed,* December 7, 2016, https://www.buzzfeed.com; Rosalind Adams, "Lawmakers Sound Alarms on UHS psychiatric hospitals," December 9, 2016, https://www.buzzfeed.com.

228   *Steve Filton:* Steve Filton, Presentation at Cowen Health Care Conference, March 4, 2013, cited in Amicus Curiae, Bazelon Center, *Universal Health Services, Inc., v. United States and Commonwealth of Massachusetts Ex Rel. Julio Escobar and Carmen Correa,* p. 4, S. Ct., no. 15-7, http://www .scotusblog.com.

229   *For nearly thirty years*: David Altimari et al., "11 Months, 23 Dead,"
      Hartford Courant, October 11, 1998, http://articles.courant.com; also see
      "Universal Health Services: Profits Over People," http://www.psy-
      chcrime.org; Service Employees International Union, Local 1107, *Failure
      to Care, A National Report on Universal Health Service's Behavioral
      Health Operations*, December 1, 2006, http://www.nappp.org.
229   *died while being restrained*: David Altimari, "11 Months, 23 Dead";
      Deaths from Restraints in Psychiatric Facilities, Hearing Before a Sub-
      committee of the Senate Committee on Appropriations, 106th Cong., 1st
      sess., April 13, 1999, 106–193, https://www.gpo.gov.
229   *burgeoning field*: Matt Shea, "Teens Are Being Trapped in Abusive 'Drug
      Rehab Centers,'" *Vice*, May 22, 2013, https://www.vice.com.
229   *as many as 200,000 kids*: GAO, "Residential Facilities: Improved Data
      and Enhanced Oversight Would Help Safeguard the Well-Being of Youth
      with Behavioral and Emotional Challenges," GAO-08-346, May 2008,
      http://www.gao.gov.
230   *earlier settled two lawsuits*: Levine, "Dark Side of a Bain Success."
230   *complaints about abusive staff conduct*: Levine, "Dark Side of a Bain Suc-
      cess"; [Pseudonym for Toni Thayer], "Utah Does It Their Way," October
      2, 2006, http://www.fornits.com/phpbb/index.php?topic=7205.15; Jonny
      Bonner, "Torture Alleged at Utah Treatment Center," citing alleged inci-
      dents in 2005, *Courthouse News Service*, June 27, 2012, http://www.cour-
      thousenews.com/torture-alleged-at-utah-treatment-center/.
231   *4,000 scattered facilities*: The Community Alliance for the Ethical Treat-
      ment of Youth (CAFETY) nationwide facilities' Excel spreadsheet, June
      25, 2011, provided with permission of Brian Lombrowski, former
      CAFETY president; Email correspondence with Lombrowski, February
      2014, online at https://www.scribd.com/document/343567772/Number-
      of-Teen-Treatment-Facilities; Angela Smith, *It's All the Rage! An In-depth
      Look at Behavior Modification in the United States*, (Seattle: HEAL,
      2010), http://www.heal-online.org/ebook.pdf.
231   *145 facilities nationwide*: CRC Health Group, website, http://www
      .crchealth.com/about-us.
231   *industry-leading patient care*: "CRC Health Group to Be Acquired by
      Acadia Healthcare," PR Newswire, October 29, 2014, http://www
      .prnewswire.com.

Chapter 13: Recipe for Disaster?

233   *finalized its takeover*: Acadia Healthcare Company, Inc., 10-K, February
      27, 2015, 1, available at http://www.acadiahealthcare.com/investors
      /sec-filings.
233   *responsible for cleaning up the legal mess*: Acadia Healthcare Company,
      Inc., 8-K, July 2, 2015, 25–26, available at http://www.acadiahealthcare
      .com/investors/sec-filings.
233   *two drug treatment patients died*: Walter Roche, Jr., "New Life Lodge Set-

tles Suit Over Woman's Death," *Tennessean*, December 26, 2013, http://www.tennessean.com; "Lawsuit Filed Against Drug Rehab Center in Death," *Daily Report,* November 30, 2012, http://www.dailyreporton-line.com; Nate Rau and Walter Roche, Jr., "Death Prompts New Probe of Rehab Center," *Tennessean*, October 27, 2011.

233 *froze all new admissions*: Walter F. Roche, Jr. and Nate Rau, "New Life Lodge Investigated," *Tennessean*, April 2, 2013, see online at https://static1.squarespace.com.

234 *won a $9.25 million settlement*: Walter F. Roche, Jr., "New Life Lodge Agrees to Settle Charges," *Tennessean*, April 16, 2014.

234 *prioritize profit margins*: DOJ, "Tennessee Substance Abuse Treatment Facility Agrees to Resolve False Claims Act Allegations for $9.25 Million," news release, April 16, 2014; Nate Rau and Walter F. Roche, Jr., "New Life Lodge to Reopen in April, Accept Only Adults," *Tennessean*, March 24, 2012.

235 *barred by the state from accepting Medicaid or Medicare*: DOJ, "Tennessee Substance Abuse Treatment Facility...," https://www.justice.gov; confirmed by author via phone call to facility, April 17, 2017.

235 *doing business as Mirror Lake*: See Mirror Lake Recovery website at http://www.mirrorlakerecovery.com.

235 *8-K filing*: Acadia Healthcare Company, Inc., 8-K, July 2, 2015; Jim Higgins, "New Life Lodge Rehab Center Faces Lawsuit Over Death of Second Patient," The Higgins Firm, September 22, 2011, https://www.tennesseelawblog.com.

235 *conference call*: "CRC Health Group to Be Acquired by Acadia Healthcare," PR Newswire, October 29, 2014, http://www.prnewswire.com.

235 *"sexualized role play"*: Maia Szalavitz, "Really Special Education: State Investigation Confirms 'Lap Dance Therapy' Allegations," *HuffPost*, March 18, 2010, http://www.huffingtonpost.com; Levine, "Dark Side of a Bain Success"; Michelle Cole, "State Suspends License From Central Oregon School for Troubled Teens," *Oregonian*, November 3, 2009, http://www.oregonlive.com.

235 *potentially costly counter-claim*: CRC Health Group et al. and the State of Oregon, Settlement Agreement and Release, September 28, 2010, http://www.theinvestigativefund.org; Alliance for the Safe, Therapeutic, & Appropriate Use of Residential Treatment, "Case Charging Abuse of Students at Mount Bachelor Academy Closes," December 2010, http://astartforteens.org.

235 *claimed the allegations*: Shelby R. King, "Lawsuit Against Mount Bachelor Academy Moving Forward," *Bulletin* (Bend, OR), January 7, 2014, http://www.bendbulletin.com; Claire Withycombe, "Mount Bachelor Academy Suits Resolved Privately," *Bulletin*, January 22, 2015, http://www.bendbulletin.com.

236 *settled three separate lawsuits*: Withycombe, "Mount Bachelor Academy Suits Resolved."

236 *died of heatstroke*: Steve Beaven, "Portland Teen Collapses and Dies During Wilderness Camp Hike," *Oregonian*, September 1, 2009, http://www.oregonlive.com; Erin Golden, "No Closure in SageWalk Death," *Bulletin*, August 29, 2010; for Lake County Sheriff's press release, see "Homicide Charges Possible in SageWalk Student Death," WTVZ, March 30, 2010, available at http://www.heal-online.org/homicide033010.pdf.

237 *"unwelcomed bumps in the road"*: Levine, "Dark Side of a Bain Success."

238 *reviewed 911 log data*: Incidents at Specific Address, 3192 Glen Canyon Road, January 2008–August 2011, Santa Cruz Regional 911, 9-page report, http://www.theinvestigativefund.org.

238 *scathing report*: John Hill, *Rogue Rehabs: State Failed to Police Drug and Alcohol Homes, With Deadly Results*, California Senate Rules Committee, Office of Outcomes and Oversight, September 4, 2012, http://sooo.senate.ca.gov.

238 *felon-run treatment centers*: California State Auditor Report 2013–119, August 2014, https://www.auditor.ca.gov; Christina Jewett and Will Evans, "Rehab Racket," series by Center for Investigative Reporting, http://cironline.org/rehabracket.

238 *eleven criminal cases*: Christina Jewett, "Two Years Later, California Is Still Cleaning Up Drug Rehab System," *Reveal* from The Center for Investigative Reporting, November 12, 2015, https://www.revealnews.org.

238 *sweeping anti-fraud investigation*: Julie Miller, "Health Net Looking for Fraud Among Treatment Centers," *Behavioral Healthcare Executive*, January 28, 2016, http://www.behavioral.net/article/health-net-looking-fraud-among-treatment-centers.

238 *unlicensed psychiatric evaluations*: Hill, *Rogue Rehabs*, 31.

239 *dozen young people*: Jesse Hyde, "Life and Death in a Troubled Teen Boot Camp," *Rolling Stone*, November 12, 2015.

239 *"were not faking it"*: U.S. House, 110th Congress, no. 110–68, *Cases of Child Neglect and Abuse at Private Residential Treatment Facilities, Hearing Before the Committee on Education and Labor*, October 10, 2007 (Washington, DC: GPO, 2008), 31, https://www.gpo.gov.

239 *never investigated the deaths*: Levine, "Dark Side of a Bain Success"; Department of Alcohol and Drug Programs Reported Narcotic Treatment Program (NTP) Patient Deaths FY 2006–2007, September 15, 2011, http://www.theinvestigativefund.org.

240 *failing to properly screen patients*: Sydney P. Freeberg, "Drug Users Turn Death Dealers as Methadone From Bain Hits Street," *Bloomberg*, February 8, 2013, https://www.bloomberg.com.

240 *over eighty methadone clinics*: See at CRC Health website, http://www.crchealth.com.

240 *loosely regulated*: Freeberg, "Drug Users Turn Death Dealers."

240 *lowers overdose mortality by 75 percent*: Maia Szalavitz, *Unbroken Brain: A Revolutionary New Way of Understanding Addiction* (New York: St. Martins, 2016).

242 *criticized the Joint Commission*: Andis Robeznieks with Matthew DoBias, "Joint Commission Under Fire," *Modern Healthcare*, March 12, 2007, http://www.modernhealthcare.com.

242 *notorious chains*: Cult Education Institute, "Straight Inc.," news articles 1983–2007, https://www.culteducation.com/group/1274-straight-inc.html.

242 *as many as ninety lawsuits*: Wesley M. Fager, "Some Civil Suits and Criminal Cases Against Straight, Inc. and Straight-Descendent Programs," *The Straights*, May 27, 2002, http://thestraights.net.

242 *remained in their executive posts*: "CRC Health Group CEO to Step Down; Announces Search for Successor," CRC Health, press release, June 28, 2010, http://www.crchealth.com.

242 *remains in her post*: Trina Quinney-Packard, Executive Director, bio, http://www.youthcare.com/about/staff/trina-packard/.

242 *down to just four treatment facilities*: Aspen Education Group, "Help for Troubled Teens: Residential and Wilderness Programs," http://aspeneducation.crchealth.com.

243 *two lawsuits*: Sebastian Murdock, "The Troubled Teen Industry Has Been a Disaster for Decades," *HuffPost*, Aug 23, 2016, *http://testkitchen .huffingtonpost.com/island-view/*.

243 *Seroquel and other antipsychotics*: Murdock, "Troubled Teen Industry Has Been a Disaster."

  NOTE: CRC's reply to the author's July 2012 *Salon* article and my response can be read online at https://www.scribd.com/document/344435519/CRC-Reply-to-2012-Salon-Article.

244 *lobbied for by HEAL*: Washington State House of Representatives, 2016 Regular Session, House Bill 2746-S.PL, online at https://www.scribd.com; also see HEAL, State Action Campaign[s], http://www.heal-online.org /action2.htm.

244 *oversight law*: *Stop Child Abuse in Residential Programs for Teens Act of 2008*, H.R. 5876 (110th Cong.), https://www .govtrack.us.

244 *including religious schools*: *Private Alternative Boarding Schools and Outdoor Programs*, Senate (State of California), SB-524, approved September 30, 2016, https://leginfo.legislature.ca.gov.

244 *Survivors of Institutional Abuse*: For SIA website, go to http://www .sia-now.org.

245 *"regulate this rogue industry"*: Los Angeles LGBT Center, "Protecting Youth From Institutional Abuse Act," press release, Sept 1, 2016, https://lalgbtcenter.org.

Chapter 14: Florida/Free-Fire Zone for Killing, Abusing and Raping Kids?

246 *'I was raped.'*: Art Levine, "Alleged Rapes Show How Failed Oversight Endangers Florida's Most Vulnerable Children," *Miami New Times*, November 11, 2014, http://www.miaminewtimes.com.

247 *the same day*: See excerpt LWPD incident report, March 4, 2011, https://www.scribd.com.

248 *Richard Straughn*: Letter from Richard Straughn, November 3, 2014, https://www.scribd.com.

249 *National Association of Therapeutic Schools and Programs (NATSAP)*: Testimony of Jan Moss, Executive Director, *Cases of Child Abuse and Neglect at Private Residential Treatment Facilities*, House Committee on Education and Labor, October 10, 2007, 44–75, https://www.gpo.gov.

250 *ninety-six children died*: Nina Berman and Michael Mechanic, "It Was Kind of Like Slavery," *Mother Jones*, February 19, 2014.

250 *unmonitored Christian academies*: Alexandra Zayas et al., "In God's Name: Unlicensed Religious Children's Homes," *Tampa Bay Times*, October 2012, http://www.tampabay.com/faccca/.

250 *nearly five hundred children*: Carol Marbin Miller and Audra D. S. Burch, "Preserving Families but Losing Children," *Miami Herald*, March 16, 2014, part I of series, "Innocents Lost," http://media.miamiherald.com.

253 *fired in January 2012*: Phil Attinger, "Capt. James Foy Fired From Police Force," *The Ledger* (Lakeland, Florida), January 14, 2012, http://www.theledger.com.

Chapter 15: Karen's Story and The Mental Health System That Never Was

257 *$444 billion a year*: Liz Szabo, "Cost of Not Caring: Nowhere to Go," *USA Today*, May 12, 2014.

257 *reduce relapses*: SAMHSA, DHHS, *Family Psychoeducation: The Evidence*, pub. no. SMA-09-4422, Center for Mental Health Services, 2009, https://store.samhsa.gov/; William R. McFarlane et al., "Clinical and Functional Outcomes After 2 Years in the Early Detection and Intervention for the Prevention of Psychosis Multisite Effectiveness Trial," *Schizophrenia Bulletin* 41, no. 1 (2015): 30–43, https://academic.oup.com/schizophreniabulletin.

261 *800 percent more likely to develop schizophrenia*: Pekka Tienari et al., "Genotype-environment Interaction in Schizophrenia-Spectrum Disorder," *British Journal of Psychiatry* 184, no. 3 (February 2004): 216–222, http://bjp.rcpsych.org.

Chapter 16: Why Can't We Just Do What Works?

271 *pioneered a work program*: Liz Szabo, "'Bleak Picture' for Mentally Ill: 80% Are Jobless," *USA Today*, July 10, 2014; "About IPS," The IPS Employment Center, The Rockville Institute, https://www.ipsworks.org/about-ips/.

271 *A little over half*: NAMI, "Mental Health by the Numbers," http://www.nami.org.

271 *unemployment rate*: NAMI, "Road to Recovery," July 1, 2014, 17, https://www.nami.org/.

272 *two-thirds of people*: Gary Bond et al., "Making the Case for IPS Supported Employment," *Administration and Policy in Mental Health* 41, no. 1 (January 2014): 69–73, researchers' copy online at https://www.researchgate.net.

272   *No one is excluded*: K. Campbell et al., "Who Benefits From Supported Employment: A Meta-Analytic Study," *Schizophrenia Bulletin*, 37, no. 2 (March 2011), https://academic.oup.com.

272   *Cornerstone Montgomery*: Vocational Department at Cornerstone Montgomery, Inc., http://www.cornerstonemontgomery.org/vocational.

274   *$166,000*: P. W. Bush et al., "The Long-Term Impact of Employment on Mental Health Service Use and Costs for Persons With Severe Mental Illness," *Psychiatric Services* 60, no. 8 (August 2009), http://ps.psychiatryonline.org.

274   *portions of approximately twenty states*: Johnson & Johnson Dartmouth Community Mental Health Program, "Johnson & Johnson–Dartmouth Community Mental Health Program: The IPS Learning Community," January 25, 2016, https://www.ipsworks.org; update by Robert Drake, phone interview with author, April 2017.

274   *billions wasted on medications*: Art Levine, "Follow the Money," *American Prospect*, June 20, 2008, http://prospect.org/article/follow-money.

275   *mandated reforms*: Disability Rights Center, New Hampshire, "Federal Judge Approves Class Action Settlement Expanding Mental Health Services," February 12, 2014, http://www.drcnh.org/mentalhealthcrisis.html.

276   *didn't make the toolkits available*: SAMHSA Publications Ordering, http://store.samhsa.gov/list/series?name=Evidence-Based-Practices-KITs.

276   *published in 2007*: Gregory McHugo et al., "Fidelity Outcomes in the National Implementing Evidence-Based Practices Project," *Psychiatric Services* 58, no. 10 (October 2007), http://ps.psychiatryonline.org.

277   *blamed*: Reply from SAMHSA on Delays in Evidence-Based Toolkits, Implementation, February 5, 2016, 3–4, online at https://www.scribd.com.

Chapter 17: Putting People Before Big Pharma

284   *illnesses develop by age twenty-four*: Child Mind Institute, *Children's Mental Health Report*, 2015,http://www.speakupforkids.org/report.html.

284   *Dr. Peter Breggin*: Peter R. Breggin, *Medication Madness: The Role of Psychiatric Drugs in Cases of Violence, Suicide, and Crime* (New York: St. Martin's Griffin, 2008).

285   *appeared to worsen prospects*: Thomas Insel, "Antipsychotics: Taking the Long View," NIMH, August 28, 2013, https://www.nimh.nih.gov.

285   *either/or debate*: Sarah Glazer, "Are Antipsychotic Drugs the Best Treatment?" *CQ Researcher* 24, no. 43 (December 5, 2014), http://library.cq-press.com.

285   *few people*: Liz Szabo, "Solutions to Woes of Mentally Ill Exist but Aren't Used," *USA Today,* December 22, 2014, http://www.usatoday.com.

286   *biology doubtlessly plays a key*: Eric R. Kandel, "The New Science of Mind," *New York Times*, September 6, 2013, http://www.nytimes.com; P. F. Sullivan et al., "Schizophrenia as a Complex Trait: Evidence From a Meta-Analysis of Twin Studies," *Archives of General Psychiatry* 60 no. 2 (December 2003): 1187–1192, https://www.ncbi.nlm.nih.gov; Benedict

Carey, "Scientists Move Closer to Understanding Schizophrenia's Cause," *New York Times,* January 27, 2016, https://www.nytimes.com.

286 *"The Village," a successful program*: Art Levine, "Abilify Is Top-Selling U.S. Drug—But New Reports Question Long-Term Antipsychotic Use, Cite Need for Personalized Services," *HuffPost,* December 12, 2014, http://www.huffingtonpost.com; MHALA The Village outcomes are online at https://www.scribd.com.

286 *compassionate psychiatrist*: Mark Ragins, "Dr. Mark's Writings," MHA The Village, http://mhavillage.squarespace.com/writings.

289 *Hearing Voices Network*: Benedict Carey, "An Alternative Form of Mental Health Care Gains a Foothold," *New York Times,* August 8, 2016, https://www.nytimes.com.

290 *best*: Full Service Partnership Program, program brochure, Los Angeles County Department of Mental Health, http://file.lacounty.gov.

291 *Alameda County in California*: Alameda County–Dartmouth Collaborative, Behavioral Health Care Services, Alameda County (CA), http://www.acbhcs.org.

291 *smeared by critics*: D. J. Jaffe, "SAMHSA Slammed by Congress...and for Good Reason," *HuffPost,* May 24, 2013, http://www.huffingtonpost.com; for an opposing view, see October 16, 2013 reply letter from members of National Coalition for Mental Health Recovery to Torrey and Jaffe *National Review* article, August 15, 2013, http://www.ncmhr.org.

292 *Dr. Elinore McCance-Katz*: McCance-Katz, "New Hope for the Mentally Ill," *National Review,* November 22, 2016, http://amp.nationalreview.com; McCance-Katz, "The Federal Government Ignores the Treatment Needs of Americans With Serious Mental Illness," *Psychiatric Times,* April 21, 2016, http://www.psychiatrictimes.com.

293 *Commission on Care report*: Commission on Care, *Final Report,* June 30, 2016, https://s3.amazonaws.com.

294 *suicides down to zero*: M. Justin Coffey, M.D. and C. Edward Coffey, M.D., "How We Dramatically Reduced Suicide," *NEJM Catalyst,* April 20, 2016, http://catalyst.nejm.org/dramatically-reduced-suicide/.

295 *results are striking*: Robert Drake et al., "Longitudinal Course of Clients With Co-occurring Schizophrenia-Spectrum and Substance Use Disorders in Urban Mental Health Centers: A 7-Year Prospective Study," *Schizophrenia Bulletin* 42, no. 1 (2016): 202–211, https://academic.oup.com.

296 *one in ten mental health clinics*: Mark P. McGovern et al., "Dual Diagnosis Capability in Mental Health and Addiction Treatment Services: An Assessment of Programs Across Multiple State Systems," *Administration and Policy in Mental Health* 41, no. 2 (March 2014): 205–214, https://www.ncbi.nlm.nih.gov; though out of date, a partial list of facilities measured for minimal dual diagnosis (DD) quality around 2012 is available online at https://www.scribd.com; a list is also available for Connecticut facilities, see "CT List: Prepared for the Hazelden Directory of Co-Occurring Programs (DDC or DDE), 2009–2012," at https://www.scribd.com.

296 *"Right Care" initiative*: "We Must Lift Up Our Voices: Lown and RCA Respond to Election Results," *The Messenger*, December 2016, http://rightcarealliance.org.

297 *reduce re-arrests*: Maia Szalavitz, "Five Studies: Mental Health Courts Are Finding Their Footing," *Pacific Standard,* November 25, 2015, https://psmag.com.

297 *slashes re-arrest rates*: Blueprints for Healthy Youth Development, "MST® for Juvenile Offenders," http://www.blueprintsprograms.com; Shields for Families, MST, https://www.shieldsforfamilies.org.

297 *funding*: NAMI, Our Finances, http://www.nami.org; Mental Health America (MHA), Financial Information and Annual Reports, http://www.mentalhealthamerica.net; Replies from NAMI and MHA regarding drug industry support, August 2016, online at https://www.scribd.com.

ASSISTANCE, ADVOCACY AND INFORMATION RESOURCE GUIDE

(NOTE: Inclusion on this ideologically diverse list doesn't imply endorsement.)

National Suicide Prevention Lifeline:
1-800-273-TALK (8255)
https://suicidepreventionlifeline.org
This hotline website also offers sources for finding local support and therapists.

American Foundation for Suicide Prevention: It conducts research and prevention initiatives, while offering support for those affected by suicide. (http://afsp.org)

The Judge David L. Bazelon Center for Mental Health Law: A nonprofit advocacy and legal organization that protects the rights of people with mental illnesses; its website is packed with information on lawsuits and reforms. (http://bazelon.org)

Blueprints for Healthy Youth Development: The University of Colorado's Center for the Study of Prevention and Violence has evaluated 1,400 programs claiming to promote the health and well-being of kids, but only 5 percent have been designated as model or promising. Here are the best: http://www.blueprintsprograms.com.

Case Western Reserve University, Center for Evidence-Based Practices: This academic center offers training and a clear resource guide on an array of well-proven methods.
(http://www.centerforebp.case.edu/practices)

The Child Mind Institute: An independent organization that provides research, advocacy and clinical care for children and teens who suffer from psychiatric and learning disorders. Although downplaying the dangers of medications, the institute's website offers a symptom checker and mental health guides that can be useful: https://childmind.org/topics-a-z/.

Drug Information:
Independent websites, such as *The Carlat Psychiatry Report*, are often behind paywalls. Most popular health websites are subsidized by drug companies,

so for laymen, the most honest research can be found at *Consumer Reports*'s Best Buy Drugs (http://www.consumerreports.org/drugs), while psych med users can share unvarnished information and resources at *CrazyMeds*: https://www.crazymeds.us. The website https://rxisk.org/ helps consumers learn about side-effects, but it could needlessly scare some people who may benefit from psychiatric drugs.

Foundation for Excellence in Mental Health Care: A philanthropy that promotes innovative alternative treatments through grants and education. (http://www.mentalhealthexcellence.org)

Hearing Voices Network (HVN) USA: The alliance offers support for those taking an alternative view on hearing voices and other extreme experiences. (http://www.hearingvoicesusa.org)

Mad in America: Founded by author Robert Whitaker, this is the nation's most influential news and commentary website critical of drug-oriented psychiatry. In recent years, it has expanded its mission to include continuing education online courses about alternative approaches, taught by experts. (https://www.madinamerica.com)

Mental Health America: The nation's leading community-based nonprofit offering both mental health services and advocacy, it has more than two hundred affiliates in forty-one states. It also provides invaluable information about mental illness, including this personal resource guide: http://www.mentalhealthamerica.net/finding-help.

National Alliance on Mental Illness: A grassroots organization that provides advocacy for access to services and support for mentally ill people across the United States. With more than 1,000 affiliate organizations across America, it's best known for providing training and support for parents of mentally ill people. (http://www.nami.org/)

National Association of State Mental Health Program Directors: The organization also promotes best practices that should be widely used: https://www.nasmhpd.org/content/technical-assistance-programs.

National Child Traumatic Stress Network: A national collaboration of providers and families, this is a good starting place to look for a skilled trauma therapist: http://www.nctsn.org/about-us/affiliated-members.

National Empowerment Center: A consumer-driven organization that provides peer-oriented training and resources. Its toll-free information and referral line is 1800-POWER2U (800-769-3728), but it's not a crisis line. (www.power2u.org) Affiliated groups can be found here: http://www.power2u.org/consumerrun-statewide.html.

National Institute of Mental Health: In addition to research, it offers helpful resources. (https://www.nimh.nih.gov/health/find-help/index.shtml)

National Mental Health Consumers' Self-Help Clearinghouse: A tiny but dedicated group that offers information and guidance to individuals with mental health conditions and mental health professionals. (http://www.mh-selfhelp.org) It has a useful, if incomplete, consumer-driven services directory here: http://www.cdsdirectory.org.

Online Mental Health Resources, prepared by Susan Rogers, Director, National Mental Health Consumers' Self-Help Clearinghouse, available here: https://www.scribd.com/document/345564979/MH-Resources. Her list combines mainstream and alternative groups addressing reform and providing assistance.

Treatment Advocacy Center: Founded by the controversial champion of mandated outpatient treatment laws, schizophrenia researcher Dr. E. Fuller Torrey, the group works to overcome barriers to treatment while offering compelling reports on the social impact of untreated mental illness. (http://www.treatmentadvocacycenter.org)

Valuable publications:
Xavier Amadour, *I Am Not Sick, I Don't Need Help*: *How to Help Someone With Mental Illness Accept Treatment* (10th Anniversary Edition), Peconic, NY: Vida Press, 2011, excerpt online at NAMI, https://www.nami.org.

Pete Earley's blog: The author of the investigative book, *Crazy*, has an informative pro-medication blog covering mental health controversies. (http://www.peteearley.com/blog/)

Sarah Glazer, "Treating Schizophrenia," *CQ Researcher*, December 5, 2014, http://library.cqpress.com/cqresearcher/document.php?id=cqresrre 2014120500. A balanced look at schizophrenia and meds, it also offers an organizational guide (article purchase may be required).

ACKNOWLEDGMENTS

Reporting and writing this book wouldn't have been possible without the support, assistance and cooperation of many individuals. I am grateful to all those people who generously shared their time and whom I quote in the book. But I'm especially indebted to these families and individuals who agreed to tell me their personal stories about the tragedies they endured in the hope of spurring reform. Among them: Stan and Shirley White, Darla Grese, Marvin Simcakoski and Jason's wife, Heather Simcakoski, Janette Layne and Marisa Conover. Equally important in shaping this book were the insights and histories of the survivors of reckless prescribing or dangerous residential treatment programs, including Scott Barber, Paul Walton, Colleen Davidson and Erin Rodriguez. A key person who enabled me to reach out to victims of abusive "troubled teen" programs was Angela Smith of HEAL, a survivor who has become the nation's best-informed activist on this issue. Heroic Brandon Coleman was my guide to VA whistleblowers.

My reporting on effective and promising mental health programs was guided by the research and insights of numerous academics, joined by ground-breaking clinicians and program administrators. Some of them were quoted directly, while others' writings also helped me address the question: How can we do a better job of providing treatment to people grappling with serious mental illness, substance abuse and PTSD? These innovators include Robert Drake, William McFarlane, Tamara Sale, Lisa Dixon, Mary Vieten, Michael Cornwall, Stephen Xenakis, J. Douglas Bremner, Mark McGovern, Susan Rogers, Daniel Carlat, Robert Rosenheck, Christopher Bellonci, David Healy, Anthony Lehman, David Pilon, Richard Van Horn, Mark Ragins— and all the important researchers, including Douglas Ziedonis, supported by the unique Foundation for Excellence in Mental Health Care. My understanding of effective and abusive treatments, and the pharmaceutical industry, clearly owes a great debt to the work of Anne Fletcher, Maia Szalavitz and especially Robert Whitaker, who has demonstrated how powerful reporting can change long-held views, as well as to Martha Rosenberg. Lobbyist Debbie Plotnick of Mental Health America was my indispensable policy expert. Maria Bamford's artistry on mental illness and stigma was a great inspiration.

My own reporting, especially in Los Angeles County and on residential programs, couldn't have happened without the support of the leaders of key journalism foundations. Among them were Margaret Engel of the Alicia Patterson Foundation; Sandy Bergo of the Fund for Investigative Journalism; and Joe Conason and Esther Kaplan of the Nation Institute's Investigative Fund. Joe and especially Esther, superb investigative reporters themselves, also helped me sharpen and deepen the emotional depth of the stories I told about CRC Health for *Salon* in 2012. Dave Daley played a key role in ensuring the article's publication.

In publishing and editing my reporting on mental health and other investigative topics, both before and after I was given the opportunity to write this book by The Overlook Press, talented and supportive magazine, policy and weekly newspaper editors gave me the encouragement and guidance that proved invaluable to me. These include Jake Cline of South Florida's *City Link* weekly, who backed me in 2001 on my first major article on this topic; David Kendall of the Progressive Policy Institute; Harold Meyerson, Tara McKelvey and the then-publisher Diane Strauss of *The American Prospect*; Strauss, now the publisher of *The Washington Monthly*, continues to support reform in a magazine that has been a journalistic home for me, first under Charlie Peters and now edited by Paul Glastris; Ryan Grim, the Washington bureau chief of *The Huffington Post*, who has supported and showcased my reporting while assigning Sasha Belenky to help me transform an investigative project into a powerful narrative; Don Hazen and Jan Frel of AlterNet; and the editors of *Newsweek*, especially James Impoco, Bob Roe, Ross Schneiderman, Matt McAllester and Barclay Palmer, who featured my article "The Jesus Gulag."

I count journalists among the friends and family members who supported and encouraged my work in ways they know well. I am especially grateful to my sister Susan Levine Houston and her husband, novelist and retired judge Julian Houston; James Fallows; Mark Stricherz; Sheila Kaplan; Alan Pell Crawford; Tom D'Antoni; David Dennie; Susan Murray; Diane Dodson; Keshini Ladduwahetty; Timothy Noah; and so many others.

Finally, this book wouldn't have seen the light of day without the aid of literary agent Jill Marsal; the dedicated Overlook editor Chelsea Cutchens, and publicist Shannon McCain; consulting editor Ed Robertson and researcher Cathy Kreyche; and independent publicist Elizabeth Shreve.

For everyone's support and wise counsel, I will be forever grateful.